Omega-3 Fatty Acids: Keys to Nutritional Health

Omega-3 Fatty Acids: Keys to Nutritional Health

Editor: Chester Cooke

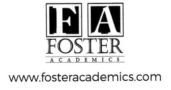

www.fosteracademics.com

www.fosteracademics.com

Cataloging-in-Publication Data

Omega-3 fatty acids : keys to nutritional health / edited by Chester Cooke.
   p. cm.
Includes bibliographical references and index.
ISBN 978-1-64646-587-3
1. Omega-3 fatty acids. 2. Omega-3 fatty acids--Nutritional aspects.
3. Essential fatty acids in human nutrition. 4. High-omega-3 fatty acid diet.
5. Omega-3 fatty acids--Physiological effect. I. Cooke, Chester.
QP752.O44 O44 2023
612.397--dc23

Foster Academics,
118-35 Queens Blvd., Suite 400,
Forest Hills, NY 11375, USA

ISBN 978-1-64646-587-3 (Hardback)

Contents

Preface

Omega-3 fatty acids are polyunsaturated fatty acids (PUFAs) that play an important role in human diet and physiology. They are classified into three types, which include α-linolenic acid (ALA), eicosapentaenoic acid (EPA) and docosahexaenoic acid (DHA). The primary source of omega-3 fatty acids are marine algae and phytoplankton. Walnuts, edible seeds and flaxseeds are common sources of plant oils containing ALA, while EPA and DHA are found in fish and fish oils. DHA is considered the most vital omega-3 fatty acid in the body, as it is the principal structural component of brain, retina and other body parts. It is essential for pregnant and breastfeeding women to get adequate DHA because it can affect the health and cognitive abilities of an infant. This book contains some path-breaking studies on the nutritional importance of omega-3 fatty acids. It is a collective contribution of a renowned group of international experts. Those in search of information to further their knowledge will be greatly assisted by this book.

This book is the end result of constructive efforts and intensive research done by experts in this field. The aim of this book is to enlighten the readers with recent information in this area of research. The information provided in this profound book would serve as a valuable reference to students and researchers in this field.

At the end, I would like to thank all the authors for devoting their precious time and providing their valuable contribution to this book. I would also like to express my gratitude to my fellow colleagues who encouraged me throughout the process.

Editor

Effects of Omega-3 Fatty Acids on Muscle Mass, Muscle Strength and Muscle Performance among the Elderly

Ya-Hui Huang [1,2,†], Wan-Chun Chiu [3,4,†], Yuan-Pin Hsu [1,5], Yen-Li Lo [6] and Yuan-Hung Wang [1,7,*]

1   Graduate Institute of Clinical Medicine, College of Medicine, Taipei Medical University, Taipei 11031, Taiwan; A0634@tpech.gov.tw (Y.-H.H.); koakoahsu@gmail.com (Y.-P.H.)
2   Department of Dietetics and Nutrition, Heping Fuyou Branch, Taipei City Hospital, Taipei 10065, Taiwan
3   School of Nutrition and Health Sciences, College of Nutrition, Taipei Medical University, Taipei 11031, Taiwan; wanchun@tmu.edu.tw
4   Research Center of Geriatric Nutrition, College of Nutrition, Taipei Medical University, Taipei 11031, Taiwan
5   Emergency Department, Wan Fang Hospital, Taipei Medical University, Taipei 11696, Taiwan
6   Department of Biomedical Engineering, National Yang-Ming University, Taipei 11221, Taiwan; doma1118@gmail.com
7   Department of Medical Research, Shuang Ho Hospital, Taipei Medical University, New Taipei City 23561, Taiwan
*   Correspondence: d508091002@tmu.edu.tw
†   These authors contributed equally to this work.

Abstract: There is increasing evidence showing the role of fatty acids and their derived lipid intermediates in the regulation of skeletal muscle mass synthesis and function. However, the role of omega-3 fatty acids remains unclear. Therefore, we conducted a meta-analysis to evaluate the potential effects of omega-3 fatty acids on sarcopenia-related performances among the elderly. Eligible literature and reports of randomized controlled trials were comprehensively searched from the PubMed, Cochrane Library, ClinicalTrials.gov, and Cumulative Index to Nursing and Allied Health Literature (CINAHL) databases until July 2018. A total of 10 articles were available for the meta-analysis. There were minor benefits for muscle mass gain (0.33 kg; 95% CI: 0.05, 0.62) and timed up and go performance (−0.30 s; 95% CI: −0.43, −0.17). Subgroup analyses regarding muscle mass and walk speed indicated that omega-3 fatty acid supplements at more than 2 g/day may contribute to muscle mass gain (0.67 kg; 95% CI: 0.16, 1.18) and improve walking speed, especially for those receiving more than 6 months of intervention (1.78 m/sec; 95% CI: 1.38, 2.17). Our findings provide some insight into the effects of omega-3 fatty acids on muscle mass, especially for those taking supplements at more than 2 g/day. We also observed that a long period of omega-3 fatty acids supplementation may improve walking speed.

Keywords: docosahexaenoic acid (DHA); elderly; eicosapentaenoic acid (EPA); omega-3 fatty acid; n-3 PUFAs; sarcopenia

1. Introduction

Age-related musculoskeletal decline presents a significant risk for falls in the elderly [1] and is becoming a major public health concern with fast-growing aging populations [2]. Sarcopenia (a loss of skeletal muscle mass and function) is common with advancing age [3], and along with frailty, is associated with severe adverse outcomes, including falls, fractures, hospitalization, and early death [4,5]. Furthermore, people with sarcopenia need substantially more medical care and incur more health-related costs [6]. As such, sarcopenia prevention is crucial in reducing the burden on social care systems and the associated costs.

Physical exercise and nutritional supplementation are currently recommended as preventive measures against the loss of muscle mass, muscle strength, or physical performance [7]. Healthy older persons are advised to maintain a daily protein intake of 1.2–1.5 g/kg body weight, and emphasis is placed on stimulating skeletal muscle anabolism [8]. However, the source and amount of protein intake also affect muscle synthesis and metabolism. Studies have shown that high protein consumption may increase the development of insulin resistance and diabetes [9–11], so a high protein intake may not be the best way to prevent sarcopenia in some cases. Such recommendations should be informed by individual dietary patterns and daily lifestyles.

In addition to protein recommendation, several observational studies and randomized controlled trials (RCTs) report the association of muscle mass and performance with specific nutrients, such as fish-derived n-3 polyunsaturated fatty acids (n-3 PUFAs) [12–15]. Given that sarcopenia is associated with increased inflammatory responses and impaired glucose homeostasis, recent research suggests that n-3 PUFAs have anti-inflammatory properties, which may be exploited for the prevention or treatment of sarcopenia [16]. Most studies have focused on three main types of n-3 PUFAs: alpha-linolenic acid (ALA, C18:3 n-3), eicosapentaenoic acid (EPA, C20:5 n-3), and docosahexaenoic acid (DHA, C22:6 n-3). Previous evidence [17] showed that n-3 PUFAs from fish, which are high in EPA and DHA, have beneficial effects on cardiovascular health due to their anti-inflammatory properties. An association between n-3 PUFAs intake and musculoskeletal health has also been reported in RCTs [18,19], which showed that supplementation with n-3 PUFAs enhanced the rate of muscle protein synthesis in the elderly; in a strength-training trial [20], fish-oil supplementation resulted in significantly improved muscle strength and functional capacity, compared with those in non-supplemented controls. Furthermore, there is some observational evidence that supports the benefits of fish-oil-derived n-3 PUFAs, from either supplementation with 1.86 g of EPA and 1.5 g of DHA or fatty fish consumption, for muscle mass, muscle strength, and physical function in older people [21,22]. By contrast, a three-year follow-up trial suggested that low-dose n-3 PUFAs (0.225 g of EPA and 0.8 g of DHA) supplementation had no effect on muscle strength in elderly people [23]. ALA is a plant-derived n-3 fatty acid that mainly exists in flaxseed, soybean, perilla, walnut, and canola oils. In healthy adults, only 5–10% and 2–5% of ALA can be converted into EPA and DHA, respectively [24]. A study [25] showed that ALA decreases the levels of plasma inflammatory cytokines, such as tumor necrosis factor (TNF)-alpha and interleukin (IL)-6, which may further improve muscle mass and strength in the elderly. As a modifiable lifestyle factor, n-3 PUFA supplementation is a potential target for preventing sarcopenia in the elderly [26]. The possible mechanism is shown in Figure 1.

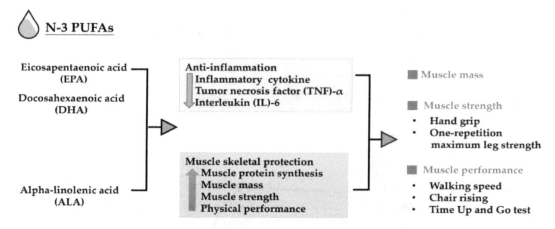

Figure 1. Impact of n-3 polyunsaturated fatty acids (n-3 PUFAs) on muscle mass, muscle strength, and muscle performance.

The musculoskeletal health benefits of n-3 PUFAs remain inconclusive; thus, the present systematic review and meta-analysis assesses the probable effects of increasing n-3 PUFAs (through supplementation or dietary ingestion) on key skeletal muscle outcomes in adults aged 60 years or older. The investigated outcomes are muscle mass, muscle strength, and muscle performance.

2. Materials and Methods

2.1. Data Sources and Searches

This systematic review and meta-analysis was performed in accordance with the Preferred Reporting Items for Systematic Reviews and Meta-Analyses (PRISMA) guidelines [27]. We searched PubMed, ClinicalTrials.gov, Cumulative Index to Nursing and Allied Health Literature (CINAHL), and the Cochrane Central Register of Controlled Trials (CENTRAL) in any language, from the date of inception until 31 July 2018. The search included the keywords 'elderly', 'muscle mass', 'muscle performance', 'muscle strength', 'dynapenia', 'frailty', 'sarcopenia', 'polyunsaturated fatty acids', 'fish oil', and synonyms.

2.2. Selection Criteria

We included RCTs that evaluated the effect of increasing n-3 PUFAs (through diet or supplementation), on the skeletal muscle mass, muscle strength, or muscle performance of older subjects. The participants included adults aged 60 years or older. A study was eligible for inclusion if it reported changes from the baseline to the last available follow-up for one or more of the following outcomes—muscle mass, muscle strength (such as hand grip), or physical performance including gait speed or time up and go test. Studies were excluded if they did not contain primary data (conference abstracts, meta-analyses, reviews, letters to the editor, and case reports).

2.3. Data Extraction and Quality Assessment

The data extracted include the authors, year of publication, study design, sample size, mean age, gender, population, duration of follow-up, period of intervention, exercise, type of n-3 PUFAs and dosage (g/day), muscle mass, muscle strength, and muscle performance outcomes. The primary outcomes of the trials were mean differences in the absolute changes in any measurements of skeletal muscle mass, muscle strength, or physical performance.

The methodological quality of included studies was evaluated according to the Cochrane Collaboration risk-of-bias tool [28]. The level of bias was considered to be high, low, or unclear based on seven domains, namely, (i) random sequence generation, (ii) allocation concealment, (iii) the blinding of the participants and personnel, (iv) the blinding of the outcome assessment, (v) incomplete outcome data, (vi) selective reporting, and (vii) other sources of bias. The result was depicted with a summarized risk-of-bias graph.

The quality of the evidence and strength of recommendation were assessed according to the Grading of Recommendations Assessment, Development, and Evaluation methodology (GRADE). The quality of evidence was classified as high, moderate, low, or very low based on judgments of risk-of-bias, inconsistency, imprecision, indirectness, and publication bias [29].

2.4. Data Synthesis and Statistical Analysis

Meta-analyses were performed using Review Manager Version 5.3 (RevMan). The primary analyses assessed the effects of n-3 PUFAs on the primary outcomes. The effect sizes were estimated as mean differences (MDs) or standardized mean differences (SMDs) when different scales were used with their 95% confidence intervals (CIs) and graphs created with a random-effects model. The MD was the absolute difference between the mean values in the two groups. The SMD was calculated as the difference in the mean outcome between groups divided by the standard deviation of outcome among participants [30]. We performed the analyses using a random-effects model to yield more conservative results. For all the analyses, $p < 0.05$ was considered statistically significant.

The forest plot is a graphic representation of the overall pooled results of the meta-analysis. The horizontal lines are the 95% CIs representing the probability that these estimates would occur in 95% of included studies. In addition, we need to assign weights, which were obtained by calculating the inverse of the variance of the treatment effect for individual studies based on their contributions to the pooled estimates. The MD was generally used for continuous outcomes under the inverse-variance (IV) method. Heterogeneity estimates between the studies were described by using Cochran Q (Chi-square test) and I^2 statistics, with values of 25–49% considered low, 50–74% considered moderate, and 75–100% considered high heterogeneity. For the chi-square test, the degrees of freedom (df) are equal to the number of studies minus one. The RevMan software presents an estimate (Tau^2) of the between-study variance in a random-effects meta-analysis. The Z test was used to examine the statistical significance of the overall effect. Furthermore, we performed subgroup analyses to explore the heterogeneity of the effect estimates according to participant characteristics (e.g., sex), intervention components (e.g., dosage of n-3 PUFAs over and below 2 g per day), and the duration of intervention. Sensitivity analysis was performed by using the one-study-out method and by restricting the synthesis of the findings to RCTs with low risks of bias. Publication bias was assessed by the visual inspection of funnel plots and the Egger bias test. The latter was performed using StataMP, version 14 (StataCorp; 2015; Stat Statistical Software: Release14; College Station, TX, USA; StataCorp LP).

3. Results

The screening and selection processes for the included studies are shown in Figure 2. We identified 230 potentially relevant records through multiple database searches (n = 226) and manual searching (n = 4). After excluding duplicate records (n = 11) and irrelevant articles by screening the titles and abstracts (n = 181), thirty-eight studies were evaluated in detail, of which 12 RCTs [20,21,25,31–39] (692 participants) met the inclusion criteria. Smith et al. [21] and Grenon et al. [33] were not considered for meta-analysis due to the lack of numerical data for the functional outcomes in the former and the reporting of only patient-perceived walking performance in the latter. Finally, data from 10 RCTs (552 participants) were submitted to the meta-analysis [20,25,31,32,34–39].

3.1. Characteristics of Eligible Studies

The basic characteristics of the 12 included studies are summarized in Table 1. Among them, five RCTs were conducted in Europe, three in the USA, three in Canada, and one in South America. The number of study participants ranged from 24 to 126, and the durations of the interventions spanned 10 to 24 weeks. Only two RCTs focused on specific diseases (non-small-cell lung cancer and peripheral artery disease); the remaining RCTs included healthy community elderly subjects. Six RCTs included only women, two of which considered only postmenopausal women. The mean ages of the participants across the 12 RCTs ranged from 63 to 75 years old.

Regarding the sources of n-3 PUFAs, nine RCTs provided long-chain n-3 PUFAs (EPA and/or DHA) from fish oil; one RCT provided ALA from flax oil, and two RCTs provided healthy dietary patterns (n-6/n-3 PUFAs < 2). The chemical form of fish oil is generally in the ethyl ester (EE) or triglyceride (TG) type; however, this information may not be formally labeled. Among the nine RCTs that provided n-3 PUFAs from fish oil, only two RCTs mentioned whether the PUFAs were in the EE [21] or TG [31] form.

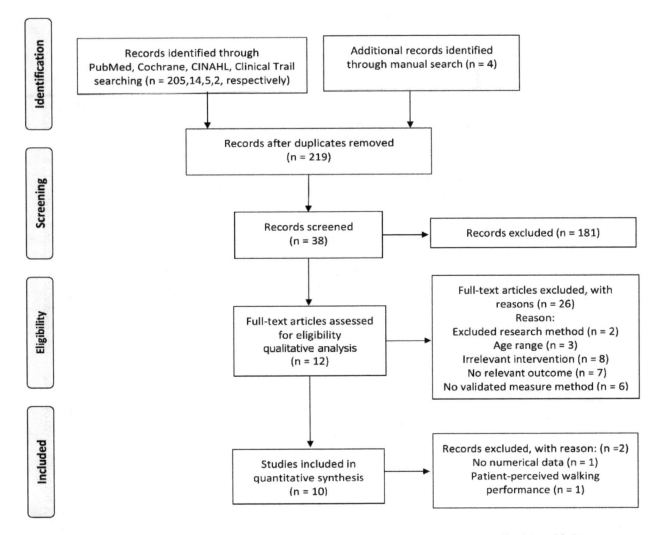

Figure 2. Flow chart of the study selection. Cumulative Index to Nursing and Allied Health Literature (CINAHL).

Strandberg et al. [38] reported a diet plan rich in fish, seafood, whole grains, and vegetables, with limited animal fat and soft drinks, while Edholm et al. [32] reported a diet based on dietary guidelines from Europe and the US; both RCTs monitored the macronutrients and n-6/n-3 PUFAs ratio using food records. Apart from the two RCTs mentioned above [32,38] with diet intervention, only three [20,31,36] of the remaining 10 RCTs requested that the study participants maintain their habitual diet. The doses ranged from 0.16 to 2.6 g/day of EPA and from 0 to 1.8 g/day of DHA. One study provided 14.0 g/day of ALA. Five RCTs reported data combining n-3 PUFA interventions with physical exercise.

Table 1. Study characteristics of the included trials.

Author (Year)	Country	Age (Years, Mean)	Subjects (n)	Sex (% Female)	Duration of Intervention (Weeks)	Exercise	Intervention: g/day, Sources	Outcome Measures
Cornish and Chilibeck (2009) [25]	Canada	65.4	Healthy (51)	45	12	RS	ALA:14 Flax oil	MM: lean tissue mass; MS: one-repetition maximum leg strength
Murphy et al. (2011) [37]	Canada	63.3	NSCLC (40)	48	~10	NA	EPA:2.2 FO capsules or liquid	MM: whole-body skeletal muscle
Rodacki et al. (2012) [20]	Brazil	64.1	Healthy (45)	100	12-20	RS	EPA:0.4 DHA:0.3 FO capsules	MS: knee flexor and extensor peak torque; MP: chair rising, Sit and reach, foot up and go, 6-min walk
Hutchins-Wiese et al. (2013) [34]	USA	75	Postmenopausal women (126)	100	24	NA	EPA:0.72 DHA:0.48 FO capsules	MS: hand grip; MP: walking speed, 8 foot walk, repeated chair rises
Krzyminska-Siemaszko et al. (2015) [35]	Poznan	74.9	Healthy (53)	100	12	NA	EPA:0.66 DHA:0.44 FO capsules	MM: ALM index, skeletal muscle mass, fat-free mass; MS: hand grip; MP: timed up and go test, 4 m walking test
Logan et al. (2015) [36]	Canada	66.1	Healthy (24)	68	12	NA	EPA:2 DHA:1 FO capsules	MM: lean mass; MS: grip strength; MP: timed up and go test, 30 s sit to stand
Strandberg et al. (2015) [38]	Sweden	67.7	Healthy (63)	100	24	RS	n-6/n-3 <2	MM: leg lean mass; MS: one-repetition maximum leg strength
Grenon et al.(2015) [33]	USA	68.5	PAD (80)	2	4	NA	EPA:2.6 DHA:1.8 FO capsules	MP: walking distance, walking speed
Smith et al. (2015) [21]	USA	68.3	Healthy (60)	66	24	NA	EPA:1.86 DHA:1.5 FO pill with EE form	MM: thigh muscle volume; MS: handgrip strength, one-repetition maximum leg strength
Strike et al. (2016) [39]	UK	66.8	Postmenopausal women (29)	100	24	NA	EPA:0.16 DHA:1.0 FO capsules	MP: habitual walking speed
Da Boit et al.(2017) [31]	UK	70.6	Healthy (58)	46	18	RS	EPA:2.1 DHA:0.6 FO capsules with TG form	MM: muscle ACSA; MS: maximal isometric torque; MP: 4 m walk time, chair-rise time
Edholm et al. (2017) [32]	Sweden	67.7	Healthy (63)	100	24	RS	n-6/n-3 <2	MM: whole body lean mass; MS: knee extension peak power one-repetition maximum; MP: five sit-to-stand, single-leg-stance tests, timed up and go Test

Abbreviations: ACSA; anatomic cross-sectional area; ALA; a-linolenic acid; NSCLC; non-small-cell lung cancer; DHA; docosahexaenoic acid; EPA; eicosapentaenoic acid; EE; ethyl esters; FO; fish oil; MM; muscle mass; MP; muscle performance; MS; muscle strength; NA, not available; PAD; peripheral artery disease; RS; resistance training; TG; triglyceride.

3.2. Risk of Bias and Evidence Certainty

The studies' risk of bias is shown in Figure 3. They were generally at low risk of bias for most domains including allocation concealment (92%), selective reporting (75%), and random sequence generation (67%) and at an unclear risk of bias for the blinding of the outcome assessment (92%). The blinding of the participants and investigators was at low risk in five studies (42%), unclear in four (33%), and at high risk in three (25%). The completeness of the outcome reporting was at low risk in four studies (33%) and high risk in eight (67%).

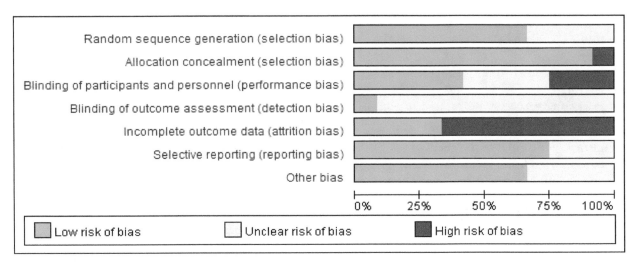

Figure 3. Summarized risk-of-bias graph for all included studies.

The evidence certainty for the primary outcomes including muscle mass, grip strength, one-repetition maximum in leg strength, walking speed, and the timed up and go test were rated from moderate to very low according to GRADE (Table 2).

Table 2. Summary effects of n-3 PUFAs on the outcomes of interest among the included studies and quality evidence of the Grading of Recommendations Assessment, Development and Evaluation (GRADE).

Outcome	No. of Studies	No. of Participants	Statistical Method	Effect Estimate	p-Value	Heterogeneity (I^2)	Certainty of the Evidence (GRADE)
Muscle mass (kg)	6	202	SMD. Random	0.33 (0.05, 0.62)	0.02	0%	⊕⊕⊕◯ MODERATE
Grip strength (kg)	3	97	SMD. Random	0.53 (−0.64, 1.69)	0.37	85%	⊕◯◯◯ VERY LOW
One-repetition maximum leg strength (kg)	3	88	SMD. Random	−0.15 (−0.93, 0.62)	0.70	69%	⊕◯◯◯ VERY LOW
Walk speed (m/sec)	5	251	SMD. Random	0.81 (−0.05, 1.67)	0.06	88%	⊕◯◯◯ VERY LOW
Time up and go test (s)	4	136	MD. Random	−0.30 (−0.43, −0.17)	<0.0001	37%	⊕◯◯◯ VERY LOW

Abbreviations: SMD: standardized mean difference; MD: mean difference.

3.3. Effects of n-3 PUFAs

A summary of the effects of the n-3 PUFAs on muscle mass, muscle strength, or muscle performance and the quality of the evidence according to GRADE are shown in Table 2.

For muscle mass, six studies with 202 participants reported measures of skeletal muscle mass based on the use of dual-energy X-ray absorptiometry, bioelectrical impedance analysis, or computed tomography, with intervention periods ranging from 10 to 24 weeks (Tables 1 and 2). There was evidence to support a beneficial effect of n-3 PUFA supplementation on the increase in skeletal muscle mass, compared with the control, with a small-to-moderate effect (SMD = 0.33, $p < 0.05$) (Figure 4).

Regarding muscle strength, the administration of n-3 PUFAs did not increase handgrip strength, the one-repetition maximum strength of the leg, and the walking speed compared with the controls (Supplementary Figure S1). However, the n-3 PUFAs group showed better performance (took less time) on the timed up and go test than the control group (MD = −0.30 s, p <0.05) (Figure 5).

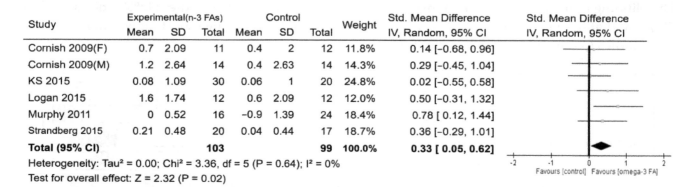

| Study | Experimental(n-3 FAs) | | | Control | | | Weight | Std. Mean Difference | Std. Mean Difference |
	Mean	SD	Total	Mean	SD	Total		IV, Random, 95% CI	IV, Random, 95% CI
Cornish 2009(F)	0.7	2.09	11	0.4	2	12	11.8%	0.14 [−0.68, 0.96]	
Cornish 2009(M)	1.2	2.64	14	0.4	2.63	14	14.3%	0.29 [−0.45, 1.04]	
KS 2015	0.08	1.09	30	0.06	1	20	24.8%	0.02 [−0.55, 0.58]	
Logan 2015	1.6	1.74	12	0.6	2.09	12	12.0%	0.50 [−0.31, 1.32]	
Murphy 2011	0	0.52	16	−0.9	1.39	24	18.4%	0.78 [0.12, 1.44]	
Strandberg 2015	0.21	0.48	20	0.04	0.44	17	18.7%	0.36 [−0.29, 1.01]	
Total (95% CI)			103			99	100.0%	0.33 [0.05, 0.62]	

Heterogeneity: Tau² = 0.00; Chi² = 3.36, df = 5 (P = 0.64); I² = 0%
Test for overall effect: Z = 2.32 (P = 0.02)

Figure 4. Forest plot of the effect of n-3 PUFA supplementation on muscle mass. IV: inverse-variance method. Random: random effect. Weight (in %), the influence of an individual study on the pooled result.

| Study | Experimental(n-3 FAs) | | | Control | | | Weight | Std. Mean Difference | Std. Mean Difference |
	Mean	SD	Total	Mean	SD	Total		IV, Random, 95% CI	IV, Random, 95% CI
Edholm 2017	−1.35	0.305	20	−1.21	0.455	17	19.1%	−0.14 [−0.39, 0.11]	
KS 2015	0.17	1.17	26	0.13	1.13	19	3.5%	0.04 [−0.64, 0.72]	
Logan 2015	−0.5	0.28	12	−0.2	0.08	12	33.0%	−0.30 [−0.46, −0.14]	
Rodacki 2012	−2.29	0.08	15	−1.89	0.22	15	44.4%	−0.40 [−0.52, −0.28]	
Total (95% CI)			73			63	100.0%	−0.30 [−0.43, −0.17]	

Heterogeneity: Tau² = 0.01; Chi² = 4.76, df = 3 (P = 0.19); I² = 37%
Test for overall effect: Z = 4.54 (P < 0.00001)

Figure 5. Forest plot of the effect of n-3 PUFA supplementation on the timed up and go test result. IV: inverse-variance method. Random, random effect. Weight (in %): the influence of an individual study on the pooled result.

Potential sources of heterogeneity between the studies were explored for the outcomes of muscle mass and walking speed. For muscle mass, we found no significant difference in the muscle mass between the subjects in the PUFA supplementation and dietary PUFA groups (Figure 6). We conducted a subgroup analysis to assess the effect of n-3 PUFA supplementation on muscle mass according to sex (Supplementary Figure S2a). There was no significant difference in the muscle mass between the n-3 PUFA group and the control group in both 61 females [25,35,38] and 14 males [25]. On the other hand, only one study by Cornish et al. [25] evaluated male participants according to n-3 PUFAs versus control. They also reported that n-3 PUFAs did not lead to an increase in muscle mass. When the subgroup analysis was based on the dosage of n-3 PUFAs, we found that only participants who received over 2 g/day of n-3 PUFAs had a significant increase in muscle mass compared to the control group (SMD = 0.67, p < 0.05) (Supplementary Figure S2b). By contrast, only one study [35] showed that participants who received n-3 PUFAs below 2 g/day exhibited no significant difference in muscle mass.

For walking speed, we found that studies with a follow-up duration of at least 24 weeks showed significant improvements in the walking speeds of subjects who received n-3 PUFAs, compared with the control group (SMD = 1.78, p < 0.05) while those with follow-up periods less than 24 weeks failed to show significant differences in walking speed (Supplementary Figure S3c). Four studies evaluated a female group, and one study by Cornish et al. [25] evaluated a male group; the results indicated that females or males who received n-3 PUFAs showed no improvement in walking speed

(Supplementary Figure S3a). Finally, when the subjects were stratified in combination with a resistance exercise intervention, the results showed no difference in walking speed (Supplementary Figure S3b).

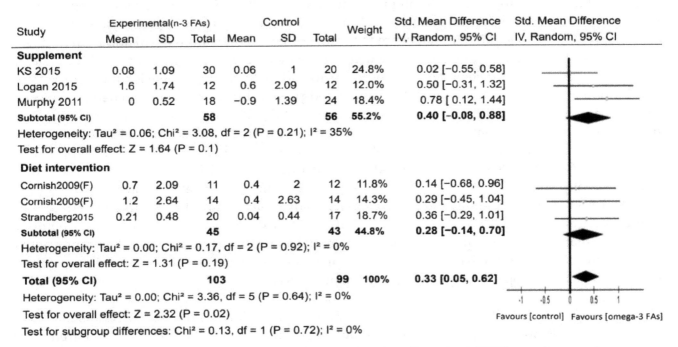

Study	Experimental(n-3 FAs)			Control			Weight	Std. Mean Difference IV, Random, 95% CI	Std. Mean Difference IV, Random, 95% CI
	Mean	SD	Total	Mean	SD	Total			
Supplement									
KS 2015	0.08	1.09	30	0.06	1	20	24.8%	0.02 [−0.55, 0.58]	
Logan 2015	1.6	1.74	12	0.6	2.09	12	12.0%	0.50 [−0.31, 1.32]	
Murphy 2011	0	0.52	18	−0.9	1.39	24	18.4%	0.78 [0.12, 1.44]	
Subtotal (95% CI)			58			56	55.2%	0.40 [−0.08, 0.88]	
Heterogeneity: Tau² = 0.06; Chi² = 3.08, df = 2 (P = 0.21); I² = 35%									
Test for overall effect: Z = 1.64 (P = 0.1)									
Diet intervention									
Cornish2009(F)	0.7	2.09	11	0.4	2	12	11.8%	0.14 [−0.68, 0.96]	
Cornish2009(F)	1.2	2.64	14	0.4	2.63	14	14.3%	0.29 [−0.45, 1.04]	
Strandberg2015	0.21	0.48	20	0.04	0.44	17	18.7%	0.36 [−0.29, 1.01]	
Subtotal (95% CI)			45			43	44.8%	0.28 [−0.14, 0.70]	
Heterogeneity: Tau² = 0.00; Chi² = 0.17, df = 2 (P = 0.92); I² = 0%									
Test for overall effect: Z = 1.31 (P = 0.19)									
Total (95% CI)			**103**			**99**	**100%**	**0.33 [0.05, 0.62]**	
Heterogeneity: Tau² = 0.00; Chi² = 3.36, df = 5 (P = 0.64); I² = 0%									
Test for overall effect: Z = 2.32 (P = 0.02)									
Test for subgroup differences: Chi² = 0.13, df = 1 (P = 0.72); I² = 0%									

Favours [control]   Favours [omega-3 FAs]

Figure 6. Forest plots of the included studies assessing the effect of n-3 PUFA supplementation on muscle mass categorized by the administration form of n-3 PUFAs. IV: inverse-variance method. Random: random effect. Weight (in %): the influence of an individual study on the pooled result.

3.4. Sensitivity Analysis and Publication Bias

To appraise the stability of the results, sensitivity analyses were carried out using the leave-one-out approach and recalculating the summary SMD. The results show that our findings are robust for muscle mass, handgrip strength, the one-repetition maximum strength of the leg, walking speed, and timed up and go performance (Supplementary Figure S4b–e). However, for muscle mass performance, the results show that the beneficial effect of n-3 PUFAs on skeletal muscle mass was not observed when the study of Murphy et al. [37] on cancer patients was excluded from the meta-analysis (Supplementary Figure S4a). In addition, no included trial was at low risk of bias, thus precluding the performance of the preplanned sensitivity analysis. The shapes of the funnel plots were symmetric, indicating that the publication bias was low in the meta-analysis (*p*-value of Egger's test > 0.05) (Supplementary Figure S5).

4. Discussion

Nutritional studies for sarcopenia-related performances had mostly focused on investigating the effects of protein supplementation. Even though studies had discussed n-3 PUFAs, outcomes with strong evidence or clear conclusions were seldom presented [15,16]. Our findings with 10 RCTs and 552 elderly participants showed that n-3 PUFA supplementation was associated with an increase in muscle mass by ~0.33 kg for the elderly, especially when more than 2 g/day of n-3 PUFAs was given. In terms of muscle strength, we found that n-3 PUFA supplementation did not elicit greater handgrip strength or one-repetition maximum strength of the leg. For muscle performance, n-3 PUFA administration slightly enhanced performance in the timed up and go test compared to that for the controls and facilitated a faster walking speed when administered for more than 24 weeks.

Our present finding that increased n-3 PUFA supplementation has a positive health effect on muscle mass is consistent with previous reports indicating that dietary ω-3 fatty acids increase the rate of muscle protein synthesis in older subjects [19], and suppresses the inflammation cascade in patients with Duchenne muscular dystrophy [40]. Muscle mass is maintained by a balance between muscle protein synthesis and breakdown. The supplementation of n-3 PUFAs increases the n-3 fatty acid composition of the phospholipids in the skeletal muscle membranes. Several muscle synthesis mechanisms involving n-3 PUFAs have been proposed, including the induction of the mTORC1-p70S6K1 signaling pathway, which leads to increased protein synthesis [41] and the downregulation of proteasome expression, thus suppressing muscle protein catabolism [42]. Concordantly, both animal [43] and human [19,40] studies have shown that n-3 PUFA supplementation enhances amino acid- and insulin-mediated increases in the rates of muscle protein syntheses. As for n-3 PUFA sources, there is a report of a strong association between EPA supplementation, increased plasma EPA levels, and elicited gains in the muscle mass of patients with non-small cell lung cancer [37]. This is consistent with evidence that lower EPA levels are associated with lower muscle mass, strength and function [44]. According to Logan et al. and Muphy et al.'s studies [36,37], when more than 2 g of n-3 PUFAs were supplied, an additional ~0.67 kg muscle mass was retained than when 1.1 g of n-3 PUFAs were given [35] according to our subgroup analysis. Although we cannot identify the effect for the elderly on taking only DHA or EPA or both based on limited studies, our meta-analysis still found that supplementation with both types of n-3 PUFAs (EPA and/or DHA) elicits a ~ 0.33 kg increase in muscle mass. Therefore, we suggest that n-3 PUFA supplementation has potential as an efficacious nutrition-based preventive or therapeutic strategy to combat the loss of muscle mass in the elderly, and the optimal dosing pattern for n-3 PUFAs for sarcopenia-associated performance needs to be confirmed by a large-scale RCT in the future.

The original definition of sarcopenia by the European Working Group on Sarcopenia in Older People (EWGSOP) was the "presence of both low muscle mass + low muscle function (strength or performance)" [3]. The recently updated consensus EWGSOP guideline for the case-finding and diagnosis of sarcopenia (EWGSOP2) focused on low muscle strength (and not low muscle mass) as a principal feature of sarcopenia [45]. Grip strength and chair stand measures are widely used for measuring muscle strength. Fish intake related to muscle strength in observational studies are not consistent [22,46]. Smith et al. [21] supplied 1.86 g of EPA and 1.5 g of DHA for older adults (aged 68.3 years old) for 6 months and observed positive outcomes in terms of sarcopenia-related performances. However, 1.3 g of n-3 PUFAs for 3 months failed to generate positive outcomes [35], and even 3-years treatment with low dose EPA (225 mg) and DHA (800 mg) resulted in no significant difference in chair stand performance according to resent RCT research [23]. We did not observe any improvement in muscle strength following the n-3 PUFA supplementation in this meta-analysis. The doses of the supplements, durations of the interventions, methodologies for assessing body composition, and characteristics of the study populations might have contributed to the inconsistency in the findings between studies.

Commonly used physical performance measures include timed up and go test performance and the gait speed. The timed up and go test is a functional mobility test that estimates the time it takes the participant to rise from an arm chair, walk 3 m away, return, and then sit down. We observed an improvement in the timed up and go test performance following n-3 PUFA supplementation, by 0.3 s, in our results. Because the percentage weight indicates the influence of an individual study on the pooled result, a larger study with a more precise effect size estimate gets a higher weight, and a smaller study gets a lower weight. For example, among these four trails (Figure 5), the percentage weight of Rodacki et al.'s trail [20], with a larger sample size, was 44.4%, which is higher than that (3.5%) of Krzyminska-Siemaszko et al.'s trail [35], with a smaller sample size. Recently, Sang-Rok's RCT trail [47] found that fish oil consumption combined with resistance training improved the strength and physical function indicators such as Timed Up and Go performance in community-dwelling older adults. Consistent with our findings, the three-city study showed that higher plasma concentrations of long-chain n-3 PUFAs were associated with a lower proportion of individuals with slow gait speed [48], but only among the elders receiving at least 6-month of n-3 PUFA supplementation in subgroups from two studies [34,39]. We found that compared with the control group, n-3 PUFAs improved the walking speed by 1.78 m/sec. This change is clinically relevant in the context of aging [49].

The limitations of this meta-analysis include the limited numbers of relevant trials. Secondly, the results were heterogeneous. The differences in the n-3 PUFAs dosage and constitution, frequency of administration, follow-up duration, study cohort and control group in each trial could have led to different supplementation efficacy. Even though we used a random-effects model in the meta-analysis, there are still possible residual confounders such as the baseline nutritional status of the cohort in each trial, which was not described. Third, data regarding the physical exercise regimens were reported for only five RCTs and thus, it was not possible to isolate the effect of n-3 PUFAs intake alone. Finally, it was mentioned that the beneficial effect of n-3 PUFAs on muscle mass was not observed after excluding from the meta-analysis a study on patients with cancer [37]. This raises the question of a cohort-/sample-specific effect of n-3 PUFAs on muscle mass and the importance of further research in this respect to clarify the issue.

5. Conclusions

The present meta-analysis based on 10 studies found moderate evidence for the beneficial effect of n-3 PUFAs on muscle mass, especially for those taking supplements at more than 2 g/day. We also observed that a long period of n-3 PUFA supplementation may improve walking speed. The appropriate supplementation of n-3 PUFAs may have benefits on muscle mass and performances among the elderly.

Supplementary Materials
Figure S1. Forest plots of the effect of n-3 PUFA supplementation on handgrip (a), one-repetition maximum strength of the leg (b), and walking speed (c). Figure S2. Forest plots of the included studies assessing the effect of n-3 PUFA supplementation on muscle mass categorized by sex (a) and the dosage of n-3 PUFAs (b). Figure S3. Forest plots of the included studies assessing the effect of n-3 PUFA supplementation on walking speed categorized by sex (a), resistance training intervention (b), and the duration of supplementation (c). Figure S4. Sensitivity analyses by muscle mass (a), handgrip strength (b), one-repetition maximum strength of the leg (c), walking speed (d), and the timed up and go test result (e). Figure S5. Charts of Egger's test of muscle mass (a), handgrip strength (b), one-repetition maximum strength of the leg (c), walking speed (d), and the timed up and go test result (e).

Author Contributions: Conceptualization, Y.-H.W.; design, Y.-H.W.; supervision, Y.-H.W.; materials, Y.-H.H. Y.-P.H. and Y.-L.L.; data collection and/or processing, Y.-H.H., Y.-P.H. and W.-C.C.; analysis and/or interpretation Y.-H.H., Y.-P.H., W.-C.C. and Y.-L.L.; literature search, Y.-H.H. and Y.-L.L.; writing manuscript, Y.-H.H. and W.-C.C.; critical review, Y.-H.W. All authors have read and agreed to the published version of the manuscript.

Acknowledgments: We thank Oluwaseun Adebayo Bamodu of the Department of Medical Research and Education, Taipei Medical University-ShuanFg Ho Hospital, for his constructive criticism, kind proofreading, and English language editing of the manuscript.

References

1. Gale, C.R.; Westbury, L.D.; Cooper, C.; Dennison, E.M. Risk factors for incident falls in older men and women: The English longitudinal study of ageing. *BMC Geriatr.* 2018, 18, 117. [CrossRef] [PubMed]

2. United Nations, Department of Economic and Social Affairs, Population Division. *World Population Prospects: The 2017 Revision, Key Findings and Advance Tables*; Working Paper No. ESA/WP/248; United Nations: New York, NY, USA, 2017.

3. Cruz-Jentoft, A.J.; Baeyens, J.P.; Bauer, J.M.; Boirie, Y.; Cederholm, T.; Landi, F.; Martin, F.C.; Michel, J.P.; Rolland, Y.; Schneider, S.M.; et al. Sarcopenia: European consensus on definition and diagnosis: Report of the European Working Group on Sarcopenia in Older People. *Age Ageing* 2010, 39, 412–423. [CrossRef] [PubMed]

4. Woo, J.; Leung, J.; Morley, J.E. Defining sarcopenia in terms of incident adverse outcomes. *J. Am. Med. Dir. Assoc.* 2015, 16, 247–252. [CrossRef]

5. Fried, L.P.; Guralnik, J.M. Disability in older adults: Evidence regarding significance, etiology, and risk. *J. Am. Geriatr. Soc.* 1997, 45, 92–100. [CrossRef]

6. Bruyere, O.; Beaudart, C.; Ethgen, O.; Reginster, J.Y.; Locquet, M. The health economics burden of sarcopenia: A systematic review. *Maturitas* 2019, 119, 61–69. [CrossRef]

7. Beaudart, C.; Dawson, A.; Shaw, S.C.; Harvey, N.C.; Kanis, J.A.; Binkley, N.; Reginster, J.Y.; Chapurlat, R.; Chan, D.C.; Bruyere, O.; et al. Nutrition and physical activity in the prevention and treatment of sarcopenia: Systematic review. *Osteoporos. Int.* 2017, 28, 1817–1833. [CrossRef]

8.   Traylor, D.A.; Gorissen, S.H.M.; Phillips, S.M. Perspective: Protein Requirements and Optimal Intakes in Aging: Are We Ready to Recommend More Than the Recommended Daily Allowance? *Adv. Nutr.* **2018**, *9*, 171–182. [CrossRef]

9.   Wang, E.T.; de Koning, L.; Kanaya, A.M. Higher protein intake is associated with diabetes risk in South Asian Indians: The Metabolic Syndrome and Atherosclerosis in South Asians Living in America (MASALA) study. *J. Am. Coll. Nutr.* **2010**, *29*, 130–135. [CrossRef]

10.   Tinker, L.F.; Sarto, G.E.; Howard, B.V.; Huang, Y.; Neuhouser, M.L.; Mossavar-Rahmani, Y.; Beasley, J.M.; Margolis, K.L.; Eaton, C.B.; Phillips, L.S.; et al. Biomarker-calibrated dietary energy and protein intake associations with diabetes risk among postmenopausal women from the Women's Health Initiative. *Am. J. Clin. Nutr.* **2011**, *94*, 1600–1606. [CrossRef]

11.   Sluijs, I.; Beulens, J.W.; Spijkerman, A.M.; Grobbee, D.E.; van der Schouw, Y.T. Dietary intake of total, animal, and vegetable protein and risk of type 2 diabetes in the European Prospective Investigation into Cancer and Nutrition (EPIC)-NL study. *Diabetes Care* **2010**, *33*, 43–48. [CrossRef]

12.   Cangussu, L.M.; Nahas-Neto, J.; Orsatti, C.L.; Bueloni-Dias, F.N.; Nahas, E.A. Effect of vitamin D supplementation alone on muscle function in postmenopausal women: A randomized, double-blind, placebo-controlled clinical trial. *Osteoporos. Int.* **2015**, *26*, 2413–2421. [CrossRef] [PubMed]

13.   Verreijen, A.M.; Verlaan, S.; Engberink, M.F.; Swinkels, S.; de Vogel-van den Bosch, J.; Weijs, P.J. A high whey protein-, leucine-, and vitamin D-enriched supplement preserves muscle mass during intentional weight loss in obese older adults: A double-blind randomized controlled trial. *Am. J. Clin. Nutr.* **2015**, *101*, 279–286. [CrossRef] [PubMed]

14.   Bloom, I.; Shand, C.; Cooper, C.; Robinson, S.; Baird, J. Diet Quality and Sarcopenia in Older Adults: A Systematic Review. *Nutrients* **2018**, *10*, 308. [CrossRef] [PubMed]

15.   Tessier, A.J.; Chevalier, S. An Update on Protein, Leucine, Omega-3 Fatty Acids, and Vitamin D in the Prevention and Treatment of Sarcopenia and Functional Decline. *Nutrients* **2018**, *10*, 1099. [CrossRef]

16.   Dupont, J.; Dedeyne, L.; Dalle, S.; Koppo, K.; Gielen, E. The role of omega-3 in the prevention and treatment of sarcopenia. *Aging Clin. Exp. Res.* **2019**, *31*, 825–836. [CrossRef]

17.   Abdelhamid, A.S.; Brown, T.J.; Brainard, J.S.; Biswas, P.; Thorpe, G.C.; Moore, H.J.; Deane, K.H.; Summerbell, C.D.; Worthington, H.V.; Song, F.; et al. Omega-3 fatty acids for the primary and secondary prevention of cardiovascular disease. *Cochrane Database Syst. Rev.* **2020**, *3*, CD003177. [CrossRef]

18.   Lalia, A.Z.; Dasari, S.; Robinson, M.M.; Abid, H.; Morse, D.M.; Klaus, K.A.; Lanza, I.R. Influence of omega-3 fatty acids on skeletal muscle protein metabolism and mitochondrial bioenergetics in older adults. *Aging* **2017**, *9*, 1096–1129. [CrossRef]

19.   Smith, G.I.; Atherton, P.; Reeds, D.N.; Mohammed, B.S.; Rankin, D.; Rennie, M.J.; Mittendorfer, B. Dietary omega-3 fatty acid supplementation increases the rate of muscle protein synthesis in older adults: A randomized controlled trial. *Am. J. Clin. Nutr.* **2011**, *93*, 402–412. [CrossRef]

20.   Rodacki, C.L.; Rodacki, A.L.; Pereira, G.; Naliwaiko, K.; Coelho, I.; Pequito, D.; Fernandes, L.C. Fish-oil supplementation enhances the effects of strength training in elderly women. *Am. J. Clin. Nutr.* **2012**, *95*, 428–436. [CrossRef]

21.   Smith, G.I.; Julliand, S.; Reeds, D.N.; Sinacore, D.R.; Klein, S.; Mittendorfer, B. Fish oil-derived n-3 PUFA therapy increases muscle mass and function in healthy older adults. *Am. J. Clin. Nutr.* **2015**, *102*, 115–122. [CrossRef]

22.   Robinson, S.M.; Jameson, K.A.; Batelaan, S.F.; Martin, H.J.; Syddall, H.E.; Dennison, E.M.; Cooper, C.; Sayer, A.A.; Hertfordshire Cohort Study Group. Diet and its relationship with grip strength in community-dwelling older men and women: The Hertfordshire cohort study. *J. Am. Geriatr Soc.* **2008**, *56*, 84–90. [CrossRef] [PubMed]

23.   Rolland, Y.; Barreto, P.S.; Maltais, M.; Guyonnet, S.; Cantet, C.; Andrieu, S.; Vellas, B. Effect of Long-Term Omega 3 Polyunsaturated Fatty Acid Supplementation with or without Multidomain Lifestyle Intervention on Muscle Strength in Older Adults: Secondary Analysis of the Multidomain Alzheimer Preventive Trial (MAPT). *Nutrients* **2019**, *11*, 1931. [CrossRef] [PubMed]

24.   Wijendran, V.; Hayes, K.C. Dietary n-6 and n-3 fatty acid balance and cardiovascular health. *Annu. Rev. Nutr.* **2004**, *24*, 597–615. [CrossRef] [PubMed]

25.   Cornish, S.M.; Chilibeck, P.D. Alpha-linolenic acid supplementation and resistance training in older adults. *Appl. Physiol. Nutr. Metab.* **2009**, *34*, 49–59. [CrossRef]

26. Gray, S.R.; Mittendorfer, B. Fish oil-derived n-3 polyunsaturated fatty acids for the prevention and treatment of sarcopenia. *Curr. Opin. Clin. Nutr. Metab. Care* **2018**, *21*, 104–109. [CrossRef]

27. Liberati, A.; Altman, D.G.; Tetzlaff, J.; Mulrow, C.; Gotzsche, P.C.; Ioannidis, J.P.; Clarke, M.; Devereaux, P.J.; Kleijnen, J.; Moher, D. The PRISMA statement for reporting systematic reviews and meta-analyses of studies that evaluate health care interventions: Explanation and elaboration. *J. Clin. Epidemiol.* **2009**, *62*, e1–e34. [CrossRef]

28. Higgins, J.P.; Altman, D.G.; Gotzsche, P.C.; Juni, P.; Moher, D.; Oxman, A.D.; Savovic, J.; Schulz, K.F.; Weeks, L.; Sterne, J.A.; et al. The Cochrane Collaboration's tool for assessing risk of bias in randomised trials. *BMJ* **2011**, *343*, d5928. [CrossRef]

29. Guyatt, G.; Oxman, A.D.; Akl, E.A.; Kunz, R.; Vist, G.; Brozek, J.; Norris, S.; Falck-Ytter, Y.; Glasziou, P.; DeBeer, H.; et al. GRADE guidelines: 1. Introduction-GRADE evidence profiles and summary of findings tables. *J. Clin. Epidemiol.* **2011**, *64*, 383–394. [CrossRef]

30. Cochrane Handbook for Systematic Reviews of Interventions Version 6.1 (Updated September 2020). Available online: www.training.cochrane.org/handbook (accessed on 10 September 2020).

31. Da Boit, M.; Sibson, R.; Sivasubramaniam, S.; Meakin, J.R.; Greig, C.A.; Aspden, R.M.; Thies, F.; Jeromson, S.; Hamilton, D.L.; Speakman, J.R.; et al. Sex differences in the effect of fish-oil supplementation on the adaptive response to resistance exercise training in older people: A randomized controlled trial. *Am. J. Clin. Nutr.* **2017**, *105*, 151–158. [CrossRef]

32. Edholm, P.; Strandberg, E.; Kadi, F. Lower limb explosive strength capacity in elderly women: Effects of resistance training and healthy diet. *J. Appl. Physiol (1985)* **2017**, *123*, 190–196. [CrossRef]

33. Grenon, S.M.; Owens, C.D.; Nosova, E.V.; Hughes-Fulford, M.; Alley, H.F.; Chong, K.; Perez, S.; Yen, P.K.; Boscardin, J.; Hellmann, J.; et al. Short-Term, High-Dose Fish Oil Supplementation Increases the Production of Omega-3 Fatty Acid-Derived Mediators in Patients With Peripheral Artery Disease (the OMEGA-PAD I Trial). *J. Am. Heart Assoc.* **2015**, *4*, e002034. [CrossRef] [PubMed]

34. Hutchins-Wiese, H.L.; Kleppinger, A.; Annis, K.; Liva, E.; Lammi-Keefe, C.J.; Durham, H.A.; Kenny, A.M. The impact of supplemental n-3 long chain polyunsaturated fatty acids and dietary antioxidants on physical performance in postmenopausal women. *J. Nutr. Health Aging* **2013**, *17*, 76–80. [CrossRef] [PubMed]

35. Krzyminska-Siemaszko, R.; Czepulis, N.; Lewandowicz, M.; Zasadzka, E.; Suwalska, A.; Witowski, J.; Wieczorowska-Tobis, K. The Effect of a 12-Week Omega-3 Supplementation on Body Composition, Muscle Strength and Physical Performance in Elderly Individuals with Decreased Muscle Mass. *Int. J. Environ. Res. Public Health* **2015**, *12*, 10558–10574. [CrossRef] [PubMed]

36. Logan, S.L.; Spriet, L.L. Omega-3 Fatty Acid Supplementation for 12 Weeks Increases Resting and Exercise Metabolic Rate in Healthy Community-Dwelling Older Females. *PLoS ONE* **2015**, *10*, e0144828. [CrossRef]

37. Murphy, R.A.; Mourtzakis, M.; Chu, Q.S.; Baracos, V.E.; Reiman, T.; Mazurak, V.C. Nutritional intervention with fish oil provides a benefit over standard of care for weight and skeletal muscle mass in patients with nonsmall cell lung cancer receiving chemotherapy. *Cancer* **2011**, *117*, 1775–1782. [CrossRef]

38. Strandberg, E.; Edholm, P.; Ponsot, E.; Wahlin-Larsson, B.; Hellmen, E.; Nilsson, A.; Engfeldt, P.; Cederholm, T.; Riserus, U.; Kadi, F. Influence of combined resistance training and healthy diet on muscle mass in healthy elderly women: A randomized controlled trial. *J. Appl. Physiol (1985)* **2015**, *119*, 918–925. [CrossRef]

39. Strike, S.C.; Carlisle, A.; Gibson, E.L.; Dyall, S.C. A High Omega-3 Fatty Acid Multinutrient Supplement Benefits Cognition and Mobility in Older Women: A Randomized, Double-blind, Placebo-controlled Pilot Study. *J. Gerontol. Biol. Sci. Med. Sci.* **2016**, *71*, 236–242. [CrossRef]

40. Rodríguez-Cruz, M.; Cruz-Guzmán, O.D.R.; Almeida-Becerril, T.; Solís-Serna, A.D.; Atilano-Miguel, S.; Sánchez-González, J.R.; Barbosa-Cortés, L.; Ruíz-Cruz, E.D.; Huicochea, J.C.; Cárdenas-Conejo, A.; et al. Potential therapeutic impact of omega-3 long chain-polyunsaturated fatty acids on inflammation markers in Duchenne muscular dystrophy: A double-blind, controlled randomized trial. *Clin. Nutr.* **2018**, *37*, 1840–1851. [CrossRef]

41. You, J.S.; McNally, R.M.; Jacobs, B.L.; Privett, R.E.; Gundermann, D.M.; Lin, K.H.; Steinert, N.D.; Goodman, C.A.; Hornberger, T.A. The role of raptor in the mechanical load-induced regulation of mTOR signaling, protein synthesis, and skeletal muscle hypertrophy. *FASEB J.* **2019**, *33*, 4021–4034. [CrossRef]

42. Whitehouse, A.S.; Smith, H.J.; Drake, J.L.; Tisdale, M.J. Mechanism of attenuation of skeletal muscle protein catabolism in cancer cachexia by eicosapentaenoic acid. *Cancer Res.* **2001**, *61*, 3604–3609.

43.   Gingras, A.A.; White, P.J.; Chouinard, P.Y.; Julien, P.; Davis, T.A.; Dombrowski, L.; Couture, Y.; Dubreuil, P.; Myre, A.; Bergeron, K.; et al. Long-chain omega-3 fatty acids regulate bovine whole-body protein metabolism by promoting muscle insulin signalling to the Akt-mTOR-S6K1 pathway and insulin sensitivity. *J. Physiol.* **2007**, *579*, 269–284. [CrossRef] [PubMed]

44.   Ter Borg, S.; Luiking, Y.C.; van Helvoort, A.; Boirie, Y.; Schols, J.M.G.A.; de Groot, C.P.G.M. Low Levels of Branched Chain Amino Acids, Eicosapentaenoic Acid and Micronutrients Are Associated with Low Muscle Mass, Strength and Function in Community-Dwelling Older Adults. *J. Nutr. Health Aging* **2019**, *23*, 27–34. [CrossRef] [PubMed]

45.   Cruz-Jentoft, A.J.; Bahat, G.; Bauer, J.; Boirie, Y.; Bruyere, O.; Cederholm, T.; Cooper, C.; Landi, F.; Rolland, Y.; Sayer, A.A.; et al. Sarcopenia: Revised European consensus on definition and diagnosis. *Age Ageing* **2019**, *48*, 16–31. [CrossRef] [PubMed]

46.   Rousseau, J.H.; Kleppinger, A.; Kenny, A.M. Self-reported dietary intake of omega-3 fatty acids and association with bone and lower extremity function. *J. Am. Geriatr. Soc.* **2009**, *57*, 1781–1788. [CrossRef]

47.   Lee, S.R.; Jo, E.; Khamoui, A.V. Chronic Fish Oil Consumption with Resistance Training Improves Grip Strength, Physical Function, and Blood Pressure in Community-Dwelling Older Adults. *Sports* **2019**, *7*, 167. [CrossRef]

48.   Frison, E.; Boirie, Y.; Peuchant, E.; Tabue-Teguo, M.; Barberger-Gateau, P.; Féart, C. Plasma fatty acid biomarkers are associated with gait speed in community-dwelling older adults: The Three-City-Bordeaux study. *Clin. Nutr.* **2017**, *36*, 416–422. [CrossRef]

49.   Perera, S.; Mody, S.H.; Woodman, R.C.; Studenski, S.A. Meaningful change and responsiveness in common physical performance measures in older adults. *J. Am. Geriatr. Soc.* **2006**, *54*, 743–749. [CrossRef]

2

Expert Opinion on Benefits of Long-Chain Omega-3 Fatty Acids (DHA and EPA) in Aging and Clinical Nutrition

Barbara Troesch [1] [ID], Manfred Eggersdorfer [2], Alessandro Laviano [3] [ID], Yves Rolland [4], A. David Smith [5], Ines Warnke [1] [ID], Arved Weimann [6] and Philip C. Calder [7],*[ID]

[1]   Nutrition Science and Advocacy, DSM Nutritional Products, 4303 Kaiseraugst, Switzerland; barbara.troesch@dsm.com (B.T.); ines.warnke@dsm.com (I.W.)
[2]   Department of Internal Medicine, University Medical Center Groningen, 9713 GZ Groningen, The Netherlands; dr.eggersdorfer@gmail.com
[3]   Department of Translational and Precision Medicine, Sapienza University, 00185 Rome, Italy; alessandro.laviano@uniroma1.it
[4]   Gérontopôle de Toulouse, Institut du Vieillissement, INSERM 1027, Centre Hospitalo-Universitaire de Toulouse, 31300 Toulouse, France; rolland.y@chu-toulouse.fr
[5]   Department of Pharmacology, University of Oxford, Oxford OX1 2JD, UK; david.smith@pharm.ox.ac.uk
[6]   Clinic for General, Visceral and Oncological Surgery, St. Georg gGmbH Clinic, 04129 Leipzig, Germany; Arved.Weimann@sanktgeorg.de
[7]   Faculty of Medicine, University of Southampton and NIHR Southampton Biomedical Research Centre, University Hospital Southampton NHS Foundation Trust and University of Southampton, Southampton SO16 6YD, UK
*   Correspondence: pcc@soton.ac.uk

Abstract: Life expectancy is increasing and so is the prevalence of age-related non-communicable diseases (NCDs). Consequently, older people and patients present with multi-morbidities and more complex needs, putting significant pressure on healthcare systems. Effective nutrition interventions could be an important tool to address patient needs, improve clinical outcomes and reduce healthcare costs. Inflammation plays a central role in NCDs, so targeting it is relevant to disease prevention and treatment. The long-chain omega-3 polyunsaturated fatty acids (omega-3 LCPUFAs) docosahexaenoic acid (DHA) and eicosapentaenoic acid (EPA) are known to reduce inflammation and promote its resolution, suggesting a beneficial role in various therapeutic areas. An expert group reviewed the data on omega-3 LCPUFAs in specific patient populations and medical conditions. Evidence for benefits in cognitive health, age- and disease-related decline in muscle mass, cancer treatment, surgical patients and critical illness was identified. Use of DHA and EPA in some conditions is already included in some relevant guidelines. However, it is important to note that data on the effects of omega-3 LCPUFAs are still inconsistent in many areas (e.g., cognitive decline) due to a range of factors that vary amongst the trials performed to date; these factors include dose, timing and duration; baseline omega-3 LCPUFA status; and intake of other nutrients. Well-designed intervention studies are required to optimize the effects of DHA and EPA in specific patient populations and to develop more personalized strategies for their use.

Keywords: clinical nutrition; oral nutritional supplementation; DHA and EPA; long-chain omega-3 polyunsaturated fatty acids; inflammation; Alzheimer's disease; immunonutrition; frailty; sarcopenia; cancer cachexia

1. Introduction

Life expectancy is increasing globally [1] and the prevalence of age- and lifestyle-related non-communicable diseases (NCDs), such as cancer, heart disease, respiratory disease, type 2 diabetes, obesity, chronic kidney disease and dementia is rising [2,3]. This has led patients to present with multiple co-morbidities [4,5] creating more complex needs (e.g., need for multiple medications), putting significant pressure on healthcare and social systems. Undernutrition and overnutrition can both seriously impact an individual's risk for developing an NCD [2,3]. There is therefore a growing demand for appropriate nutrition interventions and targeted medical nutrition supplements or formulas to address patient needs, improve outcomes and help to reduce the costs of healthcare. Inflammation is considered to play a central role in age- and lifestyle-related NCDs [6], in loss of muscle mass and strength (sarcopenia) in frailty and cancer [7–9], and in the response to surgery and in critical illness [10]. Hence, targeting inflammation is thought to be appropriate to disease prevention and treatment. The long-chain omega-3 polyunsaturated fatty acids (LCPUFAs) docosahexaenoic acid (DHA) and eicosapentaenoic acid (EPA) are known to have roles in supporting human health [11], with one of their primary actions being to reduce inflammation [12–14] and promote its resolution [15–17]. This suggests a broad role for DHA and EPA in prevention and treatment of disease including, but not restricted to, specific therapeutic areas such as age-related decline in muscle mass, oncology, perioperative care and cognitive health.

Humans, like all mammals, cannot synthesize the essential omega-3 fatty acid α-linolenic acid. Furthermore, endogenous synthesis of EPA and DHA from α-linolenic acid is described as being poor in most humans [18] and is influenced by a range of factors such as age, sex, genetics and disease [18]. Therefore, preformed EPA and DHA must be obtained from the diet or supplements. It is now generally accepted that an intake of at least 250 mg EPA and DHA per day is required for optimal nutrition [19–22], although the exact intake required for specific populations or health conditions is not known and in many cases is likely to be in excess of this suggested minimum intake.

Blood levels of EPA and DHA are highly related to intakes [23]. Global mapping indicated low or even very low blood levels of omega-3 LCPUFAs (i.e., DHA and EPA) in a large proportion of people for whom data were available [24], suggesting low intakes in those populations. Reliance on endogenous synthesis of EPA and DHA is challenged by the low activity of this pathway [18] which is further impaired in conditions such as insulin resistance [25]. Therefore, the benefits of DHA and EPA might be particularly pronounced in those population groups with insulin resistance or other features that limit endogenous synthesis. The anti-inflammatory and inflammation resolving effects of DHA and EPA have been shown to be relevant to improved clinical outcomes in a number of specific therapeutic areas [12–17,26]. Furthermore, evidence suggests that DHA and EPA support independence in the older population, improving quality of life and significantly lowering healthcare costs [27]. Moreover, they appear to be crucial for a well-functioning immune system [28] and play an essential role in the maintenance of muscle mass and function [29], both important considerations for older people.

Adequate supply with DHA and EPA should therefore be seen as a critical component of both the prevention and treatment of many, but particularly age-related, conditions. This review aims to summarize the available evidence for DHA and EPA to promote healthy aging and to improve prognosis in a selection of medical conditions as discussed at an expert group meeting in September 2019.

2. The Relevance of Mechanisms of Action of DHA and EPA

DHA and EPA appear to act via overlapping, as well as distinct, mechanisms of action, modifying cellular function to benefit overall health and wellbeing, as well as to reduce the risk and severity of disease; these mechanisms are discussed in detail elsewhere [11,30,31]. It is their membrane-mediated mechanisms that are most well established and understood [32–35] and it is considered that through alterations at the membrane level in different cell and tissue types, DHA and EPA play an important role in cell signaling, gene expression and lipid mediator production [36]. These mechanisms are quite well explored in the context of omega-3 LCPUFA regulation of inflammatory processes, as described in detail elsewhere [12–14] (Figure 1). For example, increased intake of EPA and DHA results in enhanced appearance of those fatty acids in the membrane phospholipids of cells involved in inflammation (see [12–14] for references). This has multiple effects. Firstly, cell membranes become more fluid, affecting the behavior of several membrane proteins, including their aggregation into signaling platforms, so-called lipid rafts (see [12–14] for references). As a result, transmission of inflammatory signals within cells, for example from lipopolysaccharide or saturated fatty acids, becomes blunted, resulting in reduced activation of pro-inflammatory transcription factors like nuclear factor kappa-light-chain-enhancer of activated B cells (NFκB) (see [12–14] for references). Such transcription factors control expression of genes encoding many cytokines, chemokines, adhesion molecules, inflammatory enzymes (e.g., cyclooxygenase-2) and proteases. Thus, though these effects are initiated at the cell membrane level, omega-3 LCPUFAs can affect multiple inflammatory mediators and their anti-inflammatory actions could be wide-ranging as a result. The second effect of increased EPA and DHA in the membranes of inflammatory cells is that they partially replace the omega-6 PUFA arachidonic acid (see [12–14] for references). Arachidonic acid is the usual substrate for cyclooxygenase, lipoxygenase and cytochrome P450 enzymes producing eicosanoids [37,38]; these eicosanoids (e.g., prostaglandin E_2, leukotriene B_4) are recognized mediators of inflammation [38]. Therefore, through the EPA- and DHA-mediated decrease in arachidonic acid availability, production of these inflammatory eicosanoids is decreased (see [12–14] for references). The third effect of increased EPA and DHA in the membranes of inflammatory cells is that they can be released upon cellular activation. The "free" EPA and DHA can then have further actions. For example, they can act as ligands and activators for anti-inflammatory transcription factors such as peroxisome proliferator activated receptors (see [12–14] for references) and they can act as substrates for synthesis of eicosanoid and docosanoid lipid mediators. Eicosanoids formed from EPA such as prostaglandin E_3 and leukotriene B_5 often have only weak pro-inflammatory activity (see [12–14] for references). However, probably more importantly, both DHA and EPA are substrates for the synthesis of highly active lipid mediators important in the resolution of inflammatory processes, including resolvins, protectins and maresins [16,17]. Together, these mediators have been termed specialized pro-resolving mediators, and they have been shown in many cell culture and animal-based models to terminate inflammatory processes by decreasing cellular activation and the production of inflammatory cytokines, chemokines, adhesion molecules, proteases and enzymes (see [16,17] for references).

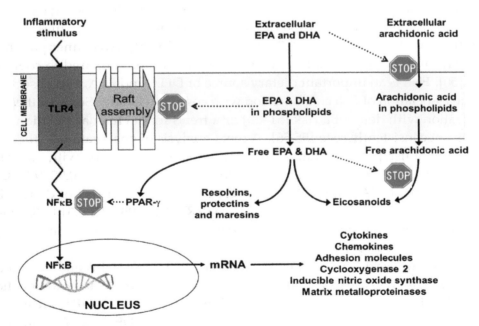

Figure 1. Overview of the key anti-inflammatory actions of EPA and DHA. DHA, docosahexaenoic acid; EPA, eicosapentaenoic acid; NFκB, nuclear factor kappa-light-chain-enhancer of activated B cells; PPAR, peroxisome proliferator activated receptor; TLR, toll-like receptor. Reproduced from Ref. [14].

The foregoing discussion has emphasized the importance of the incorporation of DHA and EPA into cell membranes in order to elicit their anti-inflammatory and inflammation resolving actions. In this regard, it is important to recognize that the incorporation of DHA and EPA into the membrane phospholipids of cells involved in inflammatory responses, and into other cells and tissues such as skeletal muscle, is dose-dependently related to their intake (see [12–14] for references). It is possible that the membrane changes induced by low intakes of DHA and EPA are insufficient to significantly alter cell and tissue function and therefore no biological or clinical impact would be observed. Thus, the dose of DHA and EPA used in human studies is likely to be important in terms of determining the effect seen and too low a dose could result in the absence of an effect.

3. Omega-3 LCPUFAs and Cognitive Decline and Dementia

With the increasingly aging population, cognitive decline has become a growing public health concern: the number of persons living with dementia is expected to nearly double every 20 years [39]. Increasing evidence indicates that poor status of essential nutrients such as omega-3 LCPUFAs is associated with increased risk of cognitive decline and of developing Alzheimer's disease [40]. DHA is a major fatty acid in membrane phospholipids in the grey matter of the brain and makes up approximately 25% of total fatty acids in the human cerebral cortex and 50% of all polyunsaturated fatty acids in the central nervous system [34,41–43]. Brain DHA levels decrease with adult age [44] and seem to be particularly low among Alzheimer's patients [45]. It is conceivable that low brain DHA contributes to the decrease in cognitive functions observed with advancing age in general and to a greater degree in dementia [43,46]. The link between low omega-3 LCPUFA status and the risk of cognitive decline is supported by the observation that a higher proportion of total omega-3 LCPUFAs in the membranes of erythrocytes, considered to be a marker of both intake and status of these fatty acids, was associated with a reduced risk of developing cognitive decline in a French cohort [47]. Assessment of individuals with Alzheimer's disease showed lower omega-3 LCPUFA intakes and plasma phosphatidylcholine levels compared to healthy controls, but the study design did not allow to draw conclusions on causality [48]. Higher DHA in plasma phosphatidylcholine was also associated with a 47% reduction in the risk of developing all-cause dementia (RR = 0.53, 95% CI 0.29–0.97; $p = 0.04$) and a 39% reduction in risk of Alzheimer's disease (RR = 0.61, 95% CI 0.31–1.18; $p = 0.14$) in a cohort from the Framingham Heart Study [49]. The study also showed that higher dietary DHA intake was associated with a non-significantly lower risk of developing dementia in general and Alzheimer's disease in particular (upper quartile versus lower three quartiles: RR = 0.56, 95% CI 0.23 to 1.40; $p = 0.22$ and RR 0.63, 95% CI 0.23 to 1.72; $p = 0.37$) [49]. Alzheimer patients were found to have lower DHA levels in their brains and cerebrospinal fluid compared to cognitively healthy elderly controls [50]. Fish is an important dietary source of DHA and EPA, and observational studies have assessed the association of fish consumption with cognitive health. Some of these studies show an inverse association with dementia risk [51–53] or a trend for such an association [54]. However, this association is not consistently seen [55,56]. A meta-analysis of observational studies showed that an additional serving of fish per week had a significant inverse association with the risk of dementia (RR = 0.95, 95% CI 0.90 to 0.99; $p = 0.042$) and Alzheimer's disease (RR = 0.93, 95% CI 0.90 to 0.95; $p = 0.003$) [57]. Similarly, DHA intake was inversely associated with risk of dementia (RR = 0.86, 95% CI 0.76 to 0.96; $p < 0.001$) and Alzheimer's disease (RR = 0.63, 95% CI 0.51 to 0.76; $p < 0.001$) [57]. A meta-analysis of observational studies showed a positive association of DHA intake or plasma levels with memory in adults in general [58].

The observational studies described above cannot establish a causal link and therefore intervention trials with omega-3 LCPUFAs are important to verify that these fatty acids can beneficially modify cognitive decline. Findings from such intervention trials with omega-3 LCPUFAs are not consistent [59]. However, there are relatively few trials and these differ in the dose of DHA and EPA and type of placebo used, the duration of supplementation, sample size, the severity of cognitive decline at baseline as well as the omega-3 LCPUFA status of the participants (where this was even assessed) and the cognitive outcomes/tests used. Supplementation with omega-3 LCPUFAs had a small effect on memory [60] and executive function [61] in non-demented older people. A meta-analysis of three randomized, placebo-controlled trials with omega-3 LCPUFA supplements found no effect on severity of dementia, quality of life or mental health in patients with mild or moderate Alzheimer's disease over 6, 12 and 18 months [62]. Intake of 600 mg EPA and 625 mg DHA per day for four months showed no effect on cognition or mood in 19 individuals with Alzheimer's disease [48,63]. However, this was a very small study and it has also been suggested that olive oil, which was used as a placebo, may have a protective effect for Alzheimer's disease [64] and might therefore have masked the effect of the supplementation with omega-3 LCPUFAs. Similarly, an intervention comparing 200 mg EPA plus 500 mg DHA daily for 24 months compared to olive oil did not find an effect on the California Verbal Learning Test in cognitively healthy older adults (mean age 75 years) [65]. Daily supplementation with 1700 mg DHA and 600 mg EPA for six months did not affect the Mini-Mental State Examination (MMSE) score in acetylcholine esterase inhibitor treated patients with Alzheimer's disease compared to a placebo [66]. However, the intervention had a significant effect on cognitive functioning measured with the Alzheimer's Disease Assessment scores as well as the sub-items, and a correlation was found with the increase in plasma omega-3 LCPUFAs [67]. This suggests that the effect of omega-3 LCPUFAs depends on the specific aspect of cognitive health assessed. Moreover, subgroup analysis showed a benefit of omega-3 LCPUFAs in the group with very mild cognitive decline (MMSE score > 27) at baseline [66]. This is in line with the results from other trials indicating that interventions with DHA and EPA are less likely to have a beneficial effect on individuals experiencing dementia that has progressed beyond the mild stage [57,68–71]. A recent systematic review also reached the conclusion that the most beneficial effect of EPA and DHA supplementation in Alzheimer's patients can be expected in the early stage of the disease [72].

While individuals with mild cognitive decline are a promising target group, it might make sense to start the intervention even earlier, in older individuals with subjective cognitive decline [73]. It has been shown that supplementation in healthy older people has a beneficial effect on white matter microstructural integrity, grey matter volume in specific brain areas and vascular parameters accompanied by improved executive function [61]. This indicates that there might be a potential for preventive uses of omega-3 LCPUFAs to maintain cognitive health in older people. However, such an effect is difficult to show as the decrease over time in the placebo group will likely be too small to show a significant difference between the groups as seen in a supplementation trial in cognitively healthy older people [74]. Therefore, careful selection of the study population is required to find the window of opportunity during which the disease has not progressed too far but is already accelerating at a sufficient speed to be able to detect a difference in the decline between the intervention and the placebo groups.

The Multidomain Alzheimer Preventive Trial (MAPT) assessed whether a multimodal intervention consisting of nutritional counseling, physical exercise and cognitive stimulation, in combination with DHA and EPA, is effective in slowing cognitive decline in older at-risk adults [75]. Three years supplementation with 800 mg DHA and 225 mg EPA showed no significant effect on cognitive decline in older people with memory complaints [76]. However, in a subgroup analysis only including individuals with low omega-3 LCPUFA status at baseline, the supplementation had a beneficial effect on cognition [77]. This indicates that people with low intakes or status of DHA and EPA should be targeted with such interventions as they may be more likely to experience the greatest benefit. Not surprisingly, the dose of DHA and EPA provided in the intervention group also plays an important role and doses below 1000 mg have not had a major effect on cognitive health in older people with some degree of cognitive decline [59].

Several trials investigating the effect of omega-3 LCPUFAs on cognitive outcomes, including decline, have been relatively short, perhaps too short to significantly affect these outcomes. It has even been suggested that the three years of supplementation evaluated in the MAPT might have been too short [78]. As neurodegeneration develops over a considerable time, longer-term intervention might be required for a benefit to manifest. A systematic review and meta-analysis of available data from animal studies suggest >10% of average total lifespan interventions had significant effects on cognitive function, neuronal loss and the amount of amyloid-beta deposits in the brain [79], but this period is considerably longer than the interventions in humans performed to date.

In addition to omega-3 LCPUFA dose, study duration and the rate of cognitive decline, other factors may also be relevant to whether an effect of these fatty acids is seen. These include the status of other nutrients and an individual's genotype. A re-analysis of the patients assessed in the OmegAD trial [65,66] found that those with low blood homocysteine, indicating good B vitamin status, benefitted cognitively and clinically from the combined DHA and EPA treatment, whereas those with high homocysteine did not [80]. Similarly, it had been shown that those older people with mild cognitive impairment who had the highest levels of plasma omega-3 LCPUFAs benefited most from supplementation with B vitamins [81,82]. In addition, adequate intake and status of antioxidants might be required for an optimal effect of DHA and EPA on cognitive health [83].

It has been well established that apolipoprotein E (ApoE) is a very important genetic risk factor for age-dependent chronic diseases, including Alzheimer's disease [84], but not all trials have controlled for this. Due to two major polymorphisms on the encoding exon 4 of this gene, three major protein isoforms, ApoE ε2, ApoE ε3 and ApoE ε4, exist [85]. Clinical and preclinical evidence suggests that carriers of ApoE ε4 are at a higher risk of low omega-3 LCPUFA status [86]. Moreover, it has been shown that homozygous carriers of the ApoE ε4 allele have a more than 10-fold increased risk of developing Alzheimer's disease, possibly due to increased cholesterol levels, altered brain development early in life [84] or increased oxidative brain damage [87]. A meta-regression by Zhang et al. [57] showed that stratification by ApoE ε4 genotype had a significant effect on the association between DHA, but not EPA, intake and cognitive impairment. Another analysis found a beneficial effect of omega-3 LCPUFA supplementation on the progression of cognitive decline at an early stage in those with the ApoE ε4 genotype [59]. Thus, individuals with certain genotypes may benefit more from omega-3 LCPUFAs than those with other genotypes.

In summary, there is good evidence from observational studies for an association between DHA and slower cognitive decline or reduced risk of Alzheimer's disease. Intervention trials are less clear, but there is some evidence that DHA and EPA can prevent or slow cognitive decline, particularly in the early stages. The inconsistent findings from trials likely relate to a number of factors including dose, duration and timing of the intervention, stage and rate of cognitive decline, status of other relevant nutrients (e.g., B vitamins) and genotype.

4. Omega-3 LCPUFAs and Sarcopenia and Frailty in Older People

With increasing age, achieving adequate intake of energy and essential nutrients becomes challenging due to alterations to appetite (anorexia of aging) and gastrointestinal physiology [88,89]. In addition, aging can affect dentition, gum and mouth health, and swallowing, so reducing food intake. Cognitive decline, systemic disease and use of some medications can also impact food intake. Reduced mobility, increased isolation and limited finances can restrict access to food in older people. As a consequence of these factors, malnutrition (i.e., undernutrition), frailty and sarcopenia are common and frequently overlapping conditions in older people [90–92]. Malnutrition is defined by ESPEN as "a state resulting from lack of intake or uptake of nutrition that leads to altered body composition (decreased fat free mass) and body cell mass leading to diminished physical and mental function and impaired clinical outcome from disease" [93]. Inflammation is an important contributor to the outcome of malnutrition. ESPEN recognizes disease-related malnutrition with inflammation as "a catabolic condition characterized by an inflammatory response, including anorexia and tissue breakdown, elicited by an underlying disease" [93]. Frailty is a state of vulnerability with limited reserve capacity in major organ systems; it involves weight loss, fatigue, low physical activity, slowness and weakness [94]. Frailty is associated with a higher risk of adverse outcomes such as falls, fractures, hospitalization and disability [94–96]. In older inpatients, frailty was found to be a risk factor for increased length of hospital stay and mortality [97,98] as well as postoperative complications [99]. Moreover, frail patients were more likely to be discharged into care homes after hospitalization [99]. A decrease in muscle mass was found to be a strong predictor of prognosis in hospitalized older people [97]. Sarcopenia is characterized by the progressive and generalized loss of skeletal muscle mass, strength and function with a consequent increased risk of adverse outcomes; the European Working Group on Sarcopenia in Older People defines sarcopenia as "a progressive and generalized skeletal muscle disorder that involves the accelerated loss of muscle mass and function" [100]. Sarcopenia is often part of the aging process preceding the onset of frailty. Age-related chronic low-grade inflammation may be an important contributor to sarcopenia [6,88,93]. Sarcopenia seems to increase the likelihood of adverse outcomes such as disability, poor quality of life and death [101–103]. Both muscle mass and strength were predictive for difficulties in performing activities of daily living after discharge from the hospital [104]. Sarcopenia and particularly sarcopenic obesity (i.e., low muscle mass in association with greater fat mass), have been linked to poorer prognosis, including survival, for a range of cancers [105–109].

Pro-inflammatory cytokines have been linked to muscle wasting [110], and consequently, the anti-inflammatory effects of omega-3 LCPUFAs may be beneficial to prevent the loss of muscle mass and strength associated with aging, sarcopenia and frailty. Furthermore, omega-3 LCPUFAs may themselves modulate muscle protein synthesis, promoting muscle strength and function [27,29], likely as a result of their incorporation into membrane phospholipids of the sarcolemma and intracellular organelles [29]. Maintenance of, or an increase in, muscle mass and function seem to be key for healthy aging [111,112], and also in recovery after surgery or during an intensive care unit (ICU) stay [113]. Long-term supplementation with DHA and EPA in older people is therefore of increasing interest as the medical community looks for safe and affordable ways to slow physical disability and improve quality of life in older individuals. Results from cross-sectional and longitudinal observational studies demonstrate that low plasma DHA and EPA levels are associated with poorer physical performance in older adults [29].

Daily supplementation with 1500 mg/d DHA and 1860 mg/d EPA for six months in healthy older men and women increased thigh muscle volume (3.6%, 95% CI 0.2% to 7.0%, $p < 0.05$), handgrip strength (2.3 kg, 95% CI 0.8 to 3.7 kg, $p < 0.05$) and one-repetition muscle strength (4.0%, 95% CI 0.8% to 7.3%, $p < 0.05$) and showed a trend towards increased average isokinetic power (5.6%, 95% CI 0.6% to 11.7%, $p = 0.075$) compared to a control group [114]. The intervention had no significant effect on body weight, total-body fat mass or the intermuscular fat content and raised no safety concerns [114]. In post-menopausal women aged > 65 years, supplementation with 720 mg/d EPA and 40 mg/d DHA for six months showed a positive effect on walking speed compared to the placebo group (3.0 ± 16% vs. −3.5 ± 14%, $p = 0.038$) [115]. Supplementation for 12 weeks with 1000 mg/d DHA and 2000 mg/d EPA in women aged 60 to 76 years resulted in a significant increase in lean body mass, increased resting metabolic rate and fat oxidation as well as decreasing time-to-get-up-and-go as a functional capacity measure [116]. However, 12 weeks supplementation with 440 mg/d DHA and 660 mg/d EPA had no effect on muscle mass or handgrip strength in community-dwelling older people (mean age 74.6 ± 8.0 years) [117]. In another study, 800 mg/d DHA and 225 mg/d EPA in combination with physical exercise, cognitive training and nutritional counseling had no effect on different measures of muscle strength in older people [118]. Based on the evidence from these trials, doses of 3000 mg/d of DHA plus EPA or more (with preferably more than 800 mg/d EPA) may be required for positive effects on physical performance in older adults [114,116] as lower doses have not had an effect [117,118]. Furthermore, the optimal ratio between DHA and EPA is not known and may differ between specific indications as different body compartments require distinct levels of omega-3 LCPUFAs (e.g., the brain is rich in DHA and poor in EPA). The scarcity of data from interventional studies [27] has prevented the development of strong recommendations on the use of omega-3 LCPUFAs in the prevention of sarcopenia so far. More randomized controlled trials, with different duration and doses, are needed to establish their effect on maintaining muscle mass in the elderly and to decrease the risk of sarcopenia and the related adverse effects on health and well-being, including the onset of frailty.

5. Omega-3 LCPUFAs for Nutritional Care of Cancer Patients

5.1. Omega-3 LCPUFAs and Cancer Cachexia

Cancer is a major public health concern and both the disease and its treatment are associated with decreased quality of life and significant economic burden due to high healthcare cost and loss of productivity. Increasing cancer incidence is due to several factors, including population growth and aging, as well as lifestyle and socio-economic factors. Various dietary behaviors are thought to be involved in the pathogenesis and progression of some cancers and they play a crucial role in tumor growth and spreading [119]. Two ways by which diet could exert effects in patients with cancer are by enhancing anticancer therapies, mitigating their side effects, and by favoring the resolution of paraneoplastic syndromes, which in turn impact outcome. Paraneoplastic syndromes are disorders triggered by an altered immune system response to new or abnormal growth of tissue. Cancer cachexia is the most frequent paraneoplastic syndrome in individuals with cancer [120]. Cachexia is a form of disease-related malnutrition with inflammation [93,121], and involves reduced appetite, altered utilization of nutrients, increased mobilization of amino acids and muscle protein turnover, loss of adipose tissue and infiltration of skeletal muscle with adipose tissue [122]. Left untreated, cachexia can progress in severity and contribute to the negative outcomes experienced by cancer patients, including mortality [123]. An international consensus of clinical experts defined cancer cachexia as "a multifactorial syndrome defined by an ongoing loss of skeletal muscle mass (with or without loss of fat mass) that cannot be fully reversed by conventional nutritional support and leads to progressive functional impairment" [124]. The importance of systemic inflammatory responses in cachexia is increasingly recognized, and it has been proposed to include this component in the definition of cancer cachexia [123,125]. Further supporting the causative role of inflammation in the pathogenesis and clinical features of cancer cachexia, it has been recently demonstrated that an elevation of the neutrophil-to-lymphocyte ratio, a simple and reliable marker of systemic inflammation, associates with greater weight loss and cachexia in patients with advanced cancer [126].

It has been proposed that current malnutrition rates in cancer patients are comparable to those >30 years ago, but they are less apparent as body mass index is often normal or even high, despite prevalence rates of cachexia and sarcopenia of 30% and 17% to 19%, respectively [122]. It is estimated that cancer cachexia affects around 50% to 80% of cancer patients and is responsible for approximately 20% of deaths in cancer patients [127,128]. Low muscle mass has a negative effect on treatment prognosis, resulting in reduced likelihood to complete at least three treatment cycles, more side effects and a lower chance of progression-free survival [129,130]. Moreover, it has a negative impact on toxicity of cancer treatment [131–134] and tumor progression during chemotherapy [133] and causes marked distress to patients and their families [135]. Still, it remains underdiagnosed and is often not treated properly as pharmacological therapies mostly fail to improve the condition significantly [136].

A review of available clinical trials showed that weight loss often starts very early in the disease progression, potentially even before the cancer itself is diagnosed [137]. The precise mechanisms are poorly understood, but chronic systemic inflammation seems to play a crucial role in most patients [123]. Inflammation is recognized as a hallmark feature of cancer development and progression [138] and targeting cancer-related inflammation at the local tumor microenvironment as well as in systemic circulation has the potential to favorably affect patient outcomes [139]. Optimal therapy should take into account the progression of the condition from pre-cachexia to cachexia and eventually refractory cachexia [140] and would ideally involve a multimodal approach including nutritional interventions targeting inflammation and reduced food intake as well as decreased physical function [126,141,142].

Given their ability to mitigate inflammation, DHA and EPA interventions in cancer patients have received increasing attention and the mechanisms are reviewed elsewhere [143–146]. There is evidence that DHA and EPA modulate the inflammatory response, measured as cytokines or C-reactive protein, and affect resting energy expenditure in cancer patients [147–152]. These findings are relevant, as increased levels of inflammation in cancer patients induce changes in pharmacokinetics of some anti-cancer drugs, resulting in slower clearance and increased treatment-related toxicities [139]. It has further been suggested that omega-3 LCPUFAs might play a role in mitigating the negative effect of disease as well as its treatment on gut health and microbiota composition [145]. In addition, observations of decreasing plasma levels indicate a depletion of EPA and DHA in cancer patients [153]. However, the effects of omega-3 LCPUFAs on nutritional status or meaningful clinical outcomes, such as quality of life, survival rates and treatment toxicity, are less well documented. Based on evidence from different systematic reviews [143,154–157], the ESPEN guidelines for nutrition in cancer patients state "in patients with advanced cancer undergoing chemotherapy and at risk of weight loss or malnourished, we suggest to use supplementation with long-chain omega-3 fatty acids or fish oil to stabilize or improve appetite, food intake, lean body mass and body weight" but the recommendation is graded as weak and the level of evidence as low [158]. A sub-group meta-analysis found a significant effect of high-protein, omega-3 LCPUFA-enriched oral nutritional supplements (ONS) when compared with isocaloric controls on body weight (+1.89 kg, 95% CI 0.51 to 3.27, $p = 0.02$) in cancer patients undergoing chemotherapy [159]. Two of the included studies reported an effect on muscle mass: supplementation with an omega-3 LCPUFA-enriched ONS (1000 mg/d DHA and 2200 mg/d EPA) resulted in a decrease in the loss of fat-free mass after three and five weeks in patients with non-small cell lung cancer ($p = 0.02$) [148], while an intervention with the same ONS resulted in a mean gain of 1.6 kg muscle mass in the intervention group versus a mean loss of 2 kg in controls ($p = 0.01$) [160]. A similar intervention resulted in an increase in skeletal muscle mass and lean body mass in cancer patients with omega-3 LCPUFA-enriched ONS ($p = 0.0002$, $p < 0.0001$, respectively), while no change was seen in these parameters in the group that received the standard ONS ($p = 0.26$, $p = 0.19$, respectively) [151]. Moreover, there are indications that supplementation with omega-3 LCPUFAs in combination with high protein might have a beneficial effect on quality of life in cancer patients [159]. Importantly, omega-3 LCPUFAs were shown to be safe and well tolerated by cancer patients [152,158].

In addition to their effect on lean mass in cancer patients, omega-3 LCPUFAs have potential use as adjuvants to cancer therapy [143]. They are thought to affect tumor activity through a range of mechanisms [144]. A review of the evidence of omega-3 LCPUFAs as an adjunct to chemotherapy found beneficial effects on tumor response to treatment, protection from therapy-related toxicity and maintenance of quality of life [145]. Further benefits of omega-3 LCPUFA supplementation might include reduction in cancer-related pain as well as a decrease in major depressive disorders, which are a frequent consequence of the stress and anxiety caused by a cancer diagnosis [161].

The lack of consensus on the definition of cachexia has led to the inclusion of patients at different stages of the condition into studies, which is expected to affect the outcomes significantly [141]. Inconsistent or negative outcomes in clinical trials, including those with omega-3 LCPUFAs, are often due to suboptimal study design regarding the selection of endpoint [137,152] or due to lack of randomization or (placebo) control group [141]. Moreover, the duration and size of the trials may have been too low in many cases to detect a relevant impact [159]. The timing of the intervention will likely also play a role, as a recent study only showed a benefit if nutritional interventions were initiated before chemotherapy started [162]. Considerable heterogeneity also exists in the pharmacological treatment as shown in a recent review that found 19 different combinations of chemotherapy used in seven studies on the effect of omega-3 LCPUFAs in cancer patients [152].

Dose selection and compliance also play an important role as shown by Fearon et al. [163] in a post-hoc analysis where there was a dose-response between reported intake of omega-3 LCPFA-enriched ONS and total ($r = 0.50$, $p < 0.001$) and lean body mass ($r = 0.33$, $p = 0.036$), as well as a correlation between plasma phospholipid EPA and change in total and lean body weight ($r = 0.50$, $p < 0.001$; $r = 0.51$, $p = 0.001$). This provides evidence that doses of 1000 mg/d DHA and 2200 mg/d EPA or even more are required for a significant effect on muscle mass. Others suggest the use of at least 2000 to

2500 mg/d DHA+EPA based on data from the available clinical trials on their use as adjuvants for chemotherapy [143,152].

It is increasingly recognized that multimodal interventions are most promising for the therapy of cancer cachexia, yet most of the clinical evidence is derived from trials using only a single therapy [141]. In a small feasibility trial, a combination of an omega-3 LCPUFA-enriched ONS (~1000 mg/d DHA and 2200 mg/d EPA), nutritional advice, 300 mg/d Celecoxib and exercise compared to standard of care resulted in a stabilization of body weight compared to weight loss in the control group [164]. The subsequent phase III study on this intervention is still ongoing [165]. Therefore, studies are needed that combine nutrition, including DHA and EPA, physical exercise as well as pharmacological interventions.

Studies highlighting cost-effectiveness might also be helpful in increasing acceptance of such interventions given the potential benefit and the low cost of omega-3 LCPUFA supplements. Due to the limited and inconclusive data available, many oncologists are yet to be convinced of the benefits that DHA and EPA have for cancer patients. Their interest in the mechanisms and possible therapies of cancer cachexia could be increased by the recent understanding that some mechanisms leading to cachexia are also involved in the process of metastasis [166]. If confirmed in clinical trials, early intervention with omega-3 LCPUFAs to prevent the development of cancer cachexia may also help to limit the spread of the tumor to distant organs. Epidemiological evidence indicates a benefit from supplementation with omega-3 LCPUFAs throughout the clinical journey of a cancer patient as higher intakes of these fatty acids in patients diagnosed with colorectal cancer were found to be associated with reduced specific mortality [167–169].

5.2. Omega-3 LCPUFAs as Components of Immunonutrition for Perioperative Care in Cancer Patients

Surgery leads to the release of stress hormones and inflammatory mediators proportional to the magnitude of the procedure, resulting in a metabolic imbalance towards increased catabolism [170,171]. While this serves to support tissue healing and the immune response, it favors the breakdown of muscle protein. This can be detrimental to the patient, especially when there is pre-existing malnutrition, sarcopenia, cachexia, obesity and myosteatosis [170] or in the presence of low-grade inflammation due to underlying conditions such as cancer or diabetes [172]. Malnutrition in surgical patients has been proposed as "a nutritional state in which nutrient intake does not match nutrient needs—due to underlying disease(s), the surgical stress response, chronic or acute inflammation, intestinal malabsorption (e.g., diarrhea) and/or patient-related factors (e.g., socio-economic status)—leading to losses in lean tissue and diminished function" [173]. Nutritional intervention can help reduce the stress of surgery, thereby preventing and treating catabolism and malnutrition [171]. This is thought to reduce the risk of complications, decrease the length of hospital stay and promote better functional recovery [170]. Considering the poor general health conditions of at-risk (e.g., many cancer) patients, nutritional conditioning (e.g., in the context of prehabilitation) may prepare individuals for an Enhanced Recovery After Surgery (ERAS) protocol [174]. Optimal timing for the introduction of nutritional therapy depends on the type of surgery and the general health status of the patient and needs further investigation [175–181].

Given their effect on inflammation mitigation, it is reasonable to expect a benefit of adding DHA and EPA to perioperative immunonutrition therapy. However, the evidence to support this is limited and most studies compared an ONS containing DHA and EPA combined with other immune modulating nutrients (i.e., arginine and nucleotides with or without glutamine) with regular hospital diet rather than with a standard ONS.

5.2.1. Pre-Operative Immunonutrition in Cancer Patients

A recent meta-analysis focusing on patients with gastrointestinal cancer included 16 studies with 1387 patients, where the control group received either no supplements or an isonitrogenous standard ONS [182]. The preoperative administration of immunonutrition resulted in significantly decreased postoperative infectious complications in the combined studies (OR 0.52, 95% CI 0.38–0.71, $p < 0.0001$) as well as the studies with a standard ONS as a control (OR 0.49, 95% CI 0.28–0.85, $p = 0.01$). For length of hospital stay, significance was only reached in the combined studies (−1.57 days, 95% CI −2.48 to −0.66, $p < 0.0001$) but there was only a weak trend when compared to ONS (−1.06 days, 95% CI −2.76 to 0.63, $p = 0.22$). No significant effect was seen on non-infectious complications or mortality. Given their effect on post-operative morbidity and length of stay, the current ESPEN guideline for surgical patients advises that standard ONS are given pre-operatively to all malnourished cancer and other high-risk patients undergoing major abdominal surgery [171].

5.2.2. Post- and Eri-Operative Immunonutrition in Cancer Patients

The evidence is somewhat stronger for benefits of postoperative than for preoperative immunonutrition [183], although the optimal timing for its introduction to patient treatment plans still needs further investigation. The ESPEN recommendation is that "peri- or at least postoperative administration of specific formulae enriched with immunonutrients should be given in malnourished patients undergoing major cancer surgery" [171]. Based on the duration of supplementation in the trials with positive outcomes, immunonutrition containing DHA and EPA as well as arginine and nucleotides should start five to seven days before surgery [171]. Similarly, the recommendations from the North American Surgical Nutrition Summit include five to seven days of pre-operative immunonutrition including omega-3 LCPUFAs, which should be continued well into the postoperative period [184]. It has even been suggested that the ideal period for pre-operative nutritional support is seven to 10 days—or longer for severely malnourished patients—in addition to postoperative nutritional support [185]. Patients who are severely compromised (e.g., due to cancer) should ideally receive preoperative nutrition support for more than 10 days [171]. Moreover, attenuation of the metabolic response to the stress of surgery through a range of measures including immunonutrition in the perioperative period is increasingly being recommended [184,186] as the combination of different elements, rather than a single one of them, is thought to produce the optimal outcome for patients [187].

While many of the trials in this area did not follow an ERAS program, adherence to such a protocol might further increase the benefits of immunonutrition. This is supported by evidence from a multicenter study in well-nourished cancer patients undergoing colorectal resection comparing peri-operative use of an ONS with immune-nutrients compared to a standard ONS as part of a more comprehensive ERAS protocol [188]. Immunonutrition including omega-3 LCPUFAs for seven days pre- and five days post-surgery was compared to a standard high caloric ONS and led to a decrease in the total number of complications, primarily due to a reduction in infectious complications (23.8% vs. 10.7%, $p = 0.0007$) [188].

It is evident that DHA and EPA play a role in perioperative immunonutrition in cancer patients, but more well-designed trials comparing standard to specialized (immunonutrition) ONS could provide clearer evidence for their use and confirm the optimal timing. A recent survey among gastrointestinal and oncologic surgeons in the U.S. showed the use of post-operative nutrition support was more common than pre-operative and the use of immune-nutrients was reported by approximately 25% of responders (versus approximately 80% use of protein-containing supplements) and lack of awareness was given as the major hurdle to a more widespread use [189].

6. Omega-3 LCPUFAs in the Nutritional Management of Critically Ill Patients

6.1. Omega-3 LCPUFAs in Sepsis

Sepsis is a severe clinical syndrome defined as "a life-threatening organ dysfunction due to a dysregulated host response to infection" [190]. In septic patients, inflammatory cytokines trigger the release of even more cytokines, culminating in a so-called cytokine storm that will in turn cause damage to cells and organs [191]. The outcome can be multi-organ failure and death. In addition to these hyperinflammatory processes, immune suppression also seems to play a role in sepsis and the balance between the two is thought to vary depending on host-, pathogen- and therapy-related factors [192,193]. The factors leading to sepsis are still incompletely understood and attempts to dampen the cytokine storm activation or consequences have failed in clinical trials [191].

A recent meta-analysis found a lower risk for mortality in 234 patients with sepsis who received omega-3 LCPUFAs, mainly intravenously, compared to control groups (OR 0.52, 95% CI 0.28 to 0.97, $p = 0.04$), while the reduction in infectious complications was only reported in one study and was not significant (OR 0.56, 95% CI 0.12 to 2.57, $p = 0.45$) and none of the studies reported cases of new onset of organ failure [194]. A complete interpretation of the findings of this meta-analysis is limited by the low number of included studies.

6.2. Omega-3 LCPUFAs in Acute Respiratory Distress Syndrome

Acute respiratory distress syndrome (ARDS) and multiple organ failure are important complications in patients with sepsis, resulting in prolonged ICU stays [194–197]. Specialized enteral formulations containing omega-3 LCPUFAs as well as other ingredients such as antioxidants are available for critically ill patients with ARDS or acute lung injury (ALI). However, the evidence for their effect is inconsistent. Early research demonstrated positive clinical outcomes such as improved oxygenation, fewer new organ failures, more ventilator- and ICU-free days as well as lower mortality when comparing these with high omega-6 PUFA or standard formulas [198–201]. However, subsequent research could not replicate these findings [202–207]. Consequently, the 2016 SCCM/ASPEN Guidelines for critically ill patients do not recommend the use of these specialized formulas for ARDS/ALI [208]. In contrast, the Canadian Clinical Practice Guidelines recommend that clinicians consider these specialized formulas with fish or borage oil and supplemental antioxidants for patients with ARDS/ALI [209]. The disparity between the two guidelines is likely related to differences in the studies included in the evaluation and the methods used for analyzing and interpreting the data to develop recommendations.

While a recent meta-analysis of 955 patients with ARDS or ALI showed no effect of enteral nutrition enriched with fish oil [210], after the exclusion of two studies using a bolus rather than continuous dose, there was evidence that omega-3 LCPUFA-containing formulas decreased mortality in critically ill patients including those with ARDS/ALI [211]. Moreover, a recent Cochrane review of these trials identified a significant improvement in blood oxygenation and significant reductions in ventilation requirement, new organ failures, length of stay in the ICU and mortality at 28 days when omega-3 LCPUFAs were used in patients with ARDS or ALI, although all-cause mortality was not significantly affected [212]. These findings are important in the context of the current coronavirus pandemic since severe COVID-19 results in ARDS and there are suggestions that omega-3 LCPUFAs could be a viable treatment that is worth investigating [213,214].

6.3. Omega-3 LCPUFAs in Critically Ill Surgical Patients

For critically ill surgical patients who require parenteral nutrition, intravenous lipid emulsions containing omega-3 LCPUFAs are considered safe, but parenteral nutrition should only be considered in patients who cannot be adequately enterally fed [171]. International consensus exists that a dose of 0.1 to 0.2 g/kg/d of fish oil would be appropriate for patients who require parenteral nutrition [215–218]. A recent meta-analysis of 49 prospective randomized trials showed significant benefits for the fish oil containing parenteral nutrition compared to a standard lipid emulsion [219]. The risk for infection was lowered by 40% (24 studies: RR 0.60. 95% CI 0.49 to 0.72; $p < 0.00001$). Mean length of stay in the ICU was significantly shortened (10 studies: 1.95 days; 95% CI −0.42 to −3.49; $p = 0.01$) as was the length of hospital stay (26 studies: 2.14 days, 95% CI −1.36 to −2.93; $p < 0.00001$). The risk for developing sepsis was also significantly diminished by 56% (nine studies: RR 0.44, 95%CI 0.28 to 0.70, $p = 0.0004$). Mortality was lower with 16%, but the difference did not reach significance (20 studies: RR 0.84, 95% CI 0.65 to 1.07; $p = 0.15$) [216]. Moreover, fish oil was found to be more cost-effective than parenteral nutrition with a standard intravenous lipid emulsion [220].

7. Discussion and Outlook

The evidence to date indicates that the provision of DHA and EPA through capsules, oral nutrition supplements, or enteral or parenteral formulas can help to regulate the inflammatory environment in a number of medical conditions and that this is linked in many cases to improved function, clinical course and outcomes. As dysregulated inflammation is a component of many acute and chronic diseases [221], the potential application of DHA and EPA is broad in terms of prevention and treatment. There is good evidence that DHA and EPA are a safe and cost-effective treatment that could benefit multiple patient outcomes. Use of DHA and EPA in some conditions is supported by their inclusion in relevant guidelines [123,158,171,184,209], although the level of evidence has sometimes been considered to be low. This is because of inconsistent data on the effect of DHA and EPA on clinical outcomes, especially in some settings. This inconsistency has limited stronger support through guidelines and has hindered the wider acceptance of the benefits of DHA and EPA in the medical community. If omega-3 LCPUFAs are effective in disease prevention and in patient care, it is important to understand the reasons behind the inconsistent findings of studies and use this information to design and conduct better clinical trials to determine if poor results may be due to a real lack of effect or to other factors. Undoubtedly the dose of DHA and EPA used is an important factor, but this is not the sole explanation for inconsistencies. Other considerations include the timing and duration of supply of DHA and EPA, EPA to DHA ratio, baseline EPA and DHA status, intake of other nutrients including omega-6 fatty acids, B vitamins and antioxidants, clinical state, and medication use. More well-designed intervention studies are required to address the relevance of these different variables in order to properly identify the effects of DHA and EPA in specific target patient populations. Such studies may lead to more personalized approaches to the provision of DHA and EPA to achieve the maximal clinical benefit. A focus on personalized approaches and knowledge of a patient's specific nutritional and medical needs will be important to determine the route to optimal use of omega-3 LCPUFAs. This should take into account the interaction between genetics and nutrients [222] as well as the interaction among the nutrients themselves. Overall, the entirety of the evidence supports use of DHA and EPA in a range of medical conditions. Additional and good quality studies building on the experience of existing studies will strengthen the evidence base required to inform relevant guidelines in the future.

Author Contributions: This manuscript was developed with input from all authors (B.T., M.E., A.L., Y.R., A.D.S., I.W., A.W., P.C.C.) based on an expert roundtable discussion and the conclusions they reached concerning the role of DHA and EPA in aging and clinical nutrition. All authors have read and agreed to the published version of the manuscript.

References

1. Maternal, Newborn, Child & Adolescent Health. Available online: https://www.who.int/data/maternal-newborn-child-adolescent/indicator-explorer-new/mca/life-expectancy-at-birth (accessed on 7 August 2020).
2. Naghavi, M.; Abajobir, A.A.; Abbafati, C.; Abbas, K.M.; Abd-Allah, F.; Abera, S.F.; Aboyans, V.; Adetokunboh, O.; Afshin, A.; Agrawal, A.; et al. GBD 2016 Causes of Death Collaborators. Global, regional, and national age-sex specific mortality for 264 causes of death, 1980–2016: A systematic analysis for the Global Burden of Disease Study 2016. *Lancet* **2017**, *390*, 1151–1210. [CrossRef]
3. Hay, S.I.; Abajobir, A.A.; Abate, K.H.; Abbafati, C.; Abbas, K.M.; Abd-Allah, F.; Abdulkader, R.S.; Abdulle, A.M.; Abebo, T.A.; Abera, S.F.; et al. GBD 2016 DALYs and HALE Collaborators. Global, regional, and national disability-adjusted life-years (DALYs) for 333 diseases and injuries and healthy life expectancy (HALE) for 195 countries and territories, 1990–2016: A systematic analysis for the Global Burden of Disease Study 2016. *Lancet* **2017**, *390*, 1260–1344.
4. Calderón-Larrañaga, A.; Vetrano, D.L.; Onder, G.; Gimeno-Feliu, L.A.; Coscollar-Santaliestra, C.; Carfí, A.; Pisciotta, M.S.; Angleman, S.; Melis, R.J.F.; Santoni, G.; et al. Assessing and measuring chronic multimorbidity in the older population: A proposal for its operationalization. *J. Gerontol. A Biol. Sci. Med. Sci.* **2017**, *72*, 1417–1423. [CrossRef] [PubMed]

5.   Marengoni, A.; Angleman, S.; Melis, R.; Mangialasche, F.; Karp, A.; Garmen, A.; Meinow, B.; Fratiglioni, L. Aging with multimorbidity: A systematic review of the literature. *Ageing Res. Rev.* **2011**, *10*, 430–439. [CrossRef] [PubMed]

6.   Calder, P.C.; Bosco, N.; Bourdet-Sicard, R.; Capuron, L.; Delzenne, N.; Doré, J.; Franceschi, C.; Lehtinen, M.J.; Recker, T.; Salvioli, S.; et al. Health relevance of the modification of low grade inflammation in ageing (inflammageing) and the role of nutrition. *Ageing Res. Rev.* **2017**, *40*, 95–119. [CrossRef]

7.   Vatic, M.; von Haehling, S.; Ebner, N. Inflammatory biomarkers of frailty. *Exp. Gerontol.* **2020**, *133*, 110858. [CrossRef]

8.   Livshits, G.; Kalinkovich, A. Inflammaging as a common ground for the development and maintenance of sarcopenia, obesity, cardiomyopathy and dysbiosis. *Ageing Res. Rev.* **2019**, *56*, 100980. [CrossRef]

9.   Fonseca, G.; Farkas, J.; Dora, E.; von Haehling, S.; Lainscak, M. Cancer cachexia and related metabolic dysfunction. *Int. J. Mol. Sci.* **2020**, *21*, 2321. [CrossRef]

10. Ramírez, P.; Ferrer, M.; Martí, V.; Reyes, S.; Martínez, R.; Menéndez, R.; Ewig, S.; Torres, A. Inflammatory biomarkers and prediction for intensive care unit admission in severe community-acquired pneumonia. *Crit. Care Med.* **2011**, *39*, 2211–2217. [CrossRef] [PubMed]

11. Calder, P.C. Very long-chain n-3 fatty acids and human health: Fact, fiction and the future. *Proc. Nutr. Soc.* **2018**, *77*, 52–72. [CrossRef]

12. Calder, P.C. Marine omega-3 fatty acids and inflammatory processes: Effects, mechanisms and clinical relevance. *Biochim. Biophys. Acta* **2015**, *1851*, 469–484. [CrossRef] [PubMed]

13. Calder, P.C. Omega-3 fatty acids and inflammatory processes: From molecules to man. *Biochem. Soc. Trans.* **2017**, *45*, 1105–1115. [CrossRef] [PubMed]

14. Calder, P.C. Omega-3 (n-3) polyunsaturated fatty acids and inflammation: From membrane to nucleus and from bench to bedside. *Proc. Nutr. Soc.* **2020**, in press. [CrossRef] [PubMed]

15. Barnig, C.; Bezema, T.; Calder, P.C.; Charloux, A.; Frossard, N.; Garssen, J.; Haworth, O.; Dilevskaya, K.; Levi-Schaffer, F.; Lonsdorfer, E.; et al. Activation of resolution pathways to prevent and fight chronic inflammation: Lessons from asthma and inflammatory bowel disease. *Front. Immunol.* **2019**, *10*, 1699. [CrossRef] [PubMed]

16. Serhan, C.N.; Levy, B.D. Resolvins in inflammation: Emergence of the pro-resolving superfamily of mediators. *J. Clin. Investig.* **2018**, *128*, 2657–2669. [CrossRef] [PubMed]

17. Chiang, N.; Serhan, C.N. The specialised pro-resolving mediator network: An update on in vivo production and actions. *Essays Biochem.* **2020**, in press.

18. Baker, E.J.; Miles, E.A.; Burdge, G.C.; Yaqoob, P.; Calder, P.C. Metabolism and functional effects of plant-derived omega-3 fatty acids in humans. *Prog. Lipid Res.* **2016**, *64*, 30–56. [CrossRef]

19. Food and Agricultural Organization. Fats and fatty acids in human nutrition—Report of an expert consultation. In *FAO Food and Nutrition Paper*; Food and Agricultural Organization: Rome, Italy, 2010.

20. Chinese Nutrition Society. *Chinese Dietary Reference Intakes Summary (2013)*; People's Medical Publishing House: Beijing, China, 2013; p. 16.

21. Institute of Medicine Dietary Reference Intakes. *The Essential Guide to Nutrient Requirements*; Otten, J.J., Hellwig, J.P., Meyers, L.D., Eds.; The National Academies Press: Washington, DC, USA, 2006; p. 1344.

22. European Food Safety Authority. Scientific opinion on dietary reference values for fats, including saturated fatty acids, polyunsaturated fatty acids, monounsaturated fatty acids, trans fatty acids and cholesterol. *EFSA J.* **2010**, *8*, 1461.

23. Browning, L.M.; Walker, C.G.; Mander, A.P.; West, A.L.; Madden, J.; Gambell, J.M.; Young, S.; Wang, L.; Jebb, S.A.; Calder, P.C. Incorporation of eicosapentaenoic and docosahexaenoic acids into lipid pools when given as supplements providing doses equivalent to typical intakes of oily fish. *Am. J. Clin. Nutr.* **2012**, *96*, 748–758. [CrossRef] [PubMed]

24. Stark, K.D.; Van Elswyk, M.; Higgins, M.R.; Weatherford, C.A.; Salem, N., Jr. Global survey of the omega-3 fatty acids, docosahexaenoic acid and eicosapentaenoic acid in the blood stream of healthy adults. *Prog. Lipid Res.* **2016**, *63*, 132–152. [CrossRef] [PubMed]

25. Brenner, R.R. Hormonal modulation of delta6 and delta5 desaturases: Case of diabetes. *Prostaglandins Leukot Essent Fat. Acids* **2003**, *68*, 151–162. [CrossRef]

26. Molfino, A.; Amabile, M.I.; Monti, M.; Muscaritoli, M. Omega-3 polyunsaturated fatty acids in critical illness: Anti-inflammatory, proresolving, or both? *Oxid. Med. Cell Longev.* **2017**, *2017*, 5987082. [CrossRef] [PubMed]

27. Dupont, J.; Dedeyne, L.; Dalle, S.; Koppo, K.; Gielen, E. The role of omega-3 in the prevention and treatment of sarcopenia. *Aging Clin. Exp. Res.* **2019**, *31*, 825–836. [CrossRef]

28. Calder, P.C.; Carr, A.C.; Gombart, A.F.; Eggersdorfer, M. Optimal. nutritional status for a well-functioning immune system is an important factor to protect against viral infections. *Nutrients* **2020**, *12*, 1181. [CrossRef] [PubMed]

29. McGlory, C.; Calder, P.C.; Nunes, E.A. The influence of omega-3 fatty acids on skeletal muscle protein turnover in health, disuse, and disease. *Front. Nutr.* **2019**, *6*, 144. [CrossRef] [PubMed]

30. Calder, P.C. Mechanisms of action of (n-3) fatty acids. *J. Nutr.* **2012**, *142*, 592S–599S. [CrossRef]

31. Surette, M.E. The science behind dietary omega-3 fatty acids. *CMAJ* **2008**, *178*, 177–180. [CrossRef]

32. Hashimoto, M.; Hossain, S. Fatty acids: From membrane ingredients to signaling molecule. In *Biochemistry and Health Benefits of Fatty Acids*; Waisundara, V., Ed.; IntechOpen Limited: London, UK, 2018.

33. Hishikawa, D.; Valentine, W.J.; Iizuka-Hishikawa, Y.; Shindou, H.; Shimizu, T. Metabolism and functions of docosahexaenoic acid-containing membrane glycerophospholipids. *FEBS Lett.* **2017**, *591*, 2730–2744. [CrossRef]

34. Calder, P.C. Docosahexaenoic acid. *Ann. Nutr. Metab.* **2016**, *69* (Suppl. 1), 8–21. [CrossRef]

35. Swanson, D.; Block, R.; Mousa, S.A. Omega-3 fatty acids EPA and DHA: Health Benefits throughout life. *Adv. Nutr.* **2012**, *3*, 1–7. [CrossRef]

36. de Carvalho, C.; Caramujo, M.J. The various roles of fatty acids. *Molecules* **2018**, *23*, 2583. [CrossRef] [PubMed]

37. Christie, W.W.; Harwwod, J.L. Oxidation of polyunsaturated fatty acids to produce lipid mediators. *Essays Biochem.* **2020**, in press. [CrossRef] [PubMed]

38. Calder, P.C. Eicosanouds. *Essays Biochem.* **2020**, in press. [CrossRef] [PubMed]

39. Alzheimer's Disease International. Dementia statistics. Available online: https://www.alz.co.uk/research/statistics (accessed on 4 May 2020).

40. Mohajeri, M.H.; Troesch, B.; Weber, P. Inadequate supply of vitamins and DHA in the elderly: Implications for brain aging and Alzheimer-type dementia. *Nutrition* **2015**, *31*, 261–275. [CrossRef]

41. Lauritzen, L.; Hansen, H.S.; Jørgensen, M.H.; Michaelsen, K.F. The essentiality of long chain n-3 fatty acids in relation to development and function of the brain and retina. *Prog. Lipid Res.* **2001**, *40*, 1–94. [CrossRef]

42. Alessandri, J.M.; Guesnet, P.; Vancassel, S.; Astorg, P.; Denis, I.; Langelier, B.; Aïd, S.; Poumès-Ballihaut, C.; Champeil-Potokar, G.; Lavialle, M. Polyunsaturated fatty acids in the central nervous system: Evolution of concepts and nutritional implications throughout life. *Reprod. Nutr. Dev.* **2004**, *44*, 509–538. [CrossRef]

43. Bazan, N.G.; Molina, M.F.; Gordon, W.C. Docosahexaenoic acid signalolipidomics in nutrition: Significance in aging, neuroinflammation, macular degeneration, Alzheimer's, and other neurodegenerative diseases. *Annu. Rev. Nutr.* **2011**, *31*, 321–351. [CrossRef]

44. Giusto, N.M.; Salvador, G.A.; Castagnet, P.I.; Pasquaré, S.J.; Ilincheta de Boschero, M.G. Age-associated changes in central nervous system glycerolipid composition and metabolism. *Neurochem. Res.* **2002**, *27*, 1513–1523. [CrossRef]

45. Söderberg, M.; Edlund, C.; Kristensson, K.; Dallner, G. Fatty acid composition of brain phospholipids in aging and in Alzheimer's disease. *Lipids* **1991**, *26*, 421–425. [CrossRef]

46. Fotuhi, M.; Mohassel, P.; Yaffe, K. Fish consumption, long-chain omega-3 fatty acids and risk of cognitive decline or Alzheimer disease: A complex association. *Nat. Clin. Pract. Neurol.* **2009**, *5*, 140–152. [CrossRef]

47. Heude, B.; Ducimetière, P.; Berr, C. Cognitive decline and fatty acid composition of erythrocyte membranes—The EVA Study. *Am. J. Clin. Nutr.* **2003**, *77*, 803–808. [CrossRef] [PubMed]

48. Phillips, M.A.; Childs, C.E.; Calder, P.C.; Rogers, P.J. Lower omega-3 fatty acid intake and status are associated with poorer cognitive function in older age: A comparison of individuals with and without cognitive impairment and Alzheimer's disease. *Nutr. Neurosci.* **2012**, *15*, 271–277. [CrossRef] [PubMed]

49. Schaefer, E.J.; Bongard, V.; Beiser, A.S.; Lamon-Fava, S.; Robins, S.J.; Au, R.; Tucker, K.L.; Kyle, D.J.; Wilson, P.W.; Wolf, P.A. Plasma phosphatidylcholine docosahexaenoic acid content and risk of dementia and alzheimer disease: The Framingham Heart Study. *Arch. Neurol.* **2006**, *63*, 1545–1550. [CrossRef] [PubMed]

50. de Wilde, M.C.; Vellas, B.; Girault, E.; Yavuz, A.C.; Sijben, J.W. Lower brain and blood nutrient status in Alzheimer's disease: Results from meta-analyses. *Alzheimers Dement.* **2017**, *3*, 416–431. [CrossRef] [PubMed]

51. Kalmijn, S.; Launer, L.J.; Ott, A.; Witteman, J.C.; Hofman, A.; Breteler, M.M. Dietary fat intake and the risk of incident dementia in the Rotterdam study. *Ann. Neurol.* **1997**, *42*, 776–782. [CrossRef]

52. Morris, M.C.; Evans, D.A.; Bienias, J.L.; Tangney, C.C.; Bennett, D.A.; Aggarwal, N.; Schneider, J.; Wilson, R.S. Dietary fats and the risk of incident Alzheimer disease. *Arch. Neurol.* **2003**, *60*, 194–200. [CrossRef]

53. Barberger-Gateau, P.; Raffaitin, C.; Letenneur, L.; Berr, C.; Tzourio, C.; Dartigues, J.F.; Alpérovitch, A. Dietary patterns and risk of dementia: The Three-City cohort study. *Neurology* **2007**, *69*, 1921–1930. [CrossRef]

54. Barberger-Gateau, P.; Letenneur, L.; Deschamps, V.; Pérès, K.; Dartigues, J.F.; Renaud, S. Fish, meat, and risk of dementia: Cohort study. *BMJ* **2002**, *325*, 932–933. [CrossRef]

55. Engelhart, M.J.; Geerlings, M.I.; Ruitenberg, A.; Van Swieten, J.C.; Hofman, A.; Witteman, J.C.; Breteler, M.M. Diet and risk of dementia: Does fat matter? The Rotterdam study. *Neurology* **2002**, *59*, 1915–1921. [CrossRef]

56. Devore, E.E.; Grodstein, F.; van Rooij, F.J.; Hofman, A.; Rosner, B.; Stampfer, M.J.; Witteman, J.C.; Breteler, M.M. Dietary intake of fish and omega-3 fatty acids in relation to long-term dementia risk. *Am. J. Clin. Nutr.* **2009**, *90*, 170–176. [CrossRef]

57. Zhang, Y.; Chen, J.; Qiu, J.; Li, Y.; Wang, J.; Jiao, J. Intakes of fish and polyunsaturated fatty acids and mild-to-severe cognitive impairment risks: A dose-response meta-analysis of 21 cohort studies. *Am. J. Clin. Nutr.* **2016**, *103*, 330–340. [CrossRef] [PubMed]

58. Yurko-Mauro, K.; Alexander, D.D.; Van Elswyk, M.E. Docosahexaenoic acid and adult memory: A systematic review and meta-Analysis. *PLoS ONE* **2015**, *10*, e0120391. [CrossRef] [PubMed]

59. Yassine, H.N.; Braskie, M.N.; Mack, W.J.; Castor, K.J.; Fonteh, A.N.; Schneider, L.S.; Harrington, M.G.; Chui, H.C. Association of docosahexaenoic acid supplementation with alzheimer disease stage in apolipoprotein e epsilon4 carriers: A review. *JAMA Neurol.* **2017**, *74*, 339–347. [CrossRef]

60. Alex, A.; Abbott, K.A.; McEvoy, M.; Schofield, P.W.; Garg, M.L. Long-chain omega-3 polyunsaturated fatty acids and cognitive decline in non-demented adults: A systematic review and meta-analysis. *Nutr. Rev.* **2019**, *78*, 563–578. [CrossRef]

61. Witte, A.V.; Kerti, L.; Hermannstädter, H.M.; Fiebach, J.B.; Schreiber, S.J.; Schuchardt, J.P.; Hahn, A.; Flöel, A. Long-chain omega-3 fatty acids improve brain function and structure in older adults. *Cereb. Cortex* **2014**, *24*, 3059–3068. [CrossRef] [PubMed]

62. Burckhardt, M.; Herke, M.; Wustmann, T.; Watzke, S.; Langer, G.; Fink, A. Omega-3 fatty acids for the treatment of dementia. *Cochrane Database Syst. Rev.* **2016**, *4*, CD009002. [CrossRef] [PubMed]

63. Phillips, M.A.; Childs, C.E.; Calder, P.C.; Rogers, P.J. No effect of omega-3 fatty acid supplementation on cognition and mood in individuals with cognitive impairment and probable Alzheimer's Disease: A randomised controlled trial. *Int. J. Mol. Sci.* **2015**, *16*, 24600–24613. [CrossRef]

64. Román, G.C.; Jackson, R.E.; Reis, J.; Román, A.N.; Toledo, J.B.; Toledo, E. Extra-virgin olive oil for potential prevention of Alzheimer disease. *Revue Neurol.* **2019**, *175*, 705–723. [CrossRef]

65. Dangour, A.D.; Allen, E.; Elbourne, D.; Fasey, N.; Fletcher, A.E.; Hardy, P.; Holder, G.E.; Knight, R.; Letley, L.; Richards, M.; et al. Effect of 2-y n-3 long-chain polyunsaturated fatty acid supplementation on cognitive function in older people: A randomized, double-blind, controlled trial. *Am. J. Clin. Nutr.* **2010**, *91*, 1725–1732. [CrossRef]

66. Freund-Levi, Y.; Eriksdotter-Jönhagen, M.; Cederholm, T.; Basun, H.; Faxén-Irving, G.; Garlind, A.; Vedin, I.; Vessby, B.; Wahlund, L.O.; Palmblad, J. Ω-3 fatty acid treatment in 174 patients with mild to moderate alzheimer disease: OmegAD study: A randomized double-blind trial. *Arch. Neurol.* **2006**, *63*, 1402–1408. [CrossRef]

67. Eriksdotter, M.; Vedin, I.; Falahati, F.; Freund-Levi, Y.; Hjorth, E.; Faxen-Irving, G.; Wahlund, L.O.; Schultzberg, M.; Basun, H.; Cederholm, T.; et al. Plasma fatty acid profiles in relation to cognition and gender in Alzheimer's Disease patients during oral omega-3 fatty acid supplementation: The OmegAD Study. *J. Alzheimers Dis.* **2015**, *48*, 805–812. [CrossRef] [PubMed]

68. Köbe, T.; Witte, A.V.; Schnelle, A.; Lesemann, A.; Fabian, S.; Tesky, V.A.; Pantel, J.; Flöel, A. Combined omega-3 fatty acids, aerobic exercise and cognitive stimulation prevents decline in gray matter volume of the frontal, parietal and cingulate cortex in patients with mild cognitive impairment. *NeuroImage* **2016**, *131*, 226–238. [CrossRef] [PubMed]

69. Bo, Y.; Zhang, X.; Wang, Y.; You, J.; Cui, H.; Zhu, Y.; Pang, W.; Liu, W.; Jiang, Y.; Lu, Q. The n-3 polyunsaturated fatty acids supplementation improved the cognitive function in the Chinese elderly with mild cognitive impairment: A double-blind randomized controlled trial. *Nutrients* **2017**, *9*, 54. [CrossRef] [PubMed]

70. Zhang, Y.P.; Miao, R.; Li, Q.; Wu, T.; Ma, F. Effects of DHA supplementation on hippocampal volume and cognitive function in older adults with mild cognitive impairment: A 12-month randomized, double-blind, placebo-controlled trial. *J. Alzheimers Dis.* **2017**, *55*, 497–507. [CrossRef]

71. Zhang, Y.P.; Lou, Y.; Hu, J.; Miao, R.; Ma, F. DHA supplementation improves cognitive function via enhancing Aβ-mediated autophagy in Chinese elderly with mild cognitive impairment: A randomised placebo-controlled trial. *J. Neurol. Neurosurg. Psychiatry* **2018**, *89*, 382–388. [CrossRef]

72. Canhada, S.; Castro, K.; Schweigert Perry, I.; Luft, V.C. Omega-3 fatty acids' supplementation in Alzheimer's disease: A systematic review. *Nutr. Neurosci.* **2018**, *21*, 529–538. [CrossRef]

73. Coley, N.; Raman, R.; Donohue, M.C.; Aisen, P.S.; Vellas, B.; Andrieu, S. Defining the optimal target population for trials of polyunsaturated fatty acid supplementation using the erythrocyte omega-3 index: A step towards personalized prevention of cognitive decline? *J. Nutr. Health Aging* **2018**, *22*, 982–998. [CrossRef]

74. van de Rest, O.; Geleijnse, J.M.; Kok, F.J.; van Staveren, W.A.; Dullemeijer, C.; Olderikkert, M.G.; Beekman, A.T.; de Groot, C.P. Effect of fish oil on cognitive performance in older subjects: A randomized, controlled trial. *Neurology* **2008**, *71*, 430–438. [CrossRef]

75. Vellas, B.; Carrie, I.; Gillette-Guyonnet, S.; Touchon, J.; Dantoine, T.; Dartigues, J.F.; Cuffi, M.N.; Bordes, S.; Gasnier, Y.; Robert, P.; et al. MAPT study: A multidomain approach for preventing Alzheimer's disease: Design and baseline data. *J. Prev. Alzheimers Dis.* **2014**, *1*, 13–22.

76. Andrieu, S.; Guyonnet, S.; Coley, N.; Cantet, C.; Bonnefoy, M.; Bordes, S.; Bories, L.; Cufi, M.N.; Dantoine, T.; Dartigues, J.F.; et al. Effect of long-term omega 3 polyunsaturated fatty acid supplementation with or without multidomain intervention on cognitive function in elderly adults with memory complaints (MAPT): A randomised, placebo-controlled trial. *Lancet Neurol.* **2017**, *16*, 377–389. [CrossRef]

77. Hooper, C.; De Souto Barreto, P.; Coley, N.; Cantet, C.; Cesari, M.; Andrieu, S.; Vellas, B. Cognitive changes with omega-3 polyunsaturated fatty acids in non-demented older adults with low omega-3 index. *J. Nutr. Health Aging* **2017**, *21*, 988–993. [CrossRef] [PubMed]

78. Yassine, H.N.; Schneider, L.S. Lessons from the Multidomain Alzheimer Preventive Trial. *Lancet Neurol.* **2017**, *16*, 585–586. [CrossRef]

79. Hooijmans, C.R.; Pasker-de Jong, P.C.M.; de Vries, R.B.M.; Ritskes-Hoitinga, M. The effects of long-term omega-3 fatty acid supplementation on cognition and Alzheimer's pathology in animal models of Alzheimer's disease: A systematic review and meta-analysis. *J. Alzheimers Dis.* **2012**, *28*, 191–209. [CrossRef] [PubMed]

80. Jernerén, F.; Cederholm, T.; Refsum, H.; Smith, A.D.; Turner, C.; Palmblad, J.; Eriksdotter, M.; Hjorth, E.; Faxen-Irving, G.; Wahlund, L.O.; et al. Homocysteine status modifies the treatment effect of omega-3 fatty acids on cognition in a randomized clinical trial in mild to moderate Alzheimer's Disease: The OmegAD Study. *J. Alzheimers Dis.* **2019**, *69*, 189–197. [CrossRef]

81. Jernerén, F.; Elshorbagy, A.K.; Oulhaj, A.; Smith, S.M.; Refsum, H.; Smith, A.D. Brain atrophy in cognitively impaired elderly: The importance of long-chain ω-3 fatty acids and B vitamin status in a randomized controlled trial. *Am. J. Clin. Nutr.* **2015**, *102*, 215–221. [CrossRef]

82. Oulhaj, A.; Jernerén, F.; Refsum, H.; Smith, A.D.; de Jager, C.A. Omega-3 fatty acid status enhances the prevention of cognitive decline by b vitamins in mild cognitive impairment. *J. Alzheimers Dis.* **2016**, *50*, 547–557. [CrossRef]

83. Assmann, K.E.; Adjibade, M.; Hercberg, S.; Galan, P.; Kesse-Guyot, E. Unsaturated fatty acid intakes during midlife are positively associated with later cognitive function in older adults with modulating effects of antioxidant supplementation. *J. Nutr.* **2018**, *148*, 1938–1945. [CrossRef]

84. Finch, C.E. Evolution of the human lifespan and diseases of aging: Roles of infection, inflammation, and nutrition. *Proc. Natl. Acad. Sci. USA* **2010**, *107* (Suppl. 1), 1718–1724. [CrossRef]

85. Egert, S.; Rimbach, G.; Huebbe, P. ApoE genotype: From geographic distribution to function and responsiveness to dietary factors. *Proc. Nutr. Soc.* **2012**, *71*, 410–424. [CrossRef]

86. Nock, T.G.; Chouinard-Watkins, R.; Plourde, M. Carriers of an apolipoprotein E epsilon 4 allele are more vulnerable to a dietary deficiency in omega-3 fatty acids and cognitive decline. *Biochim. Biophys. Acta* **2017**, *1862*, 1068–1078. [CrossRef]

87. Ramassamy, C.; Averill, D.; Beffert, U.; Bastianetto, S.; Theroux, L.; Lussier-Cacan, S.; Cohn, J.S.; Christen, Y.; Davignon, J.; Quirion, R.; et al. Oxidative damage and protection by antioxidants in the frontal cortex of Alzheimer's disease is related to the apolipoprotein E genotype. *Free Rad. Biol. Med.* **1999**, *27*, 544–553. [CrossRef]

88. Landi, F.; Calvani, R.; Tosato, M.; Martone, A.M.; Ortolani, E.; Savera, G.; Sisto, A.; Marzetti, E. Anorexia of aging: Risk factors, consequences, and potential treatments. *Nutrients* **2016**, *8*, 69. [CrossRef] [PubMed]

89. Rémond, D.; Shahar, D.R.; Gille, D.; Pinto, P.; Kachal, J.; Peyron, M.A.; Dos Santos, C.N.; Walther, B.; Bordoni, A.; Dupont, D.; et al. Understanding the gastrointestinal tract of the elderly to develop dietary solutions that prevent malnutrition. *Oncotarget* **2015**, *6*, 13858–13898. [CrossRef] [PubMed]

90. Santos-Eggimann, B.; Cuénoud, P.; Spagnoli, J.; Junod, J. Prevalence of frailty in middle-aged and older community-dwelling Europeans living in 10 countries. *J. Gerontol. A Biol. Sci. Med. Sci.* **2009**, *64*, 675–681. [CrossRef] [PubMed]

91. Collard, R.M.; Boter, H.; Schoevers, R.A.; Oude Voshaar, R.C. Prevalence of frailty in community-dwelling older persons: A systematic review. *J. Am. Geriatr. Soc.* **2012**, *60*, 1487–1492. [CrossRef] [PubMed]

92. Vetrano, D.L.; Palmer, K.; Marengoni, A.; Marzetti, E.; Lattanzio, F.; Roller-Wirnsberger, R.; Lopez Samaniego, L.; Rodríguez-Mañas, L.; Bernabei, R.; Onder, G.; et al. Frailty and multimorbidity: A systematic review and meta-analysis. *J. Gerontol. A Biol. Sci. Med. Sci.* **2019**, *74*, 659–666. [CrossRef]

93. Cederholm, T.; Barazzoni, R.; Austin, P.; Ballmer, P.; Biolo, G.; Bischoff, S.C.; Compher, C.; Correia, I.; Higashiguchi, T.; Holst, M.; et al. ESPEN guidelines on definitions and terminology of clinical nutrition. *Clin. Nutr.* **2017**, *36*, 49–64. [CrossRef]

94. Clegg, A.; Young, J.; Iliffe, S.; Rikkert, M.O.; Rockwood, K. Frailty in elderly people. *Lancet* **2013**, *381*, 752–762. [CrossRef]

95. Ligthart-Melis, G.C.; Luiking, Y.C.; Kakourou, A.; Cederholm, T.; Maier, A.B.; de van der Schueren, M.A.E. Frailty, sarcopenia, and malnutrition frequently (co-)occur in hospitalized older adults: A systematic review and meta-analysis. *J. Am. Med. Diet. Assoc.* **2020**, in press. [CrossRef]

96. Fried, L.P.; Tangen, C.M.; Walston, J.; Newman, A.B.; Hirsch, C.; Gottdiener, J.; Seeman, T.; Tracy, R.; Kop, W.J.; Burke, G.; et al. Frailty in older adults: Evidence for a phenotype. *J. Gerontol. A Biol. Sci. Med. Sci.* **2001**, *56*, M146–M156. [CrossRef]

97. Hernández-Luis, R.; Martín-Ponce, E.; Monereo-Muñoz, M.; Quintero-Platt, G.; Odeh-Santana, S.; González-Reimers, E.; Santolaria, F. Prognostic value of physical function tests and muscle mass in elderly hospitalized patients. A prospective observational study. *Geriatr. Gerontol. Int.* **2018**, *18*, 57–64. [CrossRef] [PubMed]

98. Khandelwal, D.; Goel, A.; Kumar, U.; Gulati, V.; Narang, R.; Dey, A.B. Frailty is associated with longer hospital stay and increased mortality in hospitalized older patients. *J. Nutr. Health Aging* **2012**, *16*, 732–735. [CrossRef] [PubMed]

99. Makary, M.A.; Segev, D.L.; Pronovost, P.J.; Syin, D.; Bandeen-Roche, K.; Patel, P.; Takenaga, R.; Devgan, L.; Holzmueller, C.G.; Tian, J.; et al. Frailty as a predictor of surgical outcomes in older patients. *J. Am. Coll. Surg.* **2010**, *210*, 901–908. [CrossRef] [PubMed]

100. Cruz-Jentoft, A.J.; Bahat, G.; Bauer, J.; Boirie, Y.; Bruyère, O.; Cederholm, T.; Cooper, C.; Landi, F.; Rolland, Y.; Sayer, A.A.; et al. Writing Group for the European Working Group on Sarcopenia in Older People 2 (EWGSOP2), and the Extended Group for EWGSOP2. Sarcopenia: Revised European consensus on definition and diagnosis. *Age Ageing* **2019**, *48*, 16–31. [CrossRef]

101. Cruz-Jentoft, A.J.; Baeyens, J.P.; Bauer, J.M.; Boirie, Y.; Cederholm, T.; Landi, F.; Martin, F.C.; Michel, J.P.; Rolland, Y.; Schneider, S.M.; et al. European Working Group on Sarcopenia in Older People. Sarcopenia: European consensus on definition and diagnosis: Report of the European Working Group on Sarcopenia in Older People. *Age Ageing* **2010**, *39*, 412–423. [CrossRef]

102. de Hoogt, P.A.; Reisinger, K.W.; Tegels, J.J.W.; Bosmans, J.W.A.M.; Tijssen, F.; Stoot, J.H.M.B. Functional Compromise Cohort Study (FCCS): Sarcopenia is a strong predictor of mortality in the intensive care unit. *World J. Surg.* **2018**, *42*, 1733–1741. [CrossRef]

103. Vetrano, D.L.; Landi, F.; Volpato, S.; Corsonello, A.; Meloni, E.; Bernabei, R.; Onder, G. Association of sarcopenia with short- and long-term mortality in older adults admitted to acute care wards: Results from the CRIME study. *J. Gerontol. A Biol. Sci. Med. Sci.* **2014**, *69*, 1154–1161. [CrossRef]

104. Meskers, C.G.M.; Reijnierse, E.M.; Numans, S.T.; Kruizinga, R.C.; Pierik, V.D.; van Ancum, J.M.; Slee-Valentijn, M.; Scheerman, K.; Verlaan, S.; Maier, A.B. Association of handgrip strength and muscle mass with dependency in (instrumental) activities of daily living in hospitalized older adults—The EMPOWER Study. *J. Nutr. Health Aging* **2019**, *23*, 232–238. [CrossRef]

105. Ratnayake, C.B.; Loveday, B.P.; Shrikhande, S.V.; Windsor, J.A.; Pandanaboyana, S. Impact of preoperative sarcopenia on postoperative outcomes following pancreatic resection: A systematic review and meta-analysis. *Pancreatology* **2018**, *18*, 996–1004. [CrossRef]

106. Kamarajah, S.K.; Bundred, J.; Tan, B.H.L. Body composition assessment and sarcopenia in patients with gastric cancer: A systematic review and meta-analysis. *Gastric Cancer* **2019**, *22*, 10–22. [CrossRef]

107. Matsunaga, T.; Miyata, H.; Sugimura, K.; Motoori, M.; Asukai, K.; Yanagimoto, Y.; Takahashi, Y.; Tomokuni, A.; Yamamoto, K.; Akita, H.; et al. Prognostic significance of sarcopenia and systemic inflammatory response in patients with esophageal cancer. *Anticancer Res.* **2019**, *39*, 449–458. [CrossRef]

108. Esser, H.; Resch, T.; Pamminger, M.; Mutschlechner, B.; Troppmair, J.; Riedmann, M.; Gassner, E.; Maglione, M.; Margreiter, C.; Boesmueller, C.; et al. Preoperative assessment of muscle mass using computerized tomography scans to predict outcomes following orthotopic liver transplantation. *Transplantation* **2019**, *103*, 2506–2514. [CrossRef] [PubMed]

109. Mintziras, I.; Miligkos, M.; Wächter, S.; Manoharan, J.; Maurer, E.; Bartsch, D.K. Sarcopenia and sarcopenic obesity are significantly associated with poorer overall survival in patients with pancreatic cancer: Systematic review and meta-analysis. *Int. J. Surg.* **2018**, *59*, 19–26. [CrossRef]

110. Wang, J.; Leung, K.-S.; Chow, S.K.-H.; Cheung, W.-H. Inflammation and age-associated skeletal muscle deterioration (sarcopaenia). *J. Orthopaed. Transl.* **2017**, *10*, 94–101. [CrossRef]

111. Wolfe, R.R. The underappreciated role of muscle in health and disease. *Am. J. Clin. Nutr.* **2006**, *84*, 475–482. [CrossRef] [PubMed]

112. Newman, A.B.; Kupelian, V.; Visser, M.; Simonsick, E.M.; Goodpaster, B.H.; Kritchevsky, S.B.; Tylavsky, F.A.; Rubin, S.M.; Harris, T.B. Strength, but not muscle mass, is associated with mortality in the health, aging and body composition study cohort. *J. Gerontol. A Biol. Sci. Med. Sci.* **2006**, *61*, 72–77. [CrossRef] [PubMed]

113. Wischmeyer, P.E.; Puthucheary, Z.; San Millán, I.; Butz, D.; Grocott, M.P.W. Muscle mass and physical recovery in ICU: Innovations for targeting of nutrition and exercise. *Curr. Opin. Crit. Care* **2017**, *23*, 269–278. [CrossRef] [PubMed]

114. Smith, G.I.; Julliand, S.; Reeds, D.N.; Sinacore, D.R.; Klein, S.; Mittendorfer, B. Fish oil-derived n-3 PUFA therapy increases muscle mass and function in healthy older adults. *Am. J. Clin. Nutr.* **2015**, *102*, 115–122. [CrossRef] [PubMed]

115. Hutchins-Wiese, H.L.; Kleppinger, A.; Annis, K.; Liva, E.; Lammi-Keefe, C.J.; Durham, H.A.; Kenny, A.M. The impact of supplemental n-3 long chain polyunsaturated fatty acids and dietary antioxidants on physical performance in postmenopausal women. *J. Nutr. Health. Aging.* **2013**, *17*, 76–80. [CrossRef] [PubMed]

116. Logan, S.L.; Spriet, L.L. Omega-3 fatty acid supplementation for 12 weeks increases resting and exercise metabolic rate in healthy community-dwelling older females. *PLoS ONE* **2015**, *10*, e0144828. [CrossRef] [PubMed]

117. Krzyminska-Siemaszko, R.; Czepulis, N.; Lewandowicz, M.; Zasadzka, E.; Suwalska, A.; Witowski, J.; Wieczorowska-Tobis, K. The effect of a 12-week omega-3 supplementation on body composition, muscle strength and physical performance in elderly individuals with decreased muscle mass. *Int. J. Environ. Res. Public Health* **2015**, *12*, 10558–10574. [CrossRef] [PubMed]

118. Rolland, Y.; de Souto Barreto, P.; Maltais, M.; Guyonnet, S.; Cantet, C.; Andrieu, S.; Vellas, B. Effect of long-term omega 3 polyunsaturated fatty acid supplementation with or without multidomain lifestyle intervention on muscle strength in older adults: Secondary analysis of the Multidomain Alzheimer Preventive Trial (MAPT). *Nutrients* **2019**, *11*, 1931. [CrossRef] [PubMed]

119. Locke, A.; Schneiderhan, J.; Zick, S.M. Diets for health: Goals and guidelines. *Am. Fam. Physician* **2018**, *97*, 721–728. [PubMed]

120. Mondello, P.; Mian, M.; Aloisi, C.; Famà, F.; Mondello, S.; Pitini, V. Cancer cachexia syndrome: Pathogenesis, diagnosis, and new therapeutic options. *Nutr. Cancer* **2015**, *67*, 12–26. [CrossRef]

121. Cederholm, T.; Jensen, G.L.; Correia, M.I.T.D.; Gonzalez, M.C.; Fukushima, R.; Higashiguchi, T.; Baptista, G.; Barazzoni, R.; Blaauw, R.; Coats, A.; et al. GLIM criteria for the diagnosis of malnutrition—A consensus report from the global clinical nutrition community. *Clin. Nutr.* **2019**, *38*, 1–9. [CrossRef]

122. Ryan, A.M.; Power, D.G.; Daly, L.; Cushen, S.J.; Ní Bhuachalla, Ē.; Prado, C.M. Cancer-associated malnutrition, cachexia and sarcopenia: The skeleton in the hospital closet 40 years later. *Proc. Nutr. Soc.* **2016**, *75*, 199–211. [CrossRef]

123. Arends, J.; Baracos, V.; Bertz, H.; Bozzetti, F.; Calder, P.C.; Deutz, N.E.P.; Erickson, N.; Laviano, A.; Lisanti, M.P.; Lobo, D.N.; et al. ESPEN expert group recommendations for action against cancer-related malnutrition. *Clin. Nutr.* **2017**, *36*, 1187–1196. [CrossRef]

124. Fearon, K.; Strasser, F.; Anker, S.D.; Bosaeus, I.; Bruera, E.; Fainsinger, R.L.; Jatoi, A.; Loprinzi, C.; MacDonald, N.; Mantovani, G.; et al. Definition and classification of cancer cachexia: An international consensus. *Lancet Oncol.* **2011**, *12*, 489–495. [CrossRef]

125. Baracos, V.E.; Martin, L.; Korc, M.; Guttridge, D.C.; Fearon, K.C.H. Cancer-associated cachexia. *Nat. Rev. Dis. Primers* **2018**, *4*, 17105. [CrossRef]

126. Barker, T.; Fulde, G.; Moulton, B.; Nadauld, L.D.; Rhodes, T. An elevated neutrophil-to-lymphocyte ratio associates with weight loss and cachexia in cancer. *Sci. Rep.* **2020**, *10*, 7535. [CrossRef]

127. Argilés, J.M.; Busquets, S.; Stemmler, B.; López-Soriano, F.J. Cancer cachexia: Understanding the molecular basis. *Nat. Rev. Cancer* **2014**, *14*, 754. [CrossRef]

128. Warren, S. The immediate cause of death in cancer. *Am. J. Med. Sci.* **1932**, *184*, 610–613. [CrossRef]

129. Ross, P.J.; Ashley, S.; Norton, A.; Priest, K.; Waters, J.S.; Eisen, T.; Smith, I.E.; O'Brien, M.E. Do patients with weight loss have a worse outcome when undergoing chemotherapy for lung cancers? *Brit. J. Cancer* **2004**, *90*, 1905–1911. [CrossRef] [PubMed]

130. Prado, C.M.; Lieffers, J.R.; McCargar, L.J.; Reiman, T.; Sawyer, M.B.; Martin, L.; Baracos, V.E. Prevalence and clinical implications of sarcopenic obesity in patients with solid tumours of the respiratory and gastrointestinal tracts: A population-based study. *Lancet Oncol.* **2008**, *9*, 629–635. [CrossRef]

131. Antoun, S.; Baracos, V.E.; Birdsell, L.; Escudier, B.; Sawyer, M.B. Low body mass index and sarcopenia associated with dose-limiting toxicity of sorafenib in patients with renal cell carcinoma. *Ann. Oncol.* **2010**, *21*, 1594–1598. [CrossRef]

132. Prado, C.M.; Baracos, V.E.; McCargar, L.J.; Mourtzakis, M.; Mulder, K.E.; Reiman, T.; Butts, C.A.; Scarfe, A.G.; Sawyer, M.B. Body composition as an independent determinant of 5-fluorouracil-based chemotherapy toxicity. *Clin. Cancer Res.* **2007**, *13*, 3264–3268. [CrossRef] [PubMed]

133. Prado, C.M.; Baracos, V.E.; McCargar, L.J.; Reiman, T.; Mourtzakis, M.; Tonkin, K.; Mackey, J.R.; Koski, S.; Pituskin, E.; Sawyer, M.B. Sarcopenia as a determinant of chemotherapy toxicity and time to tumor progression in metastatic breast cancer patients receiving capecitabine treatment. *Clin. Cancer Res.* **2009**, *15*, 2920–2926. [CrossRef]

134. Barret, M.; Antoun, S.; Dalban, C.; Malka, D.; Mansourbakht, T.; Zaanan, A.; Latko, E.; Taieb, J. Sarcopenia is linked to treatment toxicity in patients with metastatic colorectal cancer. *Nutr. Cancer* **2014**, *66*, 583–589. [CrossRef]

135. Hopkinson, J.B. The emotional aspects of cancer anorexia. *Curr. Opin. Support. Palliat. Care* **2010**, *4*, 254–258. [CrossRef]

136. Advani, S.M.; Advani, P.G.; VonVille, H.M.; Jafri, S.H. Pharmacological management of cachexia in adult cancer patients: A systematic review of clinical trials. *BMC Cancer* **2018**, *18*, 1174. [CrossRef]

137. Naito, T. Evaluation of the true endpoint of clinical trials for cancer cachexia. *Asia Pac. J. Oncol. Nurs.* **2019**, *6*, 227–233. [CrossRef] [PubMed]

138. Hanahan, D.; Weinberg, R.A. Hallmarks of cancer: The next generation. *Cell* **2011**, *144*, 646–674. [CrossRef] [PubMed]

139. Diakos, C.I.; Charles, K.A.; McMillan, D.C.; Clarke, S.J. Cancer-related inflammation and treatment effectiveness. *Lancet Oncol.* **2014**, *15*, e493–e503. [CrossRef]

140. MacDonald, N. Terminology in cancer cachexia: Importance and status. *Curr. Opin. Clin. Nutr. Metab. Care* **2012**, *15*, 220–225. [CrossRef] [PubMed]

141. Solheim, T.S.; Laird, B.J. Evidence base for multimodal therapy in cachexia. *Curr. Opin. Support. Palliat. Care* **2012**, *6*, 424–431. [CrossRef]

142. Fearon, K.C. Cancer cachexia: Developing multimodal therapy for a multidimensional problem. *Eur. J. Cancer* **2008**, *44*, 1124–1132. [CrossRef]

143. de Aguiar Pastore Silva, J.; Emilia de Souza Fabre, M.; Waitzberg, D.L. Omega-3 supplements for patients in chemotherapy and/or radiotherapy: A systematic review. *Clin. Nutr.* **2015**, *34*, 359–366. [CrossRef]

144. Laviano, A.; Rianda, S.; Molfino, A.; Rossi Fanelli, F. Omega-3 fatty acids in cancer. *Curr. Opin. Clin. Nutr. Metab. Care* **2013**, *16*, 156–161. [CrossRef]

145. Morland, S.L.; Martins, K.J.B.; Mazurak, V.C. n-3 polyunsaturated fatty acid supplementation during cancer chemotherapy. *J. Nutr. Intermed. Metab.* **2016**, *5*, 107–116. [CrossRef]

146. Gorjao, R.; Momesso Dos Santos, C.M.; Afonso Serdan, T.D.; Sousa Diniz, V.L.; Alba-Loureiro, T.C.; Cury-Boaventura, M.F.; Hatanaka, E.; Levada-Pires, A.C.; Takeo Sato, F.; Pithon-Curi, T.C.; et al. New insights on the regulation of cancer cachexia by n-3 polyunsaturated fatty acids. *Pharmacol. Ther.* **2019**, *196*, 117–134. [CrossRef]

147. Wigmore, S.J.; Fearon, K.C.; Maingay, J.P.; Ross, J.A. Down-regulation of the acute-phase response in patients with pancreatic cancer cachexia receiving oral eicosapentaenoic acid is mediated via suppression of interleukin-6. *Clin. Sci.* **1997**, *92*, 215–221. [CrossRef] [PubMed]

148. van der Meij, B.S.; Langius, J.A.E.; Smit, E.F.; Spreeuwenberg, M.D.; von Blomberg, B.M.E.; Heijboer, A.C.; Paul, M.A.; van Leeuwen, P.A.M. Oral nutritional supplements containing (n-3) polyunsaturated fatty acids affect the nutritional status of patients with stage iii non-small cell lung cancer during multimodality treatment. *J. Nutr.* **2010**, *140*, 1774–1780. [CrossRef] [PubMed]

149. Mocellin, M.C.; Fernandes, R.; Chagas, T.R.; Trindade, E.B.S.M. A systematic review and meta-analysis of the n-3 polyunsaturated fatty acids effects on inflammatory markers in colorectal cancer. *Clin. Nutr.* **2016**, *35*, 359–369. [CrossRef] [PubMed]

150. Silva, J.d.A.P.; Trindade, E.B.; Fabre, M.E.; Menegotto, V.M.; Gevaerd, S.; Buss Zda, S.; Frode, T.S. Fish oil supplement alters markers of inflammatory and nutritional status in colorectal cancer patients. *Nutr. Cancer* **2012**, *64*, 267–273. [CrossRef] [PubMed]

151. Shirai, Y.; Okugawa, Y.; Hishida, A.; Ogawa, A.; Okamoto, K.; Shintani, M.; Morimoto, Y.; Nishikawa, R.; Yokoe, T.; Tanaka, K.; et al. Fish oil-enriched nutrition combined with systemic chemotherapy for gastrointestinal cancer patients with cancer cachexia. *Sci. Rep.* **2017**, *7*, 4826. [CrossRef]

152. Klassen, P.; Cervantes, M.; Mazurak, V.C. N-3 fatty acids during chemotherapy: Toward a higher level of evidence for clinical application. *Curr. Opin. Clin. Nutr. Metab. Care* **2020**, *23*, 82–88. [CrossRef]

153. Murphy, R.A.; Bureyko, T.F.; Mourtzakis, M.; Chu, Q.S.; Clandinin, M.T.; Reiman, T.; Mazurak, V.C. Aberrations in plasma phospholipid fatty acids in lung cancer patients. *Lipids* **2012**, *47*, 363–369. [CrossRef]

154. Dewey, A.; Baughan, C.; Dean, T.; Higgins, B.; Johnson, I. Eicosapentaenoic acid (EPA, an omega-3 fatty acid from fish oils) for the treatment of cancer cachexia. *Cochrane Database Syst. Rev.* **2007**, *1*, CD004597. [CrossRef]

155. Mazzotta, P.; Jeney, C.M. Anorexia-cachexia syndrome: A systematic review of the role of dietary polyunsaturated fatty acids in the management of symptoms, survival, and quality of life. *J. Pain Symptom Manag.* **2009**, *37*, 1069–1077. [CrossRef]

156. Ries, A.; Trottenberg, P.; Elsner, F.; Stiel, S.; Haugen, D.; Kaasa, S.; Radbruch, L. A systematic review on the role of fish oil for the treatment of cachexia in advanced cancer: An EPCRC cachexia guidelines project. *Palliat. Med.* **2012**, *26*, 294–304. [CrossRef]

157. Colomer, R.; Moreno-Nogueira, J.M.; García-Luna, P.P.; García-Peris, P.; García-de-Lorenzo, A.; Zarazaga, A.; Quecedo, L.; del Llano, J.; Usán, L.; Casimiro, C. N-3 fatty acids, cancer and cachexia: A systematic review of the literature. *Brit. J. Nutr.* **2007**, *97*, 823–831. [CrossRef] [PubMed]

158. Arends, J.; Bachmann, P.; Baracos, V.; Barthelemy, N.; Bertz, H.; Bozzetti, F.; Fearon, K.; Hütterer, E.; Isenring, E.; Kaasa, S.; et al. ESPEN guidelines on nutrition in cancer patients. *Clin. Nutr.* **2017**, *36*, 11–48. [CrossRef]

159. de van der Schueren, M.A.E.; Laviano, A.; Blanchard, H.; Jourdan, M.; Arends, J.; Baracos, V.E. Systematic review and meta-analysis of the evidence for oral nutritional intervention on nutritional and clinical outcomes during chemo(radio)therapy: Current evidence and guidance for design of future trials. *Ann. Oncol.* **2018**, *29*, 1141–1153. [CrossRef] [PubMed]

160. Sanchez-Lara, K.; Turcott, J.G.; Juárez-Hernández, E.; Nuñez-Valencia, C.; Villanueva, G.; Guevara, P.; De la Torre-Vallejo, M.; Mohar, A.; Arrieta, O. Effects of an oral nutritional supplement containing eicosapentaenoic acid on nutritional and clinical outcomes in patients with advanced non-small cell lung cancer: Randomised trial. *Clin. Nutr.* **2014**, *33*, 1017–1023. [CrossRef]

161. Freitas, R.D.S.; Campos, M.M. Protective effects of omega-3 fatty acids in cancer-related complications. *Nutrients* **2019**, *11*, 945. [CrossRef] [PubMed]

162. Cox, S.; Powell, C.; Carter, B.; Hurt, C.; Mukherjee, S.; Crosby, T.D. Role of nutritional status and intervention in oesophageal cancer treated with definitive chemoradiotherapy: Outcomes from SCOPE1. *Br. J. Cancer* **2016**, *115*, 172–177. [CrossRef]

163. Fearon, K.C.H.; Von Meyenfeldt, M.F.; Moses, A.G.; Van Geenen, R.; Roy, A.; Gouma, D.J.; Giacosa, A.; Van Gossum, A.; Bauer, J.; Barber, M.D.; et al. Effect of a protein and energy dense n-3 fatty acid enriched oral supplement on loss of weight and lean tissue in cancer cachexia: A randomised double blind trial. *Gut* **2003**, *52*, 1479–1486. [CrossRef]

164. Solheim, T.S.; Laird, B.J.A.; Balstad, T.R.; Stene, G.B.; Bye, A.; Johns, N.; Pettersen, C.H.; Fallon, M.; Fayers, P.; Fearon, K.; et al. A randomized phase II feasibility trial of a multimodal intervention for the management of cachexia in lung and pancreatic cancer. *J. Cachexia Sarcopenia Muscle* **2017**, *8*, 778–788. [CrossRef]

165. Solheim, T.S.; Laird, B.J.A.; Balstad, T.R.; Bye, A.; Stene, G.; Baracos, V.; Strasser, F.; Griffiths, G.; Maddocks, M.; Fallon, M.; et al. Cancer cachexia: Rationale for the MENAC (Multimodal—Exercise, Nutrition and Anti-inflammatory medication for Cachexia) trial. *BMJ Supp. Palliat. Care* **2018**, *8*, 258–265. [CrossRef]

166. Biswas, A.K.; Acharyya, S. Understanding cachexia in the context of metastatic progression. *Nat. Rev. Cancer* **2020**, *20*, 274–284. [CrossRef]

167. Song, M.; Ou, F.S.; Zemla, T.J.; Hull, M.A.; Shi, Q.; Limburg, P.J.; Alberts, S.R.; Sinicrope, F.A.; Giovannucci, E.L.; Van Blarigan, E.L.; et al. Marine omega-3 fatty acid intake and survival of stage III colon cancer according to tumor molecular markers in NCCTG Phase III trial N0147 (Alliance). *Int. J. Cancer* **2019**, *145*, 380–389. [CrossRef]

168. Song, M.; Zhang, X.; Meyerhardt, J.A.; Giovannucci, E.L.; Ogino, S.; Fuchs, C.S.; Chan, A.T. Marine ω-3 polyunsaturated fatty acid intake and survival after colorectal cancer diagnosis. *Gut* **2017**, *66*, 1790–1796. [CrossRef]

169. Van Blarigan, E.L.; Fuchs, C.S.; Niedzwiecki, D.; Ye, X.; Zhang, S.; Song, M.; Saltz, L.B.; Mayer, R.J.; Mowat, R.B.; Whittom, R.; et al. Marine ω-3 polyunsaturated fatty acid and fish intake after colon cancer diagnosis and survival: CALGB 89803 (Alliance). *Cancer Epidemiol. Biomark. Prev.* **2018**, *27*, 438–445. [CrossRef] [PubMed]

170. Lobo, D.N.; Gianotti, L.; Adiamah, A.; Barazzoni, R.; Deutz, N.E.P.; Dhatariya, K.; Greenhaff, P.L.; Hiesmayr, M.; Hjort Jakobsen, D.; Klek, S.; et al. Perioperative nutrition: Recommendations from the ESPEN Expert Group. *Clin. Nutr.* **2020**, in press. [CrossRef] [PubMed]

171. Weimann, A.; Braga, M.; Carli, F.; Higashiguchi, T.; Hübner, M.; Klek, S.; Laviano, A.; Ljungqvist, O.; Lobo, D.N.; Martindale, R.; et al. ESPEN guideline: Clinical nutrition in surgery. *Clin. Nutr.* **2017**, *36*, 623–650. [CrossRef]

172. Soeters, P.B.; Schols, A.M. Advances in understanding and assessing malnutrition. *Curr. Opin. Clin. Nutr. Metab. Care* **2009**, *12*, 487–494. [CrossRef]

173. Gillis, C.; Wischmeyer, P.E. Pre-operative nutrition and the elective surgical patient: Why, how and what? *Anaesthesia* **2019**, *74* (Suppl. 1), 27–35. [CrossRef] [PubMed]

174. Ljungqvist, O.; Scott, M.; Fearon, K.C. Enhanced recovery after surgery: A review. *JAMA Surg.* **2017**, *152*, 292–298. [CrossRef]

175. Marik, P.E.; Zaloga, G.P. Immunonutrition in high-risk surgical patients. *J. Parent Ent. Nutr.* **2010**, *34*, 378–386. [CrossRef]

176. Heyland, D.K.; Novak, F.; Drover, J.W.; Jain, M.; Su, X.; Suchner, U. Should immunonutrition become routine in critically ill patients? A systematic review of the evidence. *JAMA* **2001**, *286*, 944–953. [CrossRef]

177. Beale, R.J.; Bryg, D.J.; Bihari, D.J. Immunonutrition in the critically ill: A systematic review of clinical outcome. *Crit. Care Med.* **1999**, *27*, 2799–2805. [CrossRef] [PubMed]

178. Marimuthu, K.; Varadhan, K.K.; Ljungqvist, O.; Lobo, D.N. A meta-analysis of the effect of combinations of immune modulating nutrients on outcome in patients undergoing major open gastrointestinal surgery. *Ann. Surg.* **2012**, *255*, 1060–1068. [CrossRef] [PubMed]

179. Heys, S.D.; Walker, L.G.; Smith, I.; Eremin, O. Enteral nutritional supplementation with key nutrients in patients with critical illness and cancer: A meta-analysis of randomized controlled clinical trials. *Ann. Surg.* **1999**, *229*, 467–477. [CrossRef] [PubMed]

180. Montejo, J.C.; Zarazaga, A.; López-Martínez, J.; Urrútia, G.; Roqué, M.; Blesa, A.L.; Celaya, S.; Conejero, R.; Galbán, C.; García de Lorenzo, A.; et al. Immunonutrition in the intensive care unit. A systematic review and consensus statement. *Clin. Nutr.* **2003**, *22*, 221–233. [CrossRef]

181. Waitzberg, D.L.; Saito, H.; Plank, L.D.; Jamieson, G.G.; Jagannath, P.; Hwang, T.L.; Mijares, J.M.; Bihari, D. Postsurgical infections are reduced with specialized nutrition support. *World J. Surg.* **2006**, *30*, 1592–1604. [CrossRef] [PubMed]

182. Adiamah, A.; Skořepa, P.; Weimann, A.; Lobo, D.N. The impact of preoperative immune modulating nutrition on outcomes in patients undergoing surgery for gastrointestinal cancer: A systematic review and meta-analysis. *Ann. Surg.* **2019**, *270*, 247–256. [CrossRef]

183. Osland, E.; Hossain, M.B.; Khan, S.; Memon, M.A. Effect of timing of pharmaconutrition (immunonutrition) administration on outcomes of elective surgery for gastrointestinal malignancies. *J. Parent Ent. Nutr.* **2014**, *38*, 53–69. [CrossRef]

184. McClave, S.A.; Kozar, R.; Martindale, R.G.; Heyland, D.K.; Braga, M.; Carli, F.; Drover, J.W.; Flum, D.; Gramlich, L.; Herndon, D.N.; et al. Summary points and consensus recommendations from the North American Surgical Nutrition Summit. *J. Parenter. Enter. Nutr.* **2013**, *37* (Suppl. 5), 99s–105s. [CrossRef]

185. Benoist, S.; Brouquet, A. Nutritional assessment and screening for malnutrition. *J. Visc. Surg.* **2015**, *152* (Suppl. 1), S3–S7. [CrossRef]

186. Gillis, C.; Carli, F. Promoting perioperative metabolic and nutritional care. *Anesthesiology* **2015**, *123*, 1455–1472. [CrossRef]

187. Fearon, K.C.; Jenkins, J.T.; Carli, F.; Lassen, K. Patient optimization for gastrointestinal cancer surgery. *Brit. J. Surg.* **2013**, *100*, 15–27. [CrossRef] [PubMed]

188. Moya, P.; Soriano-Irigaray, L.; Ramirez, J.M.; Garcea, A.; Blasco, O.; Blanco, F.J.; Brugiotti, C.; Miranda, E.; Arroyo, A. Perioperative standard oral nutrition supplements versus immunonutrition in patients undergoing colorectal resection in an enhanced recovery (ERAS) protocol: A multicenter randomized clinical trial (SONVI Study). *Medicine* **2016**, *95*, e3704. [CrossRef] [PubMed]

189. Williams, J.D.; Wischmeyer, P.E. Assessment of perioperative nutrition practices and attitudes: A national survey of colorectal and GI surgical oncology programs. *Am. J. Surg.* **2017**, *213*, 1010–1018. [CrossRef] [PubMed]

190. Singer, M.; Deutschman, C.S.; Seymour, C.W.; Shankar-Hari, M.; Annane, D.; Bauer, M.; Bellomo, R.; Bernard, G.R.; Chiche, J.D.; Coopersmith, C.M.; et al. The third international consensus definitions for sepsis and septic shock (Sepsis-3). *JAMA* **2016**, *315*, 801–810. [CrossRef]

191. Chousterman, B.G.; Swirski, F.K.; Weber, G.F. Cytokine storm and sepsis disease pathogenesis. *Semin. Immunopathol.* **2017**, *39*, 517–528. [CrossRef] [PubMed]

192. De Waele, E.; Malbrain, M.L.N.G.; Spapen, H. Nutrition in sepsis: A bench-to-bedside review. *Nutrients* **2020**, *12*, 395. [CrossRef]

193. Cecconi, M.; Evans, L.; Levy, M.; Rhodes, A. Sepsis and septic shock. *Lancet* **2018**, *392*, 75–87. [CrossRef]

194. Wolbrink, D.R.J.; Grundsell, J.R.; Witteman, B.; Poll, M.V.; Santvoort, H.C.V.; Issa, E.; Dennison, A.; Goor, H.V.; Besselink, M.G.; Bouwense, S.A.W.; Dutch Pancreatitis Study Group. Are omega-3 fatty acids safe and effective in acute pancreatitis or sepsis? A systematic review and meta-analysis. *Clin. Nutr.* **2020**, in press.

195. Villar, J.; Zhang, H.; Slutsky, A.S. Lung repair and regeneration in ARDS: Role of PECAM1 and Wnt signaling. *Chest* **2019**, *155*, 587–594. [CrossRef]

196. Channappanavar, R.; Perlman, S. Pathogenic human coronavirus infections: Causes and consequences of cytokine storm and immunopathology. *Semin. Immunopathol.* **2017**, *39*, 529–539. [CrossRef]

197. Wang, H.; Ma, S. The cytokine storm and factors determining the sequence and severity of organ dysfunction in multiple organ dysfunction syndrome. *Am. J. Emerg. Med.* **2008**, *26*, 711–715. [CrossRef] [PubMed]

198. Gadek, J.E.; DeMichele, S.J.; Karlstad, M.D.; Pacht, E.R.; Donahoe, M.; Albertson, T.E.; Van Hoozen, C.; Wennberg, A.K.; Nelson, J.L.; Noursalehi, M. Effect of enteral feeding with eicosapentaenoic acid, gamma-linolenic acid, and antioxidants in patients with acute respiratory distress syndrome. Enteral Nutrition in ARDS Study Group. *Crit. Care Med.* **1999**, *27*, 1409–1420. [CrossRef] [PubMed]

199. Pontes-Arruda, A.; Aragao, A.M.; Albuquerque, J.D. Effects of enteral feeding with eicosapentaenoic acid, gamma-linolenic acid, and antioxidants in mechanically ventilated patients with severe sepsis and septic shock. *Crit. Care Med.* **2006**, *34*, 2325–2333. [CrossRef]

200. Pontes-Arruda, A.; Demichele, S.; Seth, A.; Singer, P. The use of an inflammation-modulating diet in patients with acute lung injury or acute respiratory distress syndrome: A meta-analysis of outcome data. *J. Parenter. Enter. Nutr.* **2008**, *32*, 596–605. [CrossRef] [PubMed]

201. Singer, P.; Theilla, M.; Fisher, H.; Gibstein, L.; Grozovski, E.; Cohen, J. Benefit of an enteral diet enriched with eicosapentaenoic acid and gamma-linolenic acid in ventilated patients with acute lung injury. *Crit. Care Med.* **2006**, *34*, 1033–1038. [CrossRef] [PubMed]

202. Grau-Carmona, T.; Morán-García, V.; García-de-Lorenzo, A.; Heras-de-la-Calle, G.; Quesada-Bellver, B.; López-Martínez, J.; González-Fernández, C.; Montejo-González, J.C.; Blesa-Malpica, A.; Albert-Bonamusa, I.; et al. Effect of an enteral diet enriched with eicosapentaenoic acid, gamma-linolenic acid and anti-oxidants on the outcome of mechanically ventilated, critically ill, septic patients. *Clin. Nutr.* **2011**, *30*, 578–584. [CrossRef]

203. Santacruz, C.A.; Orbegozo, D.; Vincent, J.L.; Preiser, J.C. Modulation of dietary lipid composition during acute respiratory distress syndrome: Systematic review and meta-analysis. *J. Parenter. Enter. Nutr.* **2015**, *39*, 837–846. [CrossRef]

204. Li, C.; Bo, L.; Liu, W.; Lu, X.; Jin, F. Enteral immunomodulatory diet (omega-3 fatty acid, γ-linolenic acid and antioxidant supplementation) for acute lung injury and acute respiratory distress syndrome: An updated systematic review and meta-analysis. *Nutrients* **2015**, *7*, 5572–5585. [CrossRef]

205. García de Acilu, M.; Leal, S.; Caralt, B.; Roca, O.; Sabater, J.; Masclans, J.R. The role of omega-3 polyunsaturated fatty acids in the treatment of patients with acute respiratory distress syndrome: A clinical review. *BioMed Res. Int.* **2015**, *2015*, 653750. [CrossRef]

206. Rice, T.W.; Wheeler, A.P.; Thompson, B.T.; deBoisblanc, B.P.; Steingrub, J.; Rock, P.; NIH NHLBI Acute Respiratory Distress Syndrome Network of Investigators. Enteral omega-3 fatty acid, gamma-linolenic acid, and antioxidant supplementation in acute lung injury. *JAMA* **2011**, *306*, 1574–1581. [CrossRef]

207. Kagan, I.; Cohen, J.; Stein, M.; Bendavid, I.; Pinsker, D.; Silva, V.; Theilla, M.; Anbar, R.; Lev, S.; Grinev, M.; et al. Preemptive enteral nutrition enriched with eicosapentaenoic acid, gamma-linolenic acid and antioxidants in severe multiple trauma: A prospective, randomized, double-blind study. *Intens. Care Med.* **2015**, *41*, 460–469. [CrossRef] [PubMed]

208. McClave, S.A.; Taylor, B.E.; Martindale, R.G.; Warren, M.M.; Johnson, D.R.; Braunschweig, C.; McCarthy, M.S.; Davanos, E.; Rice, T.W.; Cresci, G.A.; et al. Guidelines for the provision and assessment of nutrition support therapy in the adult critically ill patient: Society of Critical Care Medicine (SCCM) and American Society for Parenteral and Enteral Nutrition (A.S.P.E.N.). *J. Parenter. Enter. Nutr.* **2016**, *40*, 159–211. [CrossRef] [PubMed]

209. Critical Care Nutrition. Canadian Clinical Practice Guidelines: Composition of Enteral Nutrition: Fish Oils, Borage Oils and Antioxidants. 2015. Available online: https://www.criticalcarenutrition.com/docs/CPGs% 202015/Summary%20CPGs%202015%20vs%202013.pdf (accessed on 22 August 2019).

210. Zhu, D.; Zhang, Y.; Li, S.; Gan, L.; Feng, H.; Nie, W. Enteral omega-3 fatty acid supplementation in adult patients with acute respiratory distress syndrome: A systematic review of randomized controlled trials with meta-analysis and trial sequential analysis. *Intens. Care Med.* **2014**, *40*, 504–512. [CrossRef]

211. Glenn, J.O.H.; Wischmeyer, P.E. Enteral fish oil in critical illness: Perspectives and systematic review. *Curr. Opin. Clin. Nutr. Metab. Care* **2014**, *17*, 116–123. [CrossRef] [PubMed]

212. Dushianthan, A.; Cusack, R.; Burgess, V.A.; Grocott, M.P.; Calder, P.C. Immunonutrition for acute respiratory distress syndrome (ARDS) in adults. *Cochrane Database Syst. Rev.* **2019**, *1*, D012041. [CrossRef]

213. Torrinhas, R.S.; Calder, P.C.; Lemos, G.O.; Waitzberg, D.L. Parenteral fish oil: An adjuvant pharmacotherapy for coronavirus disease 2019? *Nutrition* **2020**, *81*, 110900. [CrossRef]

214. Bistrian, B.R. Parenteral fish-oil emulsions in critically ill COVID-19 emulsions. *J. Parenter. Enter. Nutr.* **2020**, in press. [CrossRef]

215. Martindale, R.G.; Berlana, D.; Boullata, J.I.; Cai, W.; Calder, P.C.; Deshpande, G.H.; Evans, D.; Garcia-de-Lorenzo, A.; Goulet, O.J.; Li, A.; et al. Summary of Proceedings and Expert Consensus Statements from the International Summit "Lipids in Parenteral Nutrition". *J. Parenter. Enter. Nutr.* **2020**, *44* (Suppl. 1), S7–S20. [CrossRef]

216. Mayer, K.; Klek, S.; García-de-Lorenzo, A.; Rosenthal, M.D.; Li, A.; Evans, D.C.; Muscaritoli, M.; Martindale, R.G. Lipid use in hospitalized adults requiring parenteral nutrition. *J. Parenter. Enter. Nutr.* **2020**, *44* (Suppl. 1), S28–S38. [CrossRef]

217. Elke, G.; Hartl, W.H.; Kreymann, K.G.; Adolph, M.; Felbinger, T.W.; Graf, T.; de Heer, G.; Heller, A.R.; Kampa, U.; Mayer, K.; et al. Clinical Nutrition in Critical Care Medicine—Guideline of the German Society for Nutritional Medicine (DGEM). *Clin. Nutr. ESPEN* **2019**, *33*, 220–275. [CrossRef]

218. Singer, P.; Blaser, A.R.; Berger, M.M.; Alhazzani, W.; Calder, P.C.; Casaer, M.P.; Hiesmayr, M.; Mayer, K.; Montejo, J.C.; Pichard, C.; et al. ESPEN guideline on clinical nutrition in the intensive care unit. *Clin. Nutr.* **2019**, *38*, 48–79. [CrossRef] [PubMed]

219. Pradelli, L.; Mayer, K.; Klek, S.; Omar Alsaleh, A.J.; Clark, R.A.C.; Rosenthal, M.D.; Heller, A.R.; Muscaritoli, M. ω-3 Fatty-acid enriched parenteral nutrition in hospitalized patients: Systematic review with meta-analysis and trial sequential analysis. *J. Parenter. Enter. Nutr.* **2020**, *44*, 44–57. [CrossRef] [PubMed]

220. Pradelli, L.; Muscaritoli, M.; Klek, S.; Martindale, R.G. Pharmacoeconomics of parenteral nutrition with ω-3 fatty acids in hospitalized adults. *J. Parenter. Enter. Nutr.* **2020**, *44* (Suppl. 1), S68–S73. [CrossRef] [PubMed]

221. Chen, L.; Deng, H.; Cui, H.; Fang, J.; Zuo, Z.; Deng, J.; Li, Y.; Wang, X.; Zhao, L. Inflammatory responses and inflammation-associated diseases in organs. *Oncotarget* **2017**, *9*, 7204–7218. [CrossRef] [PubMed]

222. Grimble, R.F.; Howell, W.M.; O'Reilly, G.; Turner, S.J.; Markovic, O.; Hirrell, S.; East, J.M.; Calder, P.C. The ability of fish oil to suppress tumor necrosis factor alpha production by peripheral blood mononuclear cells in healthy men is associated with polymorphisms in genes that influence tumor necrosis factor alpha production. *Am. J. Clin. Nutr.* **2002**, *76*, 454–459. [CrossRef]

3

Increased Omega-3 Fatty Acid Intake is Inversely Associated with Sarcopenic Obesity in Women but not in Men, Based on the 2014–2018 Korean National Health and Nutrition Examination Survey

Woojung Yang [1], Jae-woo Lee [1], Yonghwan Kim [1], Jong Hun Lee [2] and Hee-Taik Kang [1,3,*]

[1] Department of Family Medicine, Chungbuk National University Hospital, Cheongju 28644, Korea; kineto@naver.com (W.Y.); shrimp0611@gmail.com (J.-w.L.); airsantajin@gmail.com (Y.K.)
[2] Department of Food Science and Biotechnology, Gachon University, Seongnam 13120, Korea; foodguy@gachon.ac.kr
[3] Department of Family Medicine, Chungbuk National University College of Medicine, Cheongju 28644, Korea
* Correspondence: kanght0818@gmail.com

Abstract: (1) Background: Omega-3 fatty acids (ω3FAs) are known to improve protein anabolism, increase the sensitivity to anabolic stimuli, decrease lipogenesis, and stimulate lipid oxidation. We aim to investigate whether ω3FAs are associated with the prevalence of sarcopenic obesity (SO). (2) Methods: Data were obtained from the 2014–2018 Korean National Health and Nutrition Examination Survey. The ratio of daily ω3FA intake to energy intake (ω3FA ratio) was categorized into four quartile groups. (3) Results: The prevalence of SO from Q1 to Q4 was 8.9%, 11.3%, 11.0%, and 9.8% respectively, in men and 17.4%, 14.0%, 13.9%, and 10.1% respectively, in women. The ω3FA ratio in individuals with and without SO were 1.0% and 0.9% in men (p-value = 0.271) respectively, and 0.8% and 1.0% in women (p-value = 0.017), respectively. Compared with Q1, odds ratios (95% confidence intervals) of Q2, Q3, and Q4 of ω3FA ratios were 1.563 (0.802–3.047), 1.246 (0.611–2.542), and 0.924 (0.458–1.864) respectively, in men and 0.663 (0.379–1.160), 0.640 (0.372–1.102), and 0.246 (0.113–0.534) respectively, in women, after fully adjusting for confounding factors. (4) Conclusions: The ω3FA ratio was significantly higher in older females without SO than in older females with SO. The ω3FA ratio was associated with the prevalence of SO in elderly females.

Keywords: omega-3 fatty acids; sarcopenic obesity; omega-3 fatty acid ratio; sarcopenia

1. Introduction

The greatest epidemiological trend in Korea in the 21st century is the unprecedented growth of the rapidly aging population. In general, aging leads to a progressive decrease in muscle mass (sarcopenia) and an increase in fat mass (obesity) [1]. Korea, with the most rapidly aging population in the world, may confront a massive increase in the prevalence of sarcopenic obesity (SO). Sarcopenia and obesity in the elderly are frequently related to physical disability and visceral fat accumulation, displaying a synergistic interaction that can lead to a vicious cycle [2,3]. As a result, concurrent sarcopenia and obesity in elderly people increase all-cause mortality and lead to worse health outcomes than sarcopenia or obesity alone [4].

Omega-3 fatty acids (ω3FAs) are known to improve net muscle protein anabolism by activating the mammalian target of rapamycin/ribosomal protein kinase S6 (mTORp/70s6k) signaling pathway [5,6]. This signaling pathway increases the sensitivity of responses to anabolic stimuli such as enhanced protein intake, resistance exercise, and insulin [5,6]. On the other hand, ω3FAs are also found to downregulate lipogenesis by inhibiting differentiation of adipocytes by competing with prostacyclin (PGI2) in downstream [7,8] and to stimulate basal lipid oxidation by increasing the activity of peroxisomal acyl-CoA oxidase [9,10].

In some recent studies, dietary supplementation with ω3FAs has been shown to significantly decrease muscle mass loss and obesity [5,6]. Furthermore, it is noteworthy that adequate protein intake above the recommended daily intake (RDI) alone cannot guarantee prevention of sarcopenia [11–13]. These previous studies, however, have some limitations in that they have been implemented only in animals and in small sample sizes of people.

Therefore, the purpose of this study is to evaluate whether the ratio of daily ω3FA consumption to daily energy intake is associated with the prevalence of SO in elderly people in Korea based on the 2014–2018 Korean National Health and Nutrition Examination Survey (KNHANES).

2. Materials and Methods

2.1. Study Population

As a nationwide representative cross-sectional survey, the KNHANES has been administered to assess the health and nutritional status of Koreans residing in Korea by the Korea Centers for Disease Control and Prevention (KCDC) since 1998, following the National Health Promotion Act. The KNHANES collects data by staged, stratified, clustered, and systematic probability sampling based on sex, age, and geographic area using household registries to represent the entire Korean population living in Korea. To date, the KNHANES has been performed in seven phases including KNHANES phases I (1998), II (2001), III (2005), IV (2007–2009), V (2010–2012), VI (2013–2015), and VII (2016–2018). Among the phases of data, we selected data from 2018 (which is the latest data) to provide timely health statistics results. However, the range of selected data was expanded to 2014 to compensate for the decreased statistical power by exclusion criteria according to the definition of sarcopenia.

To gather information such as health status, health behavior, socioeconomic demographics, laboratory test results, and nutritional status of respondents, the survey consists of three components including a health interview, a health examination, and a nutrition survey among respondents. Health interviews and health examinations are conducted by trained personnel at mobile examination centers, while nutrition surveys are conducted by dietician visits to the homes of participants [14,15].

Individuals aged 60 years or older were included in our analysis from 2014 to 2018 [2,16]. Participants who have any cancers according to the definition of sarcopenia were excluded [16]. We also excluded participants with daily protein intakes under the Recommended Daily Allowance (RDA) for Korean elderly adults (0.91 g/kg/day) to evaluate the proper effects of ω3FAs on aging-related muscle loss [17]. In the final analysis, a total of 3815 participants (1960 men and 1855 women) were included and analyzed. Approval from an institutional review board (IRB) was not required because the survey did not deal with any sensitive information, only publicly available information. Data from the KNHANES are available for free on the KNHANES website (http://knhanes.cdc.go.kr) for academic research.

2.2. Definitions of Sarcopenic Obesity, Handgrip Strength, Obesity, and ω3FA Ratio

Sarcopenic obesity (SO) is a combination of low muscle mass (sarcopenia) and obesity [18]. Sarcopenia is an aging-related loss of muscle mass or decrease in muscular function without other comorbidities such as malignancies [16,19]. Because data regarding muscle mass were not available in the 2014–2018 KNHANES, we used decreased muscular function instead of muscle mass loss to diagnose sarcopenia [16,19,20]. To assess muscular function, the handgrip strength test was utilized.

Handgrip strength was measured using a digital grip dynamometer (T.K.K.5401; Takei Scientific Instruments Co., Ltd., Niigata, Japan) and defined as the maximally measured grip strength out of three tries with the dominant hand of participants [21]. Differences in handgrip strength among races have been reported in previous studies. For instance, the mean handgrip strength of Asian subjects was significantly different from that of Caucasian subjects [22]. Based on this, the Asian Working Group for Sarcopenia (AWGS) recommends using the lower 20th percentile of handgrip strength of each country's health population as the cut-off value to identify low muscle strength for diagnosis of sarcopenia instead of adopting the European-based Europe Working Group on Sarcopenia in Older People 2 (EWGSOP2) cut-off points [16]. To date, there are no standard and nationally representative handgrip strength cut-off values for sarcopenia in Korea, although those based on single-year KNHANES data have been suggested [19]. Therefore, rather than referring to one of the existing values, we determined the cut-off point for sarcopenia in Korean subjects by analyzing the latest five years of KNHANES data in person according to AWGS recommendations to enhance the reliability of our study. The cut-off value of handgrip strength for a sarcopenia diagnosis was the lowest 20th percentile of handgrip strength of people without other comorbidities such as malignancies [16,19], aged from 19 to 80 years, in both sexes (34.5 kg in men and 20.0 kg in women) [19].

Body mass index (BMI) was calculated as body weight (kg) divided by squared height (m^2). Obesity based on BMI was defined as equal to or above 25 kg/m^2 [23].

The ratio of daily ω3FA intake to energy intake was categorized into four quartile groups: Q1, <0.4 (both sexes), Q2, 0.4–<0.7 (both sexes), Q3, 0.7–<1.1 (men), 0.7–<1.2 (women), and Q4, ≥1.1 (men), ≥1.2 (women). Hereinafter, we will refer to the ratio of daily ω3FA intake to energy intake as the ω3FA ratio.

2.3. Definitions of Other Variables

Individuals who engaged in moderate physical activity over 150 min per week or who engaged in vigorous physical activity over 75 min per week comprised the group defined as having sufficient physical activity. Men who drank more than seven alcoholic beverages and women who drank more than five alcoholic beverages more than twice a week were categorized as heavy alcohol drinkers [24]. Occupational status was classified into three groups, including (1) manual workers (clerks, service and sales workers, skilled agricultural, forestry, and fishery workers, persons who operate or assemble crafts, equipment, or machines, and elementary workers), (2) office workers (general managers, government administrators, professionals, and simple office workers), and (3) others (unemployed persons, housekeepers, and students). Educational status was divided into four groups as follows: <6 years, 6–<9 years, 9–<12 years, and ≥12 years of education. Marital status was categorized into two groups of (1) married and not separated (individuals who were married and living together with their spouse without separation) and (2) single (individuals who were unmarried, separated, divorced, or widowed). Blood pressure (BP) was measured three times in subjects by a standard mercury sphygmomanometer (Baumanometer; Baum Co., Inc., Copiague, NY, USA) and a mean value of the last two measurements was used as the final BP of subjects. Total cholesterol, glucose, and aspartate transaminase (AST) levels were measured by an enzymatic method, hexokinase ultraviolet, and International Federation of Clinical Chemistry (IFCC) techniques without pyridoxal-5-phosphate (P5P), respectively (Hitachi 7600 Automatic Analyzer, Hitachi, Ltd., Tokyo, Japan). High-sensitivity C-reactive protein (hsCRP) values were measured by immunoturbidimetry (Cobas analyzer; F. Hoffmann-La Roche Ltd., Basel, Switzerland).

2.4. Statistical Analysis

All data on continuous variables are presented as means ± standard errors (SEs). Data on categorical variables are presented as percentages ± SEs. All sampling and weight variables were stratified by sex. Statistical software SAS version 9.4 (SAS Institute Inc., Cary, NC, USA) was used for statistical analysis. This was to account for the intricate sampling design and to provide nationally representative prevalence estimates. Survey regressions and chi-squared (χ2) tests were used to compare sexes and quartiles of ω3FA ratios. p-values were calculated by multiple logistic regression analyses with weighting of the survey design (adjusted with age, body mass index (BMI), total cholesterol, systolic BP, fasting plasma glucose, AST, hsCRP, smoking status, alcohol intake, economic status, marital status, education duration, occupation, physical activity, history of diabetes mellitus, history of hypertension, and protein intake). We also estimated adjusted odds ratios (ORs) and 95% confidence intervals (CIs) by multivariate logistic regression models to investigate factors associated with the sarcopenic obesity group according to the ω3FA ratio. All statistical tests were two-tailed, and statistical significance was considered at p-values < 0.05.

3. Results

Table 1 presents population characteristics according to sex. The mean ages of men and women were 68.8 and 68.5 years, respectively. Male and female daily energy intakes were 2423.1 and 2013.3 kilocalories (kcal), respectively. Men consumed more macronutrients (carbohydrates, proteins, and fats) than women (all p-values < 0.001). However, in terms of the ω3FA ratio, the same amount was consumed (0.9%) in both sexes (p-value = 0.254).

Table 1. Population characteristics according to sex.

Characteristic	Males	Females	p-Value
Number	1960	1855	
Age, years	68.8 ± 0.2	68.5 ± 0.2	0.159
BMI, Kg/m^2	23.5 ± 0.1	23.6 ± 0.1	0.173
Energy intake, Kcal/day	2423.1 ± 18.8	2013.3 ± 17.0	<0.001
Carbohydrate intake, g/day	381.6 ± 3.4	339.0 ± 3.4	<0.001
Protein intake, g/day	88.3 ± 0.8	73.1 ± 0.6	<0.001
Fat intake, g/day	44.6 ± 0.8	38.1 ± 0.6	<0.001
Daily omega-3/energy intake, %	0.9 ± 0.0	0.9 ± 0.0	0.254
Total cholesterol, mg/dL	182.4 ± 1.0	194.6 ± 1.1	<0.001
Systolic blood pressure, mmHg	125.0 ± 0.4	127.3 ± 0.6	<0.001
Fasting plasma glucose, mg/dL	108.6 ± 0.7	104.1 ± 0.7	<0.001
AST, IU/L	24.6 ± 0.3	23.0 ± 0.2	<0.001
hsCRP, mg/L	1.5 ± 0.1	1.3 ± 0.1	0.082
Current smoking, %	21.7 ± 1.0	2.4 ± 0.4	<0.001
Heavy alcohol intake, %	12.9 ± 0.9	1.8 ± 0.3	<0.001
Economic status, %			0.006
Low	26.6 ± 1.2	31.9 ± 1.3	
Middle–low	29.2 ± 1.2	27.8 ± 1.3	
Middle–high	23.7 ± 1.0	20.8 ± 1.1	
High	20.5 ± 1.1	19.6 ± 1.3	
Marital status, %			<0.001
Married and not separated	90.9 ± 0.7	62.2 ± 1.4	
Single	9.1 ± 0.7	37.8 ± 1.4	
Education duration, %			<0.001
<6 years	30.8 ± 1.3	52.9 ± 1.5	
6–<9 years	17.8 ± 1.1	16.8 ± 1.0	
9–<12 years	29.2 ± 1.3	18.6 ± 1.1	
≥12 years	22.2 ± 1.2	11.6 ± 1.0	
Occupation, %			<0.001
Office workers	11.4 ± 0.9	4.0 ± 0.6	
Manual workers	40.9 ± 1.4	30.5 ± 1.3	
Other	47.7 ± 1.4	65.5 ± 1.3	
Sufficient physical activity, %	46.5 ± 1.4	36.8 ± 1.4	<0.001
History of diabetes mellitus, %	17.0 ± 1.0	13.0 ± 0.9	0.002
History of hypertension, %	42.1 ± 1.3	41.5 ± 1.4	0.782

All data are presented as mean ± standard errors (SEs) or percentage ± SEs. Abbreviations: BMI, body mass index; AST, aspartate transaminase; IU/L, international units per liter; hsCRP, high-sensitivity C-reactive protein.

Table 2 shows participants' characteristics according to ω3FA ratio quartile. In men, mean age was not significantly different among the four quartile groups, while daily energy intake and hsCRP levels decreased with increasing quartiles of ω3FA ratio. Daily protein intake positively correlated with ω3FA ratio quartile. In women, individuals in higher quartiles of ω3FA ratio were younger. Daily energy intake decreased with ω3FA ratio quartiles, while protein intake increased. Among the four groups, hsCRP levels were not different.

Table 2. Population characteristics according to quartiles of ω3FA ratio.

Males	Q1	Q2	Q3	Q4	p-Value
	(<0.4)	(0.4–<0.7)	(0.7–<1.1)	(≥1.1)	
Number	517	483	485	475	
Age, years	68.8 ± 0.3	69.4 ± 0.3	68.3 ± 0.3	68.8 ± 0.3	0.087
BMI, Kg/m^2	23.3 ± 0.1	23.3 ± 0.1	23.7 ± 0.1	23.6 ± 0.1	0.061
Energy intake, Kcal/day	2495.8 ± 36.6	2458.4 ± 36.8	2360.2 ± 32.6	2378.4 ± 39.8	0.024
Carbohydrate intake, g/day	403.0 ± 7.3	401.7 ± 6.3	366.2 ± 5.3	355.7 ± 5.9	<0.001
Protein intake, g/day	82.7 ± 1.3	86.5 ± 1.4	88.6 ± 1.3	95.5 ± 1.9	<0.001
Fat intake, g/day	38.6 ± 1.3	42.6 ± 1.4	43.8 ± 1.3	53.2 ± 1.7	<0.001
Daily omega-3/energy intake, %	0.3 ± 0.0	0.5 ± 0.0	0.9 ± 0.0	2.0 ± 0.1	<0.001
Total cholesterol, mg/dL	185.4 ± 1.9	181.8 ± 1.8	183.0 ± 2.1	179.3 ± 2.1	0.223
Systolic blood pressure, mmHg	126.8 ± 0.8	126.2 ± 0.8	123.4 ± 0.7	123.7 ± 0.9	0.002
Fasting plasma glucose, mg/dL	111.1 ± 1.5	106.7 ± 1.3	109.1 ± 1.5	107.6 ± 1.3	0.170
AST, IU/L	25.7 ± 0.7	24.2 ± 0.4	24.3 ± 0.4	24.2 ± 0.5	0.283
hsCRP, mg/L	1.8 ± 0.2	1.5 ± 0.2	1.6 ± 0.1	1.2 ± 0.1	0.013
Current smoking, %	26.3 ± 2.3	20.0 ± 2.0	21.5 ± 2.2	19.2 ± 2.1	0.113
Heavy alcohol intake, %	16.3 ± 1.8	12.0 ± 1.6	13.0 ± 1.8	10.4 ± 1.6	0.082
Economic status, %					0.037
Low	32.2 ± 2.4	26.1 ± 2.4	22.1 ± 2.1	25.9 ± 2.3	
Middle–low	29.4 ± 2.2	29.0 ± 2.4	28.9 ± 2.4	29.4 ± 2.4	
Middle–high	19.5 ± 2.0	22.4 ± 2.1	27.2 ± 2.2	25.8 ± 2.1	
High	18.9 ± 2.1	22.5 ± 2.4	21.8 ± 2.2	18.9 ± 1.9	
Marital status, %					0.038
Married and not separated	87.7 ± 1.6	90.9 ± 1.5	93.4 ± 1.2	91.5 ± 1.5	
Single	12.3 ± 1.6	9.1 ± 1.5	6.6 ± 1.2	8.5 ± 1.5	
Education duration, %					<0.001
<6 years	39.7 ± 2.4	29.5 ± 2.3	28.7 ± 2.3	25.1 ± 2.4	
6–<9 years	17.8 ± 1.9	18.1 ± 2.0	17.3 ± 2.1	18.0 ± 2.2	
9–<12 years	25.2 ± 2.1	28.4 ± 2.4	32.3 ± 2.5	31.1 ± 2.6	
≥12 years	17.4 ± 2.1	24.0 ± 2.3	21.7 ± 2.1	25.7 ± 2.2	
Occupation, %					0.450
Office workers	10.7 ± 1.6	10.9 ± 1.7	12.7 ± 1.9	11.3 ± 1.6	
Manual workers	46.4 ± 2.6	41.3 ± 2.7	38.8 ± 2.6	37.1 ± 2.4	
Other	42.9 ± 2.6	47.7 ± 2.7	48.4 ± 2.7	51.6 ± 2.7	
Sufficient physical activity, %	44.7 ± 2.5	49.0 ± 2.8	47.3 ± 2.6	44.8 ± 2.6	0.633
History of diabetes mellitus, %	14.4 ± 1.7	15.9 ± 1.9	20.4 ± 2.2	17.3 ± 1.8	0.172
History of hypertension, %	41.8 ± 2.4	44.5 ± 2.6	39.2 ± 2.5	42.8 ± 2.7	0.523

All data are presented as mean ± SEs or percentage ± SEs. Abbreviations: ω3FA, omega-3 fatty acid; ω3FA ratio, ratio of daily omega-3 fatty acid intake to energy intake; BMI, body mass index; AST, aspartate transaminase; hsCRP, high-sensitivity C-reactive protein.

Table 2. *Cont.*

Females	Q1	Q2	Q3	Q4	*p*-Value
	(<0.4)	(0.4–<0.7)	(0.7–<1.2)	(≥1.2)	
Number	460	479	454	462	
Age, years	69.5 ± 0.4	68.9 ± 0.3	68.0 ± 0.4	67.6 ± 0.3	<0.001
BMI, Kg/m²	23.5 ± 0.2	23.7 ± 0.1	23.7 ± 0.1	23.7 ± 0.1	0.704
Energy intake, Kcal/day	2138.0 ± 40.5	1975.8 ± 30.0	1945.5 ± 31.7	1994.2 ± 34.4	0.002
Carbohydrate intake, g/day	388.5 ± 8.7	337.8 ± 5.8	317.4 ± 5.6	312.6 ± 6.7	<0.001
Protein intake, g/day	69.5 ± 1.5	69.4 ± 1.0	74.8 ± 1.3	78.7 ± 1.3	<0.001
Fat intake, g/day	30.1 ± 1.1	34.7 ± 1.1	40.3 ± 1.2	47.2 ± 1.4	<0.001
Daily omega-3/energy intake, %	0.3 ± 0.0	0.6 ± 0.0	0.9 ± 0.0	2.0 ± 0.1	<0.001
Total cholesterol, mg/dL	194.9 ± 2.1	195.1 ± 2.2	193.9 ± 2.0	194.4 ± 2.2	0.979
Systolic blood pressure, mmHg	129.2 ± 1.2	127.1 ± 0.8	126.1 ± 0.9	126.9 ± 1.1	0.211
Fasting plasma glucose, mg/dL	102.9 ± 1.3	106.4 ± 1.9	101.6 ± 1.1	105.5 ± 1.3	0.062
AST, IU/L	22.6 ± 0.4	23.2 ± 0.7	23.1 ± 0.4	23.1 ± 0.4	0.702
hsCRP, mg/L	1.3 ± 0.1	1.4 ± 0.2	1.4 ± 0.2	1.2 ± 0.1	0.863
Current smoking, %	4.0 ± 1.2	2.6 ± 0.9	1.2 ± 0.5	2.0 ± 0.9	0.129
Heavy alcohol intake, %	2.9 ± 0.9	1.9 ± 0.7	1.6 ± 0.7	0.8 ± 0.3	0.084
Economic status, %					<0.001
Low	36.1 ± 2.6	36.9 ± 2.5	24.6 ± 2.4	29.8 ± 2.3	
Middle–low	32.9 ± 2.5	25.9 ± 2.3	26.3 ± 2.2	26.0 ± 2.3	
Middle–high	17.7 ± 2.3	18.7 ± 2.0	26.1 ± 2.6	20.6 ± 2.2	
High	13.4 ± 2.1	18.4 ± 2.4	23.0 ± 2.2	23.7 ± 2.5	
Marital status, %					<0.001
Married and not separated	55.3 ± 2.7	56.7 ± 2.7	67.6 ± 2.6	69.2 ± 2.5	
Single	44.7 ± 2.7	43.3 ± 2.7	32.4 ± 2.6	30.8 ± 2.5	
Education duration, %					<0.001
<6 years	64.2 ± 3.1	55.0 ± 2.7	45.9 ± 2.6	47.2 ± 2.8	
6–<9 years	15.2 ± 2.1	16.3 ± 1.9	17.7 ± 1.9	17.9 ± 2.4	
9–<12 years	13.8 ± 2.3	18.8 ± 2.2	22.0 ± 2.3	19.5 ± 2.0	
≥12 years	6.8 ± 1.6	9.8 ± 1.5	14.3 ± 1.9	15.3 ± 1.8	
Occupation, %					0.782
Office workers	2.9 ± 1.1	2.9 ± 0.9	5.1 ± 1.2	4.9 ± 1.0	
Manual workers	31.8 ± 2.5	34.7 ± 2.3	26.3 ± 2.3	29.3 ± 2.2	
Other	65.4 ± 2.5	62.4 ± 2.4	68.5 ± 2.4	65.9 ± 2.3	
Sufficient physical activity, %	34.6 ± 2.7	35.5 ± 2.4	39.9 ± 2.7	36.9 ± 2.6	0.547
History of diabetes mellitus, %	13.0 ± 1.9	13.5 ± 1.9	10.5 ± 1.5	14.9 ± 1.7	0.327
History of hypertension, %	41.1 ± 2.6	41.3 ± 2.5	40.1 ± 2.6	43.6 ± 2.6	0.804

All data are presented as mean ± SEs or percentage ± SEs. Abbreviations: ω3FA, omega-3 fatty acid; ω3FA ratio, ratio of daily omega-3 fatty acid intake to energy intake; BMI, body mass index; AST, aspartate transaminase; hsCRP, high-sensitivity C-reactive protein.

Table 3 demonstrates fat intake according to the presence of sarcopenic obesity. Values of ω3FA ratio in women are the only significant difference between groups with sarcopenic obesity and non-sarcopenic obesity. The ω3FA ratio in individuals without sarcopenic obesity was significantly higher than in individuals with sarcopenic obesity (0.8% in sarcopenic obesity vs. 1.0% in non-sarcopenic obesity, *p*-value = 0.017).

Table 3. Ratio of daily total fat and fatty acids intake to energy intake according to the presence of sarcopenic obesity.

Ratio of Daily Total Fat and Fatty Acids Intake to Energy Intake (%)	Sarcopenic Obesity	Non-Sarcopenic Obesity	*p*-Value
Males			
Total fat	16.5 ± 0.6	16.3 ± 0.2	0.741
SFA	4.7 ± 0.2	4.7 ± 0.1	0.853
MUFA	5.0 ± 0.2	5.0 ± 0.1	0.922
PUFA	4.9 ± 0.2	4.6 ± 0.1	0.177
Omega-3 FA	1.0 ± 0.1	0.9 ± 0.0	0.271
Omega-6 FA	3.9 ± 0.2	3.7 ± 0.1	0.270
Females			
Total fat	16.8 ± 0.6	17.1 ± 0.2	0.633
SFA	4.9 ± 0.2	4.9 ± 0.1	0.879
MUFA	5.2 ± 0.2	5.2 ± 0.1	0.995
PUFA	4.6 ± 0.2	5.0 ± 0.1	0.121
Omega-3 FA	0.8 ± 0.0	1.0 ± 0.0	0.017
Omega-6 FA	3.8 ± 0.2	4.0 ± 0.1	0.334

All data are presented as mean (± standard errors). Abbreviations: SFA, saturated fatty acids; MUFA, monounsaturated fatty acids; PUFA, polyunsaturated fatty acids; FA, fatty acids.

Figure 1 presents the prevalence of sarcopenic obesity according to quartile of ω3FA ratio. There was no significant difference in sarcopenic obesity prevalence among male quartile groups, while the female prevalence was marginally different (*p*-value = 0.055). The lowest quartile of ω3FA ratio had the highest prevalence (17.4%) of sarcopenic obesity in women, while the highest quartile of ω3FA ratio showed the lowest (10.1%).

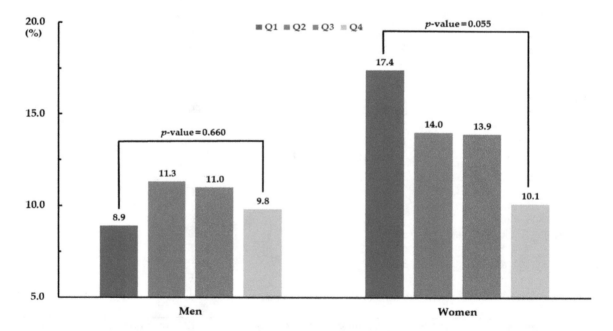

Figure 1. Prevalence of sarcopenic obesity according to quartile group of omega-3 fatty acid ratio.

Table 4 demonstrates logistic regression models according to ω3FA ratio quartile. Compared with Q1, ORs (95% CIs) for sarcopenic obesity of Q2, Q3, and Q4 of ω3FA ratio were 1.288 (0.776–2.138), 1.298 (0.804–2.097), and 1.118 (0.701–1.782) respectively, in men and 0.807 (0.534–1.221), 0.847 (0.552–1.299), and 0.603 (0.376–0.967) respectively, in women after adjusting for age. After full adjustment, ORs (95% CIs) of Q2, Q3, and Q4 of ω3FA ratio were 1.563 (0.802–3.047), 1.246 (0.611–2.542), and 0.924 (0.458–1.864) respectively, in men, and 0.663 (0.379–1.160), 0.640 (0.372–1.102), and 0.246 (0.113–0.534) respectively, in women.

Table 4. Adjusted odds ratios (ORs) and 95% confidence intervals (CIs) of sarcopenic obesity by quartiles of ω3FA ratio.

Males	Q1	Q2	Q3	Q4
	(<0.4)	(0.4–<0.7)	(0.7–<1.1)	(≥1.1)
Model 1	1 (ref)	1.288 (0.776–2.138)	1.298 (0.804–2.097)	1.118 (0.701–1.782)
Model 2	1 (ref)	1.668 (0.868–3.205)	1.160 (0.592–2.272)	1.000 (0.512–1.953)
Model 3	1 (ref)	1.563 (0.802–3.047)	1.246 (0.611–2.542)	0.924 (0.458–1.864)
Females	**Q1**	**Q2**	**Q3**	**Q4**
	(<0.4)	(0.4–<0.7)	(0.7–<1.2)	(≥1.2)
Model 1	1 (ref)	0.807 (0.534–1.221)	0.847 (0.552–1.299)	0.603 (0.376–0.967)
Model 2	1 (ref)	0.604 (0.355–1.028)	0.649 (0.394–1.072)	0.282 (0.129–0.617)
Model 3	1 (ref)	0.663 (0.379–1.160)	0.640 (0.372–1.102)	0.246 (0.113–0.534)

Odds ratios (ORs) and 95% confidence intervals (CIs) were calculated using weighted multivariate logistic regression analyses. Model 1: Adjusted for age. Model 2: Adjusted for age, BMI, total cholesterol, systolic blood pressure, fasting plasma glucose, AST, and hsCRP. Model 3: Adjusted for current smoking status, heavy alcohol intake, economic status, marital status, education duration, occupation, sufficient physical activity, history of diabetes mellitus, history of hypertension, and protein intake in addition to variables of Model 2. Abbreviation: ω3FA ratio, ratio of daily ω3FA intake to energy intake; AST, aspartate transaminase; hsCRP, high-sensitivity C-reactive protein.

4. Discussion

This study finds that the ω3FA ratio was significantly higher in women without SO than in women with SO. Logistic regression models demonstrate that the ω3FA ratio was inversely associated with the prevalence of SO in elderly females (but not in males), even after adjusting for confounding variables.

To date, resistance exercise and protein supplementation have been generally accepted as the most effective lifestyle changes to prevent sarcopenia [25,26]. Thus, the two are recommended for the prevention and management of sarcopenia [27,28]. However, resistance exercise and protein supplementation have not been shown to consistently lead to significantly positive results in all the research [28]. Anabolic resistance, which is a decreased response to anabolic stimuli such as physical exercise and ingested protein, arises in the protein metabolism of human bodies as people get older [29]. Thus, we have hypothesized that an additional approach for overcoming anabolic resistance would be necessary along with exercise and protein intake to prevent and treat sarcopenia in the elderly.

In the past, many researchers hypothesized that anti-inflammatory effects of ω3FAs were mainly related to observed prevention effects in sarcopenia such as cachexia in cancers or chronic diseases [30]. Today, overcoming age-related anabolic resistance is considered to be the main mechanism of ω3FAs in the prevention of sarcopenia [31]. On the molecular level, the mTORp/70s6k signaling pathway is considered an integral point of age-related anabolic resistance [6]. The mammalian target of rapamycin (mTOR) is a sensing effector of hormone and nutrient availability that controls two key translation initiation promoters, S6 kinase (S6K) and 4E binding protein (BP), of eukaryotic initiation factor eIF4E [5]. ω3FAs make this effector more sensitive to anabolic stimuli, and thus, promote cellular mRNA translation of proteins [5,31]. Prostaglandin I2 (prostacyclin, PGI2) triggers cyclic adenosine monophosphate (cAMP) production through prostacyclin receptors at the surface of preadipocytes. cAMP activates the protein kinase A pathway that promotes the differentiation of preadipocytes into adipocytes. ω3FAs inhibit the synthesis of PGI2 at the level of cyclooxygenases (COX) by competing with omega-6 fatty acids (ω6FAs), which are precursors of PGI2, and consequently inhibit lipogenesis [32,33].

ω3FAs are also found to increase the activity of peroxisomal and mitochondrial enzymes for β-oxidation of fatty acids. ω3FAs mainly induce gene expression of acyl-CoA oxidase, which is the key enzyme of fatty acids β-oxidation in peroxisomes [10]. Concurrently, ω3FAs elevate the activity of carnitine palmitoyltransferase II, which is a shuttle of fatty acids into mitochondria for further β-oxidation. Therefore, ω3FAs accelerate overall lipid oxidation in both peroxisomes and mitochondria [34].

As mentioned above, previous studies show that ω3FAs have the potential to prevent and treat SO. However, because most studies have explored the effects of ω3FAs either for sarcopenia [6] or obesity (but not for both [35]), previous studies alone cannot directly evaluate the beneficial effects of ω3FAs for SO. By directly investigating the association between ω3FA intake and the prevalence of SO, this study differentiates its clinical significance from previous studies to date.

A noteworthy point of our findings is that there is a significant association between ω3FA ratio and prevalence of SO in older women but not in men. Although the exact mechanism remains unknown, women might have more capacity for improvement with ω3FAs compared to men [36]. Unlike men, the muscle strength of women does not usually increase to its optimal level in response to resistance exercise; thereby, most women get greater muscle function reservoir to enhance with the intake of ω3FAs [37]. The innate biologically sexual differences in the pattern of muscle mass and strength changes with age may also explain these differences. Peak muscle mass and strength of women are lower than in men [38]. Furthermore, the muscle decline in women occurs earlier due to menopause and is steeper than in men, particularly after menopause [39]. Menopause is a major risk factor for sarcopenia and SO [40]. In the present study, only elderly individuals were included, indicating the possibility that most of the women were postmenopausal. Considering the differences in changes between men and women in the pattern of muscle mass and strength with aging, supplementation of muscle-preserving nutrients, including ω3FA, may show a greater preventive effect against SO in women than in men.

Comparing the intake of ω3FA to that in Western countries such as the US and European countries, Koreans are known to consume more ω3FA. We can compare this more reliably by measuring the blood level of eicosapentaenoic acid (EPA) and docosahexaenoic acid (DHA) than by the 24 h recall method because we can exclude the potential for reporting or recall bias [40,41]. The blood EPA and DHA levels in Koreans are more than twice those of US subjects and higher than most of those in European countries, except Scandinavia [42].

Several limitations should be considered in interpreting this study. First, we defined sarcopenia not directly by measuring muscle mass using body composition examination such as dual-energy X-ray absorptiometry, but indirectly, by measuring muscle function using a handgrip strength test. Because handgrip strength is a reliable predictor of clinical outcomes of low muscle mass, handgrip strength can be used as an indicator to diagnose sarcopenia [16,19]. Second, it is difficult to conclude causality from this study because it was cross-sectionally designed without any follow-up. Third, because we use the data of dietary ω3FA intake gathered by a 24 h recall method instead of actual measurements of ω3FAs in the red blood cell membrane or plasma of subjects, we cannot completely exclude the potential for reporting or recall bias from this study.

In spite of these limitations, this study has several strengths that distinguish our research from previous studies. First, this study is derived from a population-based sample from a complex survey design, seeking to produce estimates that accurately represent the Korean population. Second, to the best of our knowledge, this is the first Korean study to evaluate the association of ω3FA intake and ω3FA ratio with the prevalence of SO using nationally representative data. Third, to minimize confounding effects of several factors, especially protein levels, we analyzed the data not only by adjusting for variables such as daily protein intake but also by using the ω3FA ratio instead of measured amounts of ω3FAs. Fourth, the definition of sarcopenia was not quantitatively measured by muscle mass but instead was functionally evaluated using handgrip strength. To predict clinical outcomes in elderly people, muscular functionality such as handgrip strength is more important than the quantity of muscle mass [20,43].

5. Conclusions

In conclusion, this study shows that an increased ω3FA ratio-based intake is associated with a decreased prevalence of SO in elderly females. This means that interventions to increase dietary ω3FA ratio may help with the prevention and management of SO in elderly females. However, longitudinally designed cohort studies or interventional studies are further needed to confirm causality between the ω3FA ratio and the prevalence of SO and to determine whether a diet with an increased ω3FA ratio might be an effective strategy to prevent and manage SO in specific populations.

Author Contributions: Conceptualization, H.-T.K., J.-w.L., Y.K. and W.Y.; methodology, H.-T.K., J.-w.L., and W.Y.; statistical analysis, J.-w.L. and W.Y.; interpretation, H.-T.K., J.-w.L., Y.K., J.H.L., and W.Y.; writing—original draft preparation, H.-T.K., J.-w.L., Y.K., J.H.L., and W.Y.; funding acquisition, Y.K. All authors have read and agreed to the published version of the manuscript.

References

1. Saini, A.; Sharples, A.P.; Al-Shanti, N.; Stewart, C.E. Omega-3 fatty acid EPA improves regenerative capacity of mouse skeletal muscle cells exposed to saturated fat and inflammation. *Biogerontology* **2017**, *18*, 109–129. [CrossRef] [PubMed]

2. Kim, T.N.; Yang, S.J.; Yoo, H.J.; Lim, K.I.; Kang, H.J.; Song, W.; Seo, J.A.; Kim, S.G.; Kim, N.H.; Baik, S.H.; et al. Prevalence of sarcopenia and sarcopenic obesity in Korean adults: The Korean Sarcopenic Obesity Study (KSOS). *Nat. Précéd.* **2009**, *33*, 885–892. [CrossRef]

3. Riechman, S.E.; Schoen, R.E.; Weissfeld, J.L.; Thaete, F.L.; Hamman, R.F. Association of Physical Activity and Visceral Adipose Tissue in Older Women and Men. *Obes. Res.* **2002**, *10*, 1065–1073. [CrossRef]

4. Wannamethee, S.G.; Atkins, J.L. Muscle loss and obesity: The health implications of sarcopenia and sarcopenic obesity. In *Proceedings of the Nutrition Society*; Cambridge University Press (CUP): Cambridge, UK, 2015; Volume 74, pp. 405–412.

5. Gingras, A.-A.; White, P.J.; Chouinard, P.Y.; Julien, P.; Davis, T.A.; Dombrowski, L.; Couture, Y.; Dubreuil, P.; Myre, A.; Bergeron, K.; et al. Long-chain omega-3 fatty acids regulate bovine whole-body protein metabolism by promoting muscle insulin signalling to the Akt-mTOR-S6K1 pathway and insulin sensitivity. *J. Physiol.* **2007**, *579*, 269–284. [CrossRef] [PubMed]

6. Smith, G.I.; Atherton, P.; Reeds, D.N.; Mohammed, B.S.; Rankin, D.; Rennie, M.J.; Mittendorfer, B. Dietary omega-3 fatty acid supplementation increases the rate of muscle protein synthesis in older adults: A randomized controlled trial. *Am. J. Clin. Nutr.* **2011**, *93*, 402–412. [CrossRef] [PubMed]

7. Pisani, D.F.; Amri, E.-Z.; Ailhaud, G. Disequilibrium of polyunsaturated fatty acids status and its dual effect in modulating adipose tissue development and functions. *OCL* **2015**, *22*, D405. [CrossRef]

8. Simopoulos, A.P. An Increase in the Omega-6/Omega-3 Fatty Acid Ratio Increases the Risk for Obesity. *Nutrients* **2016**, *8*, 128. [CrossRef]

9. Baillie, R.; Takada, R.; Nakamura, M.; Clarke, S. Coordinate induction of peroxisomal acyl-CoA oxidase and UCP-3 by dietary fish oil: A mechanism for decreased body fat deposition. *Prostaglandins Leukot. Essent. Fat. Acids* **1999**, *60*, 351–356. [CrossRef]

10. Ukropec, J.; Reseland, J.E.; Gašperíková, D.; Demcáková, E.; Madsen, L.; Berge, R.K.; Rustan, A.C.; Klimes, I.; Drevon, C.A.; Sebokova, E. The hypotriglyceridemic effect of dietary n-3 FA is associated with increased β-oxidation and reduced leptin expression. *Lipids* **2003**, *38*, 1023–1029. [CrossRef]

11. Wolfe, R.R.; Miller, S.L. The Recommended Dietary Allowance of Protein: A misunderstood concept. *JAMA* **2008**, *299*, 2891–2893. [CrossRef]

12. Pepersack, T.; Corretge, M.; Beyer, I.; Namias, B.; Andre, S.; Benoit, F.; Mergam, A.; Simonetti, C. Examining the effect of intervention to nutritional problems of hospitalized elderly: A pilot project. *J. Nutr. Health Aging* **2002**, *6*, 306–310. [PubMed]

13. Houston, D.K.; Nicklas, B.J.; Ding, J.; Harris, T.B.; Tylavsky, F.A.; Newman, A.B.; Lee, J.S.; Sahyoun, N.R.; Visser, M.; Kritchevsky, S.B.; et al. Dietary protein intake is associated with lean mass change in older, community-dwelling adults: The Health, Aging, and Body Composition (Health ABC) Study. *Am. J. Clin. Nutr.* **2008**, *87*, 150–155. [CrossRef] [PubMed]

14. Kim, Y. The Korea National Health and Nutrition Examination Survey (KNHANES): Current Status and Challenges. *Epidemiol. Health* **2014**, *36*, e2014002. [CrossRef]

15. Kweon, S.; Kim, Y.; Jang, M.-J.; Kim, Y.; Kim, K.; Choi, S.; Chun, C.; Khang, Y.-H.; Oh, K. Data resource profile: The Korea National Health and Nutrition Examination Survey (KNHANES). *Int. J. Epidemiol.* **2014**, *43*, 69–77. [CrossRef] [PubMed]

16. Chen, L.-K.; Woo, J.; Assantachai, P.; Auyeung, T.-W.; Chou, M.-Y.; Iijima, K.; Jang, H.C.; Kang, L.; Kim, M.; Kim, S.; et al. Asian Working Group for Sarcopenia: 2019 Consensus Update on Sarcopenia Diagnosis and Treatment. *J. Am. Med. Dir. Assoc.* **2020**, *21*, 300–307.e2. [CrossRef] [PubMed]

17. Kwon, D.H.; Park, H.A.; Cho, Y.-G.; Kim, K.; Kim, N.H. Different Associations of Socioeconomic Status on Protein Intake in the Korean Elderly Population: A Cross-Sectional Analysis of the Korea National Health and Nutrition Examination Survey. *Nutrients* **2019**, *12*, 10. [CrossRef]

18. Lee, D.-C.; Shook, R.P.; Drenowatz, C.; Blair, S.N. Physical activity and sarcopenic obesity: Definition, assessment, prevalence and mechanism. *Futur. Sci. OA* **2016**, *2*, FSO127. [CrossRef] [PubMed]

19. Yoo, J.-I.; Choi, H.; Ha, Y.-C. Mean Hand Grip Strength and Cut-off Value for Sarcopenia in Korean Adults Using KNHANES VI. *J. Korean Med. Sci.* **2017**, *32*, 868–872. [CrossRef]

20. Cruz-Jentoft, A.J.; Baeyens, J.P.; Bauer, J.M.; Boirie, Y.; Cederholm, T.; Landi, F.; Martin, F.C.; Michel, J.-P.; Rolland, Y.; Schneider, S.M.; et al. Sarcopenia: European consensus on definition and diagnosis: Report of the European Working Group on Sarcopenia in Older People. *Age Ageing* **2010**, *39*, 412–423. [CrossRef]

21. Roberts, H.C.; Denison, H.J.; Martin, H.J.; Patel, H.P.; Syddall, H.; Cooper, C.; Sayer, A.A. A review of the measurement of grip strength in clinical and epidemiological studies: Towards a standardised approach. *Age Ageing* **2011**, *40*, 423–429. [CrossRef]

22. Chen, L.-K.; Liu, L.-K.; Woo, J.; Assantachai, P.; Auyeung, T.-W.; Bahyah, K.S.; Chou, M.-Y.; Hsu, P.-S.; Krairit, O.; Lee, J.S.; et al. Sarcopenia in Asia: Consensus Report of the Asian Working Group for Sarcopenia. *J. Am. Med. Dir. Assoc.* **2014**, *15*, 95–101. [CrossRef] [PubMed]

23. Paik, D.W.; Han, K.; Kang, S.W.; Ham, D.-I.; Kim, S.J.; Chung, T.-Y.; Lim, D.H. Differential effect of obesity on the incidence of retinal vein occlusion with and without diabetes: A Korean nationwide cohort study. *Sci. Rep.* **2020**, *10*, 1–9. [CrossRef] [PubMed]

24. World Health Organization. *International Guide for Monitoring Alcohol Consumption and Related Harm*; World Health Organization: Geneva, Switzerland, 2000.

25. Cruz-Jentoft, A.J.; Landi, F.; Schneider, S.M.; Zúñiga, C.; Arai, H.; Boirie, Y.; Chen, L.-K.; Fielding, R.A.; Martin, F.C.; Michel, J.-P.; et al. Prevalence of and interventions for sarcopenia in ageing adults: A systematic review. Report of the International Sarcopenia Initiative (EWGSOP and IWGS). *Age Ageing* **2014**, *43*, 748–759. [CrossRef] [PubMed]

26. Beaudart, C.; Rabenda, V.; Simmons, M.; Geerinck, A.; De Carvalho, I.A.; Reginster, J.-Y.; Thiyagarajan, J.A.; Bruyère, O. Effects of Protein, Essential Amino Acids, B-Hydroxy B-Methylbutyrate, Creatine, Dehydroepiandrosterone and Fatty Acid Supplementation on Muscle Mass, Muscle Strength and Physical Performance in Older People Aged 60 Years and Over. A Systematic Review of the Literature. *J. Nutr. Health Aging* **2018**, *22*, 117–130. [CrossRef] [PubMed]

27. Bauer, J.; Biolo, G.; Cederholm, T.; Cesari, M.; Cruz-Jentoft, A.J.; Morley, J.E.; Phillips, S.; Sieber, C.; Stehle, P.; Teta, D.; et al. Evidence-Based Recommendations for Optimal Dietary Protein Intake in Older People: A Position Paper From the PROT-AGE Study Group. *J. Am. Med. Dir. Assoc.* **2013**, *14*, 542–559. [CrossRef]

28. Beaudart, C.; Dawson, A.; Shaw, S.C.; Harvey, N.C.; Kanis, J.A.; Binkley, N.; Reginster, J.Y.; Chapurlat, R.; Chan, D.C.; Bruyère, O.; et al. Nutrition and physical activity in the prevention and treatment of sarcopenia: Systematic review. *Osteoporos. Int.* **2017**, *28*, 1817–1833. [CrossRef]

29. Dupont, J.; Dedeyne, L.; Dalle, S.; Koppo, K.; Gielen, E.E. The role of omega-3 in the prevention and treatment of sarcopenia. *Aging Clin. Exp. Res.* **2019**, *31*, 825–836. [CrossRef]

30. Yan, Y.; Jiang, W.; Spinetti, T.; Tardivel, A.; Castillo, R.; Bourquin, C.; Guarda, G.; Tian, Z.; Tschopp, J.; Zhou, R. Omega-3 Fatty Acids Prevent Inflammation and Metabolic Disorder through Inhibition of NLRP3 Inflammasome Activation. *Immunity* **2013**, *38*, 1154–1163. [CrossRef]

31. Di Girolamo, F.G.; Situlin, R.; Mazzucco, S.; Valentini, R.; Toigo, G.; Biolo, G. Omega-3 fatty acids and protein metabolism: Enhancement of anabolic interventions for sarcopenia. *Curr. Opin. Clin. Nutr. Metab. Care* **2014**, *17*, 145–150. [CrossRef]

32. Aubert, J.; Saint-Marc, P.; Belmonte, N.; Dani, C.; Negrel, R.; Ailhaud, G. Prostacyclin IP receptor up-regulates the early expression of C/EBPβ and C/EBPδ in preadipose cells. *Mol. Cell. Endocrinol.* **2000**, *160*, 149–156. [CrossRef]

33. Vassaux, G.; Gaillard, D.; Ailhaud, G.; Negrel, R. Prostacyclin is a specific effector of adipose cell differentiation. Its dual role as a cAMP- and Ca(2+)-elevating agent. *J. Biol. Chem.* **1992**, *267*, 11092–11097. [PubMed]

34. Ide, T.; Kobayashi, H.; Ashakumary, L.; Rouyer, I.A.; Takahashi, Y.; Aoyama, T.; Hashimoto, T.; Mizugaki, M. Comparative effects of perilla and fish oils on the activity and gene expression of fatty acid oxidation enzymes in rat liver. *Biochim. Biophys. Acta BBA Mol. Cell Biol. Lipids* **2000**, *1485*, 23–35. [CrossRef]

35. Couet, C.; Delarue, J.; Ritz, P.; Antoine, J.-M.; Lamisse, F. Effect of dietary fish oil on body fat mass and basal fat oxidation in healthy adults. *Int. J. Obes.* **1997**, *21*, 637–643. [CrossRef] [PubMed]

36. Da Boit, M.; Sibson, R.; Sivasubramaniam, S.; Meakin, J.R.; Greig, C.A.; Aspden, R.M.; Thies, F.; Jeromson, S.; Hamilton, D.L.; Speakman, J.R.; et al. Sex differences in the effect of fish-oil supplementation on the adaptive response to resistance exercise training in older people: A randomized controlled trial. *Am. J. Clin. Nutr.* **2017**, *105*, 151–158. [CrossRef] [PubMed]

37. Da Boit, M.; Sibson, R.; Meakin, J.R.; Aspden, R.M.; Thies, F.; Mangoni, A.A.; Gray, S.R. Sex differences in the response to resistance exercise training in older people. *Physiol. Rep.* **2016**, *4*, e12834. [CrossRef] [PubMed]

38. Neder, J.A.; Nery, L.E.; Andreoni, S.; Whipp, B.J. Maximal aerobic power and leg muscle mass and strength related to age in non-athletic males and females. *Graefe's Arch. Clin. Exp. Ophthalmol.* **1999**, *79*, 522–530. [CrossRef]

39. Greeves, J.P.; Cable, N.T.; Reilly, T.; Kingsland, C. Changes in muscle strength in women following the menopause: A longitudinal assessment of the efficacy of hormone replacement therapy. *Clin. Sci.* **1999**, *97*, 79–84. [CrossRef]

40. Fratesi, J.A.; Hogg, R.C.; Young-Newton, G.S.; Patterson, A.C.; Charkhzarin, P.; Thomas, K.B.; Sharratt, M.T.; Stark, K.D. Direct quantitation of omega-3 fatty acid intake of Canadian residents of a long-term care facility. *Appl. Physiol. Nutr. Metab.* **2009**, *34*, 1–9. [CrossRef]

41. Patterson, A.C.; Metherel, A.H.; Hanning, R.M.; Stark, K.D. The percentage of DHA in erythrocytes can detect non-adherence to advice to increase EPA and DHA intakes. *Br. J. Nutr.* **2013**, *111*, 270–278. [CrossRef]

42. Stark, K.D.; Van Elswyk, M.E.; Higgins, M.R.; Weatherford, C.A.; Salem, J.N. Global survey of the omega-3 fatty acids, docosahexaenoic acid and eicosapentaenoic acid in the blood stream of healthy adults. *Prog. Lipid Res.* **2016**, *63*, 132–152. [CrossRef]

43. Sinclair, M.; Chapman, B.; Hoermann, R.; Angus, P.W.; Testro, A.; Scodellaro, T.; Gow, P.J. Handgrip Strength Adds More Prognostic Value to the Model for End-Stage Liver Disease Score Than Imaging-Based Measures of Muscle Mass in Men with Cirrhosis. *Liver Transplant.* **2019**, *25*, 1480–1487. [CrossRef] [PubMed]

4

Potential Benefits of Omega-3 Fatty Acids in Non-Melanoma Skin Cancer

Homer S. Black [1],* and **Lesley E. Rhodes** [2]

[1] Department of Dermatology, Baylor College of Medicine, Houston, TX 77030, USA
[2] Photobiology Unit, Dermatology Centre, University of Manchester, Salford Royal Hospital, Manchester M6 8HD, UK; Lesley.E.Rhodes@manchester.ac.uk
* Correspondence: hblack@bcm.edu

Academic Editors: Lindsay Brown, Bernhard Rauch and Hemant Poudyal

Abstract: Considerable circumstantial evidence has accrued from both experimental animal and human clinical studies that support a role for omega-3 fatty acids (FA) in the prevention of non-melanoma skin cancer (NMSC). Direct evidence from animal studies has shown that omega-3 FA inhibit ultraviolet radiation (UVR) induced carcinogenic expression. In contrast, increasing levels of dietary omega-6 FA increase UVR carcinogenic expression, with respect to a shorter tumor latent period and increased tumor multiplicity. Both omega-6 and omega-3 FA are essential FA, necessary for normal growth and maintenance of health and although these two classes of FA exhibit only minor structural differences, these differences cause them to act significantly differently in the body. Omega-6 and omega-3 FA, metabolized through the lipoxygenase (LOX) and cyclooxygenase (COX) pathways, lead to differential metabolites that are influential in inflammatory and immune responses involved in carcinogenesis. Clinical studies have shown that omega-3 FA ingestion protects against UVR-induced genotoxicity, raises the UVR-mediated erythema threshold, reduces the level of pro-inflammatory and immunosuppressive prostaglandin E2 (PGE_2) in UVR-irradiated human skin, and appears to protect human skin from UVR-induced immune-suppression. Thus, there is considerable evidence that omega-3 FA supplementation might be beneficial in reducing the occurrence of NMSC, especially in those individuals who are at highest risk.

Keywords: skin cancer; omega-3 fatty acids; ultraviolet radiation; prostaglandins; immune modulation

1. Introduction

Considerable interest has been focused on the potential health benefits of omega-3 fatty acids (FA) on a range of human diseases. This interest arose from a series of reports in which high dietary intake of these unsaturated FA among Greenlandic West Coast Eskimos was specifically associated with low incidence of ischemic heart disease, and inflammatory symptoms, in general [1–3]. Whereas the major focus has been on cardiovascular disease [4–6], studies have been extended to type II diabetes and the metabolic syndrome, inflammatory bowel disease, rheumatoid arthritis, renal disease, systemic lupus erythematosus, and osteoporosis [7,8].

Dietary lipids have also been implicated in the development of several kinds of cancer, e.g., breast, lung, bowel, bladder, pancreatic, and prostate [9–12]. Whereas, omega-3 FA have generally shown positive effects on cardiovascular disease, studies are equivocal for human cancers [13,14]. Among 43 risk ratios calculated across 19 cohorts for 11 different types of cancer and 5 different ways to assess omega-3 FA consumption, only four were significant, and it was concluded that omega-3 FA do not reduce overall cancer risk [14]. A systematic review involving 20 cohorts and using up to 6 different ways to categorize omega-3 FA consumption similarly arrived at the conclusion that, overall, there was not a significant association between omega-3 FA and cancer incidence and that dietary supplementation was unlikely to prevent cancer [15].

Although women with high intake ratios of marine omega-3 FA, relative to omega-6 FA have been found to have a reduced risk of breast cancer, not all case-control and cohort studies are in agreement [16]. In the first meta-analysis previously referenced [14], five estimates of risk for breast cancer did not show a significant association, and no effects were found for cancers of the aero-digestive tract, bladder, colorectum, ovary, pancreas or stomach, or for lymphoma. While a recent study observed that high levels of serum phospholipid omega-3 FA (a biomarker) were associated with a large *increase* in the risk of high-grade prostate cancer [17], subsequent systematic review and meta-analysis, including 12 studies of self-reported dietary intake of omega-3 FA and 9 biomarker studies, failed to find an association between omega-3 FA and prostate cancer [18]. These ambiguities require clarification and undoubtedly will require randomized, double-blinded intervention trials.

Inflammatory processes are involved in initiation, promotion, and progression stages of cancer and herein rests the rationale upon which omega-3 FA might be expected to reduce cancer risk [19]. In this regard, there has accrued a considerable body of evidence, albeit circumstantial at this point, that omega-3 FA could reduce cancer risk for the most common of cancers, *i.e.*, skin cancer. The American Cancer Society [20] estimates that over 3.5 million cases of skin cancer will occur this year in the United States alone. The evidence to support a beneficial outcome for omega-3 FA supplementation on non-melanoma skin cancer (NMSC) is presented herein.

2. Essential Fatty Acids

Linoleic acid (LA) and α-linolenic acid (ALA) cannot be synthesized by humans and are, thus, considered essential and must be supplied in the diet. These essential fatty acids (EFA) are the precursors of the omega-6 and omega-3 series of FA, respectively. These FA are often abbreviated by their chemical designation, e.g., LA is 18:2n-6 where 18 indicated the length of the carbon chain, the 2 represents the number of double bonds and the n-6 indicates that the first of the double bonds begins at the sixth carbon atom from the methyl end of the carbon chain. ALA is abbreviated as 18:3n-3, the n-3 signifies that the first double bond is at the third carbon from the methyl end of the chain. Longer chain polyunsaturated FA (PUFA) can be synthesized in humans from their respective precursor EFA (LA or ALA) through a series of elongation (addition of two carbon atoms) and desaturation (addition of a double bond) enzymatic reactions. The two series of EFA cannot be inter-converted in humans and thus compete for these enzymes. Because Western diets may contain 15–20 times more LA than ALA, greater levels of long- chain omega-6 FA (Arachidonic acid, 20:4n-6) result. Consequently under certain dietary conditions supplementation with EPA (Eicosapentaenoic acid, 20:5n-3) and DHA (Docosahexaenoic acid, 22:6n-3) may be essential for maintenance of good health.

Not only do these two series of EFA compete for elongase and desaturase enzymes, but they also compete with the cyclooxygenase (COX) and lipoxygenase (LOX) enzymes and differentially influence the flux of metabolites through these pathways. These oxidative metabolites differ in hormonal potency. The omega-6 FA derived products are more active than their omega-3 FA counterparts. Some of these metabolites are known to influence tumor biology. PGE_2, derived from omega-6 FA oxidation via the COX pathway, acts as a tumor promoter and has been associated with aggressive tumor growth patterns in both basal cell carcinoma (BCC) and squamous cell carcinoma (SCC) in humans [21]. On the other hand, omega-3 FA compete with omega-6 FA for binding sites on COX and inhibit the production of PGE_2, resulting in higher levels of the less potent PGE3. Omega-3 FA may also shunt potential PG precursors through the LOX pathway, resulting in products that inhibit tumor growth and in products that are involved in immune surveillance [21–23]. A simplified schema of eicosanoid metabolism is illustrated in Figure 1. Thus, the COX and LOX pathways, with their bioactive intermediates, provide a strong rational foundation for the cancer preventive potential of omega-3 FA [24].

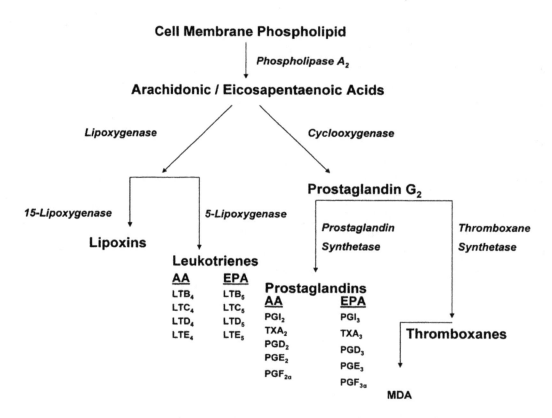

Figure 1. Differential eicosanoid metabolism from omega-6 and omega-3 FA sources. Arachidonic acid, 20:4n-6 (AA), is metabolized via lipoxygenase and cyclooxygenase pathways. Eicosapentaenoic acid, 20:5n-3 (EPA) acts as a competitive inhibitor to the cyclooxygenase enzyme complex with AA and produces different leukotriene and prostaglandin oxidation products. Malondialdehyde (MDA) is a product of prostaglandin and thromboxane metabolism and is commonly used as a measure of lipid peroxidation.

3. Evidence for Participation of Dietary PUFA in UVR-Induced Skin Cancer

3.1. Animal Studies

The first report that dietary fat could potentiate UVR-carcinogenesis came in 1939 [25]. With the advent of World War II, this avenue of research lay fallow for nearly 45 years until this lead was followed-up in a series of studies that demonstrated that an approximate linear relationship occurred between PUFA (dietary corn oil that contained roughly 50% omega-6 FA) and UVR-carcinogenic expression [26,27]. Increasing dietary levels of omega-6 FA shortened the tumor latent period and increased tumor multiplicity. Partial hydrogenation of the PUFA resulted in a marked inhibition of carcinogenesis [26]. Reeve *et al.* [28] found that feeding a totally hydrogenated PUFA completely abolished UVR-carcinogenic expression while those animals fed the normal PUFA exhibited 100% tumor incidence. Furthermore, when the diet of animals fed the hydrogenated fat was reconstituted with a normal mixed fat, large numbers of tumors rapidly appeared. The authors suggested that UVR initiation of tumors had not been prevented by lack of PUFA, but that the EFA deficiency held the appearance of tumors in abeyance, probably at the promotion stage of carcinogenesis. Confirmation that omega-6 FA exerted their influence principally at the post-initiation stage of carcinogenesis came from cross-over feeding studies [29]. Animals were placed on a defined, isocaloric diet containing high (12% w/w) and low (0.75%, w/w) levels of corn oil. At completion of a regimen of UVR, and before tumors appeared, some diets were crossed to the contravening diet, e.g., high to low fat and low to high fat. Incidence curves and tumor multiplicity analysis provided confirmation that diets containing high levels of omega-6 FA enhanced UVR-carcinogenic expression and that enhancement occurred during the post-initiation, or promotion/progression, stages of carcinogenesis. Importantly, crossing from a high fat to a low fat diet after a cancer causing dose of UVR had already been administered, negated the exacerbating influence of high fat diets. This finding provided the rationale upon which a low-fat dietary intervention might act to ameliorate cancer expression.

Contrary to the tumor promoting effects of omega-6 FA, animals fed a diet containing menhaden oil as lipid source exhibited a marked *inhibition* of UVR-carcinogenic expression [30]. Menhaden oil is rich in omega-3 FA. Unlike omega-6 FA, cross-over feeding studies indicated that omega-3 FA exert their principal anti-cancer effects during the initiation stage of carcinogenesis. Animals fed with the omega-3 FA diet throughout the study exhibited an increased tumor latent period and decreased tumor multiplicity compared to animals receiving an equivalent level of corn oil (rich in omega-6 FA).

As noted previously, omega-3 FA compete with omega-6 FA for active sites on COX, a major enzyme in the eicosanoid cascade [24,31]. As such, the level of pro-inflammatory and immune modulating omega-6 FA metabolites is reduced. As dietary omega-6 FA increase, the plasma PGE_2 level increases. Omega-3 FA intake reduces PGE_2 levels approximately 7-fold in comparison to an equivalent level of omega-6 FA [32]. These data support the thesis that omega-6 and omega-3 PUFA differentially influence not only PGE_2 levels, but other pro-inflammatory and immune-modulating intermediates of the COX and LOX pathways.

Supporting evidence for a role of omega-3 FA in carcinogenesis has recently been acquired from studies with a transgenic mouse model designated *fat-1* [33]. The *fat-1* transgenic mice are capable of producing omega-3 FA from omega-6 FA, *i.e.*, the transgenic has received a gene encoding an omega-3 FA desaturase that converts omega-6 FA to omega-3 FA. This results in abundant omega-3 FA and reduced omega-6 FA in the animals' tissues without the need for omega-3 FA supplementation and eliminates many of the confounding variables encountered in dietary studies. With regard to skin tumorigenesis, Xia *et al.* [34] showed that there was a dramatic reduction of melanoma formation and growth when *fat-1* mice were injected with B16 melanoma cells, compared to their non-transgenic littermates. The levels of omega-3 FA and metabolite PGE_3 were much higher in the transgenic animals and the omega-6/omega-3 FA ratio much lower. This transgenic model should be invaluable in future studies to elucidate the role and mechanism(s) of effects of omega-3 FA in NMSC.

As alluded to earlier, previous studies had indicated that carcinogenesis might be modulated immunologically and that this influence might occur at the promotion stage [32]. Notably, the systemic alteration induced by UVR that suppresses an animal's ability to reject highly antigenic UVR-induced allergens occurs during the chemical promotion stage of carcinogenesis [35]. Reeve *et al.* [28] had already shown that feeding mice an EFA (omega-6 FA) deficient diet inhibited the appearance of UVR-induced tumors and suggested that this inhibition might be due to the lack of eicosanoid precursors that, in turn, might prevent UVR induction of the immune state. In the case of omega-6 FA, this would be deficient levels of PGE_2, the gate-keeper for other eicosanoids. This would account for protection observed from UVR-initiated tumor outgrowth. Chung *et al.* [36] had shown that T-cell function was PGE_2 dependent and that UVR-induced suppression of contact hypersensitivity (CHS) was abrogated by treatment with an inhibitor of PG synthesis.

It was subsequently shown that plasma PGE_2 levels were directly related to omega-6 FA dietary intake, *i.e.*, the highest level of PGE_2 occurring with the highest level of omega-6 FA intake [32]. This, in turn, induced the greatest exacerbation of UVR carcinogenic expression. Importantly, omega-3 FA provided striking protection against UVR-induced immunosuppression. This observation was subsequently confirmed [37]. Delayed type hypersensitivity (DTH) and CHS are both regulated by T-cell function and share common pathways with immunological tumor rejection. DTH in UVR-irradiated animals is dramatically suppressed in animals fed high levels of omega-6 FA when compared to those receiving low levels of the FA or those receiving omega-3 FA [32,38].The ability of an animal to reject a transplanted tumor was related to the level of omega-6 FA intake. Moreover, the tumor rejection time for animals fed high levels of omega-6 FA was three times longer than animals fed low levels of the omega-6 FA and occurred at a time when high omega-6 FA had been shown to exacerbate primary tumor expression [38].These studies suggest that one potential mechanism of omega-3 FA inhibition of carcinogenic expression is via immune modulation [31].

In summary, the following sequence of observations support the thesis that omega-6, -3 PUFA metabolism, through the LOX and COX pathways, leads to differential metabolites that influence inflammatory and immune responses involved in UVR-carcinogenesis:

1. Increasing levels of dietary omega-6 FA *exacerbate* UVR carcinogenic expression, with respect to both shortened tumor latent period and increased tumor multiplicity.
2. Dietary omega-3 FA *inhibit* UVR carcinogenic expression.
3. Omega-6 FA exert their principal effect upon the post-initiation, or promotion/progression stages of UVR carcinogenesis.
4. Omega-3 FA appear to exert their principal effects during the initiation stage of the carcinogenic continuum.
5. Pro-inflammatory and immunosuppressive PGE_2 levels are increased linearly as dietary omega-6 FA levels increase.
6. Pro-inflammatory and immunosuppressive PGE_2 levels are dramatically reduced by dietary omega-3 FA intake.
7. Dietary omega-6 FA suppress the immunologic responses involved in tumor transplant rejection and the immunologic pathways involved in DTH and CHS.
8. Dietary omega-3 FA inhibit UVR-induced suppression of DTH and CHS.

3.2. Clinical Studies

The experimental studies employing a high-fat diet to low-fat diet cross-over, even after a cancer causing dose of UVR had been administered, negated the exacerbating influence of the high-fat diet and provided a rationale for undertaking a clinical intervention trial. This trial, involving 133 skin cancer patients, of whom 115 completed the two year study, clearly demonstrated that a low-fat intervention reduced the occurrence of NMSC [39,40]. The cumulative rate of occurrence of NMSC (cumulative NMSC/patient/time period) was 0.21 and 0.19 during the first 8-month period of the study and 0.26 and 0.02 ($p \leqslant 0.02$) during the last 8-month period for control and intervention arms, respectively. The dietary parameters involved only a reduction in the calories consumed as fat, while maintaining total calorie intake and body weight. Efforts were made to maintain the P/S ratio (polyunsaturated/saturated fat ratio) of patients' diets going into the trial and there were no increases in omega-3 FA intake. Thus, the influence of fat on MNSC occurrence was primarily that resulting from lowering fat intake, primarily omega-6 FA. Furthermore, the influence of this low-fat intervention was observed early in the study as a significant difference in the number of actinic keratoses (pre-malignant lesions) between control and low-fat diets occurred [41]. Patients in the control arm of the study (no dietary modifications introduced) were found to be at 4.7 times greater risk of having one or more actinic keratoses during the two-year study period than patients in the low-fat intervention arm.

Whereas lower intake of omega-6 FA reduces the risk of NMSC occurrence in skin cancer patients, a population based case-control study showed a consistent tendency toward a lower risk of SCC with higher intakes of omega-3 FA [42]. Their data also suggested a tendency for a lower risk of SCC with diets containing high omega-3/omega-6 FA ratios. Although this study was suggestive that omega-3 FA could influence NMSC risk, a number of human studies have provided a physiological rationale to support such a hypothesis. Encouraged by the experimental animal results, a short term supplementation study of mixed omega-3 FA was conducted in humans [43]. The patients received oral capsules of either 4 g/day of mixed omega-3 FA (2.8 g EPA + 1.2 g DHA) or a gelatin placebo. After four weeks there was a statistically significant increase in the minimal erythema dose (MED) to UVB in the active group. Serum triglyceride levels decreased by 40 mg/dL. A second study examined the effects of omega-3 FA supplementation on UVB-induced erythema and lipid peroxidation [44]. This study employed a supplement of 3 g/day of mixed omega-3 FA (1.8 g EPA + 1.2 g DHA) administered over a

3–6 month period. The MED rose progressively with increasing time of omega-3 FA supplementation, and had more than doubled at six months. This increase in MED was accompanied by an increase in epidermal omega-3 FA composition and increased susceptibility to lipid peroxidation. The MED had returned to baseline two and a half months after omega-3 FA supplementation was halted.

As noted earlier, a number of cytokines and PG have been shown to be modulated by omega-3 FA. When human keratinocytes were cultured in the presence of omega-3 FA, TNF-α and IL-1α secretion was induced and PGE$_2$ and IL-6 level reduced [45]. Subsequently, further *in vitro* keratinocyte studies showed that EPA and DHA each inhibited basal and UVR-induced IL-8, a chemokine pivotal to UVR-induced skin inflammation and which exhibits pro-carcinogenic activity [46]. However, a double-blind, randomized trial of 28 patients supplemented with 4 g/day of 95% of ethyl esters of EPA or oleic acid for three months found no evidence that the MED response evoked by omega-3 FA was mediated by the pro-inflammatory cytokines IL-8, TNF-α, IL-6 or IL-1β. In contrast, there was a notable and significant reduction in cutaneous PGE$_2$, the pro-inflammatory and immune-suppressor mediator [47]. Further, lipidomic analysis was performed in a human intervention trial of EPA-rich omega-3 FA, quantifying impact of supplement on eicosanoid levels in skin blister fluid [48]. This showed a significant reduction in the ratio of PGE$_2$: PGE$_3$ in UVR-exposed skin, accompanied by a reduction in the ratio of the pro-inflammatory and tumor promoting 12-LOX product 12-hydroxyeicosatetraenoic acid (12-HETE): 12-hydroxyeicosapentaenoic acid (12-HEPE), EPA-derived homologue of 12-HETE [48].

A double-blind, randomized intervention examined the impact of oral omega-3 FA on UVR suppression of cell-mediated immunity, assessed through the nickel CHS response [49]. Seventy-nine nickel-sensitive adult females consumed encapsulated omega-3 FA (3.5 g EPA + 1.5 g DHA) or control lipid daily for 3 months, with compliance and skin bioavailability of omega-3 FA assessed by blood [49] and skin [48] assay, respectively. This indicated apparent abrogation of the photo-immunosuppression induced by low level solar simulated ultraviolet radiation (SSR; 95% UVA, 5% UVB) exposure. Following SSR exposure equivalent to ~15 min of midday summer sunlight in Manchester, UK (latitude 53.5° N), on 3 consecutive days, the UVR-suppression of the CHS response was 50% lower in the subjects taking omega-3 FA compared to those taking control.

Previous discussion provides clear evidence that omega-3 FA protect against the clinical sunburn response. Yet, there was no evidence of an EPA effect on direct UVR-induced DNA damage to DNA, *i.e.*, cyclobutane pyrimidine dimer formation in skin [50]. There was, however, protection against UVR induction of cutaneous p53, considered to be a biomarker of DNA damage and which acts as a tumor suppressor gene. In addition, in *ex vivo* UVR-treated peripheral blood lymphocytes, omega-3 FA protected against DNA single-strand breaks [50].

Thus, human studies (and cell culture studies employing human cells) have shown:

1. Omega-3 FA supplementation significantly increases the erythema threshold to UVR.
2. Omega-3 FA modulate a number of cytokines (in human cells *in vitro* only) and eicosanoids that mediate inflammatory and immune responses.
3. Omega-3 FA inhibit certain genotoxic markers of UVR-induced DNA damage, e.g., UVR- induced cutaneous p53.
4. Omega-3 FA abrogate UVR-induced immunosuppression of cell mediated immunity assessed as nickel CHS

4. Conclusions

In Toto, the results of experimental studies, and the influence of omega-3 FA on UVR-induced erythema, early genotoxic markers and immune-suppression in human trials, suggest that supplementation of these photoprotective nutrients [51] could result, in the longer term, in a reduction in NMSC in humans. Based upon age-adjusted cancer incidence/UVR exposure plots, an omega-3 FA enhanced sun protection factor (SPF), even of the low reported magnitude could reduce incidence of NMSC by as much as 30% [50–52]. Neither have observational studies, case-control or prospective cohort studies, provided clear evidence that dietary omega-6 FA or omega-3 FA reduces the risk of

NMSC. A recent meta-analysis has been suggestive, but lacked adequate data due to scarcity of trials in this area, to support the hypothesis that omega-3 FA protect against NMSC [53]. For the most part, both case-control and prospective cohort studies have failed to find a relationship between skin cancer incidence with dietary fat intake. Indeed these types of studies are fraught with methodological difficulties resulting from: (1) the complexity of the human diet in a free living population; (2) the difficulties in measuring food intake and analyzing dietary information; (3) the epidemiologist requires assess of dietary patterns that are stable over long periods, *i.e.*, usually years if cancer induction is under study [54].

The authors have previously proposed that the most direct evidence for the preventive potential of omega-3 FA would be achieved through intervention trials in populations with high, and known, risk for NMSC—much in the manner that reduction in the percentage of calories consumed as fat was shown to influence NMSC occurrence in skin cancer patients [24,39–41,55]. Caveats to the design of such a study will include consideration of baseline omega-3 FA nutrition at study inclusion [56] and careful monitoring of the diets of study patients to assure that any potential benefits of omega-3 FA supplementation is not diminished by increasing omega-6 FA intake. The relative omega-6/omega-3 FA ratios will determine response and could be monitored by an easily determined parameter such as red blood cell membrane omega-6/omega-3 FA ratios [48,56]. This parameter could also be used to determine adherence to the supplement protocol. It is also important that an adequate level of omega-3 FA supplementation be employed. Omega-3 FA have a high safety profile and a daily intake of *circa* 4 g/day as employed in previous photoprotection studies is envisaged to be adequate. Because of the promising evidence from animal and clinical studies, it is imperative that the potential of omega-3 FA as a preventive agent for NMSC be fully explored.

Acknowledgments: LER acknowledges the financial support of the Association for International Cancer Research and the European Commission.

References

1.   Bang, H.O.; Dyerberg, J. Plasma lipid and lipoprotein pattern in Greenlandic West Coast Eskimos. *Lancet* **1971**, *1*, 1143–1145. [CrossRef]

2.   Bang, H.O.; Dyerberg, J.; Hjorne, N. The composition of food consumed by Greenland Eskimos. *Acta Med. Scand.* **1976**, *200*, 69–73. [CrossRef] [PubMed]

3.   Bang, H.O.; Dyerberg, J.; Sinclair, H.M. The composition of the Eskimo food in North Western Greenland. *Am. J. Clin. Nutr.* **1980**, *33*, 2657–2661. [PubMed]

4.   Jordan, H.; Matthan, N.; Chung, M.; Balk, E.; Chew, P.; Kupelnick, B.; Lawrence, A.; Lichtenstein, A.; Lau, J. *Effects of Omega-3 Fatty Acids on Arrhythmogenic Mechanisms in Animal and Isolated Organ/Cell Culture Studies*; Evidence Report/Technology Assessment No. 92; Publication No. 04-EO11-2. Agency for Healthcare Research and Quality: Rockville, MD, USA, 2004.

5.   Balk, E.; Chung, M.; Lichtenstein, A.; Chew, P.; Kupelnick, B.; DeVine, D.; Lawrence, A.; Lau, J. *Effects of Omega-3 Fatty Acids on Cardiovascular Risk Factors and Intermediate Markers of Cardiovascular Disease*; Evidence Report/Technology Assessment No. 93; Publication No. 04-EO10-2. Agency for Healthcare Research and Quality: Rockville, MD, USA, 2004.

6.   Wang, C.; Chung, M.; Lichtenstein, A.; Balk, E.; Kupelnick, B.; DeVine, D.; Lawrence, A.; Lau, J. *Effects of Omega-3 Fatty Acids on Cardiovascular Disease*; Evidence Report/Technology Assessment No. 94; Publication No. 04-EO09-2. Agency for Healthcare Research and Quality: Rockville, MD, USA, 2004.

7.   Schacter, H.; Reisman, J.; Tran, K.; Dales, B.; Kourad, K.; Barnes, D.; Sampson, M.; Morrison, A.; Gaboury, I.; Blackman, J. *Health Effects of Omega-3 Fatty Acids on Asthma*; Evidence Report/Technology Assessment No. 94; Publication No. 04-EO13-2. Agency for Healthcare Research and Quality: Rockville, MD, USA, 2004.

8.   MacLean, C.H.; Mojica, W.A.; Morton, S.C.; Pencharz, J.; Hasenfeld Garland, R.; Tu, W.; Newberry, S.J.; Jungvig, L.K.; Khanna, P.; Rhodes, S.; *et al. Effects of Omega-3 Fatty Acids on Lipids and Glycemic Control in Type II Diabetes and the Metabolic Syndrome and on Inflammatory Bowel Disease, Rheumatoid Arthritis, Renal Disease, Systemic Lupus Erythematosus, and Osteoporosis*; Evidence Report/Technology Assessment No. 89; Publication No. 04-EO12–2. Agency for Healthcare Research and Quality: Rockville, MD, USA, 2004.

9. Nixon, D.W.; Rodgers, K. Breast Cancer. In *Nutritional Oncology*, 2nd ed.; Heber, D., Blackburn, G.L., Go, V.L.W., Eds.; Academic Press: San Diego, CA, USA, 1999; pp. 447–452.

10. Aronson, W.; Yip, I.; Dekernion, J. Prostate Cancer. In *Nutritional Oncology*, 2nd ed.; Heber, D., Blackburn, G.L., Go, V.L.W., Eds.; Academic Press: San Diego, CA, USA, 1999; pp. 453–461.

11. Clinton, S.K.; Michaud, D.; Giovannucci, E. Nutrition and Bladder Cancer. In *Nutritional Oncology*, 2nd ed.; Heber, D., Blackburn, G.L., Go, V.L.W., Eds.; Academic Press: San Diego, CA, USA, 1999; pp. 463–475.

12. Harris, D.M.; Kang, S.Y.; Go, V.L.W. Nutrient-Gene Interactions and Prevention of Colorectal, Liver, and Pancreatic Cancer. In *Nutritional Oncology*, 2nd ed.; Heber, D., Blackburn, G.L., Go, V.L.W., Eds.; Academic Press: San Diego, CA, USA, 1999; pp. 469–500.

13. Caygill, C.P.J.; Charlett, A.; Hill, M.J. Fat, fish, fish oil and cancer. *Br. J. Cancer* **1996**, *74*, 159–164. [CrossRef] [PubMed]

14. MacLean, C.H.; Newberry, S.J.; Mojica, W.A.; Issa, A.; Khanna, P.; Lim, Y.S.W.; Morton, S.C.; Suttorp, M.; Tu, W.; Hilton, L.G.; *et al. Effects of Omega-3 Fatty Acids on Cancer*; Evidence Report/Technology Assessment No. 113; Publication No. 05-EO10-1. Agency for Healthcare Research and Quality: Rockville, MD, USA, 2006.

15. MacLean, C.H.; Newberry, S.J.; Mojica, W.A.; Khanna, P.; Issa, A.M.; Suttorp, M.J.; Lim, Y.W.; Traina, S.B.; Hilton, L.; Garland, R.; *et al.* Effects of omega-3 fatty acids on cancer risk: a systematic review. *JAMA* **2006**, *295*, 403–415. [CrossRef] [PubMed]

16. Fabian, C.J.; Kimler, B.F.; Hursting, S.D. Omega-3 fatty acids for breast cancer prevention and survivorship. *Breast Cancer Res.* **2015**, *17*, 62–77. [CrossRef] [PubMed]

17. Brasky, T.M.; Darke, A.K.; Song, X.; Tangen, C.M.; Goodman, P.J.; Thompson, I.M.; Mayskens, F.L., Jr.; Goodman, G.E.; Minasian, L.M.; Parnes, H.L.; *et al.* Plasma phospholipid fatty acids and prostate cancer risk in the SELECT trial. *J. Natl. Cancer Inst.* **2013**, *105*, 1132–1141. [CrossRef] [PubMed]

18. Alexander, D.D.; Bassett, J.K.; Weed, D.L.; Barrett, E.C.; Watson, H.; Harris, W. Meta-analysis of long-chain omega-3 polyunsaturated fatty acids (LCω-3 PUFA) and prostate cancer. *Nutr. Cancer* **2015**, *67*, 543–554. [CrossRef] [PubMed]

19. Lu, H.; Ouyang, W.; Huang, C. Inflammation, a key event in cancer development. *Mol. Cancer Res.* **2006**, *4*, 221–233. [CrossRef] [PubMed]

20. American Cancer Society. Cancer Facts and Figures, Atlanta, GA. 2014. Available online: http://www.cancer.org (accessed on 8 November 2015).

21. Vanderveen, E.; Grekin, R.; Swanson, N.; Kragballe, K. Arachidonic acid metabolites in cutaneous carcinomas. Evidence suggesting that elevated levels of prostaglandins in basal cell carcinomas are associated with aggressive growth pattern. *Arch Dermatol.* **1986**, *122*, 407–412. [CrossRef] [PubMed]

22. Malmsten, C. Leukotrienes: Mediators of inflammation and immediate hypersensitivity reactions. *Crit. Rev. Immunol.* **1984**, *4*, 307–334. [PubMed]

23. Werner, E.; Walenga, R.; Dubowy, R.; Boone, S.; Stuart, M. Inhibition of human malignant neuroblastoma cell DNA synthesis by lipoxygenase metabolites of arachidonic acid. *Cancer Res.* **1985**, *45*, 561–563. [PubMed]

24. Black, H.S.; Rhodes, L.E. The potential of omega-3 fatty acids in the prevention of non- melanoma skin cancer. *Cancer Det. Prev.* **2006**, *30*, 224–232. [CrossRef] [PubMed]

25. Baumann, C.; Rusch, H. Effect of diet on tumors induced by ultraviolet light. *Am. J. Cancer* **1939**, *35*, 213–221.

26. Black, H.S.; Lenger, W.; Phelps, A.W.; Thornby, J.I. Influence of dietary lipid upon ultraviolet-light carcinogenesis. *Nutr. Cancer* **1983**, *5*, 59–68. [CrossRef] [PubMed]

27. Black, H.S.; Lenger, W.A.; Gerguis, J.; Thornby, J.I. Relation of antioxidants and level of dietary lipid to epidermal lipid peroxidation and ultraviolet carcinogenesis. *Cancer Res.* **1985**, *45*, 6254–6259. [PubMed]

28. Reeve, V.; Bosnic, M.; Boehm-Wilcox, C. Dependence of photocarcinogenesis and photoimmunosuppression in the hairless mouse on dietary polyunsaturated fat. *Cancer Lett.* **1966**, *108*, 271–279. [CrossRef]

29. Black, H.S.; Thornby, J.I.; Gerguis, J.; Lenger, W. Influence of dietary omega-6, -3 fatty acid sources on the initiation and promotion stages of photocarcinogenesis. *Photochem. Photobiol.* **1992**, *56*, 195–199. [CrossRef] [PubMed]

30. Orengo, I.F.; Black, H.S.; Kettler, A.H.; Wolf, J.E., Jr. Influence of dietary menhaden oil upon carcinogenesis and various cutaneous responses to ultraviolet radiation. *Photochem. Photobiol.* **1989**, *49*, 71–77. [CrossRef] [PubMed]

31. Black, H.S. Omega-3 fatty acids and non-melanoma skin cancer. In *Handbook of Diet, Nutrition and the Skin*; Preedy, V.R., Ed.; Wageningen Academic Publishers: Wageningen, The Netherlands, 2012; pp. 367–378.

32. Fischer, M.A.; Black, H.S. Modification of membrane composition, eicosanoid metabolism, and immunoresponsiveness by dietary omega-3 and omega-6 fatty acid sources, modulators of ultraviolet-carcinogenesis. *Photochem. Photobiol.* **1991**, *54*, 381–387. [CrossRef] [PubMed]

33. Kang, J.X. Fat-1 transgenic mice: A new model for omega-3 research. *Prostaglandins Leukot Essent Fatty Acids* **2007**, *77*, 263–267. [CrossRef] [PubMed]

34. Xia, S.; Lu, Y.; Wang, J.; He, C.; Hong, S.; Serhan, C.N.; Kang, J.X. Melanoma growth is reduced in fat-1 transgenic mice: Impact of omega-6/omega-3 essential fatty acids. *Proc. Natl. Acad. Sci. USA* **2006**, *103*, 12499–12504. [CrossRef] [PubMed]

35. Strickland, P.; Creasia, D.; Kripke, M. Enhancement of two-stage skin carcinogenesis by exposure of distant skin to UV-radiation. *J. Natl. Cancer Inst.* **1985**, *74*, 1129–1134. [PubMed]

36. Chung, H.; Burnham, D.; Robertson, B.; Roberts, I.; Daynes, R. Involvement of prostaglandins in the immune alterations caused by exposure of mice to ultraviolet radiation. *J. Immunol.* **1986**, *137*, 2478–2884. [PubMed]

37. Moison, R.; Beijersbergen Van Henegouwen, G. Dietary eicosapentaenoic acid prevents systemic immunosuppression in mice induced by UVB radiation. *Radiat. Res* **2001**, *156*, 36–44. [CrossRef]

38. Black, H.S.; Okotie-Eboh, G.; Gerguis, J.; Urban, J.I.; Thornby, J.I. Dietary fat modulates immunoresponsiveness in UV-irradiated mice. *Photochem. Photobiol.* **1995**, *62*, 964–969. [CrossRef] [PubMed]

39. Black, H.S.; Thornby, J.I.; Wolf, J.E.; Goldberg, L.H.; Herd, J.A.; Rosen, T.; Bruce, S.; Tschen, J.A.; Scott, L.W.; Jaax, S.; *et al.* Evidence that a low-fat diet reduces the occurrence of non-melanoma skin cancer. *Int. J. Cancer* **1995**, *62*, 165–169. [CrossRef] [PubMed]

40. Jaax, S.; Scott, L.W.; Wolf, J.E.; Thornby, J.I.; Black, H.S. General guidelines for a low-fat diet effective in the management and prevention of nonmelanoma skin cancer. *Nutr. Cancer* **1997**, *27*, 150–156. [CrossRef] [PubMed]

41. Black, H.S.; Herd, J.A.; Goldberg, L.H.; Wolf, J.E.; Thornby, J.I.; Rosen, T.; Bruce, S.; Tschen, J.A.; Foreyt, J.P.; Scott, L.W.; *et al.* Effect of a low-fat diet on the incidence of actinic keratosis. *N. Engl. J. Med.* **1994**, *330*, 1272–1275. [CrossRef] [PubMed]

42. Hakim, I.A.; Harris, R.B.; Ritenbaugh, C. Fat intake and risk of squamous cell carcinomas of the skin. *Nutr. Cancer* **2000**, *36*, 155–162. [CrossRef] [PubMed]

43. Orengo, I.F.; Black, H.S.; Wolf, J.E. Influence of fish oil supplementation on the minimal erythema dose in humans. *Arch. Dermatol.* **1992**, *284*, 219–221. [CrossRef]

44. Rhodes, L.E.; O'Farrell, S.; Jackson, M.J.; Friedmann, P.S. Dietary fish-oil supplementation in humans reduces UVB-erythemal sensitivity but increases epidermal lipid peroxidation. *J. Investig. Dermatol.* **1994**, *103*, 151–154. [CrossRef] [PubMed]

45. Pupe, A.; Moison, R.; De Haes, P.; Beijersbergen van Henegouwen, G.; Rhodes, L.E.; Degreef, H.; Garmyn, M. Eicosapentaenoic acid, a *n*-3 polyunsaturated fatty acid differentially modulates TNF-α, IL-1α, IL-6 and PGE$_2$ expression in UVB-irradiated human keratinocytes. *J. Investig. Dermatol.* **2002**, *118*, 692–698. [CrossRef] [PubMed]

46. Storey, A.; McArdle, F.; Friedmann, P.S.; Jackson, M.J.; Rhodes, L.E. Eicosapentaenoic acid and docosahexaenoic acid reduce UVB- and TNF-alpha-induced IL-8 secretion in keratinocytes and UVB-induced IL-8 in fibroblasts. *J. Investig. Dermatol.* **2005**, *124*, 248–255. [CrossRef] [PubMed]

47. Shahbakhti, H.; Watson, R.; Azurdia, R.; Ferreira, R.; Garmyn, M.; Rhodes, L.E. Influence of eicosapentaenoic acid, an omega-3 fatty acid, on ultraviolet B generation of prostaglandin E2 and proinflammatory cytokines interleukin-1 beta, tumor necrosis factor-alpha, interleukin-6 and interleukin-8 in human skin *in vivo*. *Photochem. Photobiol.* **2004**, *80*, 231–235. [CrossRef] [PubMed]

48. Pilkington, S.M.; Rhodes, L.E.; Al-Aasswad, N.M.I.; Massey, K.A.; Nicolaou, A. Impact of EPA ingestion on COX- and LOX-mediated eicosanoid synthesis in skin with and without a pro- inflammatory UVR challenge. Report of a randomised controlled study in humans. *Mol. Nutr. Food Res.* **2014**, *58*, 580–590. [CrossRef] [PubMed]

49. Pilkington, S.M.; Massey, K.A.; Bennett, S.P.; Al-Aasswad, N.M.; Roshdy, K.; Gibbs, N.K.; Friedmann, P.S.; Nicolaou, A.; Rhodes, L.E. Randomized controlled trial of oral omega-3 PUFA in solar-simulated radiation-induced suppression of human cutaneous immune responses. *Am. J. Clin. Nutr.* **2013**, *97*, 646–652. [CrossRef] [PubMed]

50. Rhodes, L.E.; Shahbakhti, H.; Azurdia, R.; Moison, R.; Steenwinkel, M.-J.S.T.; Homburg, M.; Dean, M.; McArdle, F.; Beijersbergen van Henegouwen, G.; Epe, B.; *et al.* Effect of eicosapentaenoic acid, an omega-3 polyunsaturated fatty acid, on UVR-related cancer risk in humans. An assessment of early genotoxic markers. *Carcinogenesis* **2003**, *24*, 919–925. [CrossRef] [PubMed]
51. Pilkington, S.M.; Watson, R.E.B.; Nicolaou, A.; Rhodes, L.E. Omega-3 Polyunsaturated Fatty Acids: Photoprotective Macronutrients. *Exp. Dermatol.* **2011**, *20*, 537–543. [CrossRef] [PubMed]
52. Rhodes, L.E. Preventive oncology. *Lancet* **2004**, *363*, 1736–1737. [CrossRef]
53. Noel, S.E.; Stoneham, A.C.S.; Olsen, C.M.; Rhodes, L.E.; Green, A.C. Consumption of omega-3 fatty acids and the risk of skin cancers: A systemic review and meta-analysis. *Int. J. Cancer* **2014**, *135*, 149–156. [CrossRef] [PubMed]
54. Lyon, J.Y.; Gardner, J.W.; West, D.W.; Mahoney, A.M. Methodological issues in epidemiological studies of the diet and cancer. *Cancer Res.* **1992**, *52*, 2040–2048.
55. Black, H.S. Skin Cancer. In *Nutritional Oncology*, 2nd ed.; Heber, D., Blackburn, G.L., Go, V.L.W., Eds.; Academic Press: San Diego, CA, USA, 1999; pp. 405–422.
56. Wallingford, S.C.; Pilkington, S.M.; Massey, K.A.; Al-Aasswad, N.M.I.; Ibiebele, T.I.; Hughes, M.C.; Bennett, S.; Nicolaou, A.; Rhodes, L.E.; Green, A.C. Three-way assessment of long chain omega-3 polyunsaturated fatty acid nutrition: By questionnaire and matched blood and skin samples. *Br. J. Nutr.* **2013**, *109*, 701–708. [CrossRef] [PubMed]

5

Cancer Risk and Eicosanoid Production: Interaction between the Protective Effect of Long Chain Omega-3 Polyunsaturated Fatty Acid Intake and Genotype

Georgia Lenihan-Geels [1,*], Karen S. Bishop [2] and Lynnette R. Ferguson [2]

[1] Wageningen University and Research Centre, 6708 PB Wageningen, the Netherlands
[2] Auckland Cancer Society Research Centre, University of Auckland; Private Bag 92019, Auckland 1142, New Zealand; k.bishop@auckland.ac.nz (K.S.B.); l.ferguson@auckland.ac.nz (L.R.F.)
* Correspondence: g.lenihangeels@gmail.com

Academic Editors: Lindsay Brown, Bernhard Rauch and Hemant Poudyal

Abstract: Dietary inclusion of fish and fish supplements as a means to improve cancer prognosis and prevent tumour growth is largely controversial. Long chain omega-3 polyunsaturated fatty acids (LCn-3 PUFA), eicosapentaenoic acid and docosahexaenoic acid, may modulate the production of inflammatory eicosanoids, thereby influencing local inflammatory status, which is important in cancer development. Although *in vitro* studies have demonstrated inhibition of tumour cell growth and proliferation by LCn-3 PUFA, results from human studies have been mainly inconsistent. Genes involved in the desaturation of fatty acids, as well as the genes encoding enzymes responsible for eicosanoid production, are known to be implicated in tumour development. This review discusses the current evidence for an interaction between genetic polymorphisms and dietary LCn-3 PUFA in the risk for breast, prostate and colorectal cancers, in regards to inflammation and eicosanoid synthesis.

Keywords: long chain omega-3 polyunsaturated fatty acid; cancer; single nucleotide polymorphism; eicosanoids; genotype

1. Introduction

Cancer is a multifactorial, widely spread, variable and largely non-communicable disease, affecting populations in all parts of the world. Currently, some of the most significant cancers throughout the Western world include breast, colorectal and prostate cancers [1]. The role of nutrition in cancer risk and development is becoming increasingly recognised, particularly in regards to dietary intake of fresh fruit and vegetables, meat and meat products, and fish or fish oils, which may be related to their effects on inflammatory processes [2–6]. Intake of animal sources of fat, saturated and trans-unsaturated fatty acids are associated with all-cause mortality and death due to colorectal, breast and prostate cancers. On the other hand, plant based oils and fish oils are associated with a decrease in the risk and death due to the aforementioned cancers [7–9].

The predominant omega-6 (*n*-6) and omega-3 (*n*-3) fatty acids (FA) in the typical Western diet are linoleic acid (LA) (18:2*n*-6) and alpha-linolenic acid (ALA) (18:3*n*-3), respectively, known as the essential fatty acids. Through elongation and desaturation, these FA are converted to longer and more desaturated FAs via the *n*-6 and *n*-3 pathways (Figure 1). However, the conversion of LA and ALA to longer-chain FAs is limited by the enzymatic capacity of the desaturases, as well as dietary levels of LA and ALA, which compete for the same enzymes. For example, the conversion of ALA to eicosapentaenoic acid (EPA) (20:5*n*-3) ranges from between 0.2% and 21% [10].

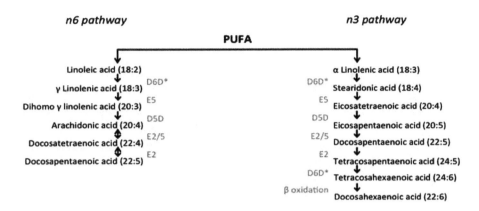

Figure 1. Synthesis of polyunsaturated fatty acids through the *n*-3 and *n*-6 pathways. Polyunsaturated fatty acid elongation from ALA and LA begins with desaturation by the D6D enzyme. Subsequent elongation and desaturation by the corresponding enzymes (orange) generates longer chain PUFA such as AA and EPA. *n*-3 and *n*-6 PUFA compete for the D6D, E5, D5D and E2 enzymes [11–15]. D5D: Delta 5 desaturase; D6D: Delta 6 desaturase; E: Elongase.*: Rate limiting step.

Long chain (LC) polyunsaturated fatty acids (PUFA) play a significant role in inflammatory processes, as they act as precursors for inflammatory mediators called eicosanoids. Eicosanoids are potent signaling molecules synthesized during inflammation and include leukotrienes, thromboxanes and prostaglandins [16]. A diverse set of enzymes are responsible for the synthesis of eicosanoids from PUFA, some of which are outlined in Figure 2. Cyclooxygenases catalyse the formation of series 2 and series 3 prostaglandins and thromboxanes, while lipoxygenases synthesise lipoxins and leukotrienes, which are further metabolized by glutathione transferases [16]. Additionally, dietary EPA and docosahexaenoic acid (DHA) are precursors for mainly anti-inflammatory eicosanoids, while arachidonic acid (AA) (20:4*n*-6) is a precursor for mainly pro-inflammatory compounds and is in competition with EPA for eicosanoid production. Furthermore, the ratio of AA to EPA/DHA in cell membranes is thought to be informative in regards to inflammatory status. In fact, studies clearly show lower levels of circulating pro-inflammatory compounds such as cytokines and adhesion molecules with higher levels of membrane-bound and free EPA and DHA [17–20].

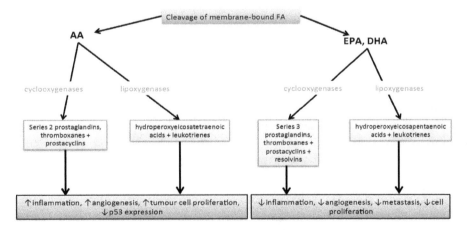

Figure 2. Effects of eicosanoids derived from AA and EPA/DHA. Cyclooxygenases and lipoxygenases act on AA, EPA and DHA to synthesise a range of different eicosanoids during an inflammatory response. AA-derived eicosanoids often generate pro-inflammatory compounds that enhance tumour growth, while EPA/DHA-derived eicosanoids often have anti-inflammatory properties and inhibit tumour growth [21,22]. FA: fatty acids; AA: arachidonic acid; EPA: eicosapentanoic acid; DHA: docosahexanoic acid.

Inflammation is a key event in the development of tumours and is known to promote tumour growth, angiogenesis and metastasis [23]. For example, the metabolism of AA to pro-inflammatory eicosanoids is characteristic of some colorectal and breast cancer cells [24–26]. Therefore, dietary LCn-3 PUFA intake is of great interest in the prevention and treatment of these cancers and as agents in reducing inflammation, although the topic remains largely controversial [9,27–29]. Discrepancies in both observational and experimental data may arise from multiple sources including: heterogeneity of cancers; confounding in epidemiological data; environmental contaminants, particularly from LCn-3 PUFA-rich marine sources; accuracy of dietary intake data; bioavailability; and/or genetic variation [9,12,30–33]. One challenging aspect in cancer epidemiology is that any factor reducing cancer risk will usually promote life-expectancy, which in itself is a risk for cancer [34].

It has come to light that efficiency of conversion of LA and ALA to LC PUFA is partially determined by the genotype of the *fatty acid desaturase (FADS)* family of genes, which code for the delta-5 and delta-6 desaturases that catalyse the rate limiting steps of the *n*-3 and *n*-6 pathways, which may therefore impact downstream eicosanoid production [9,14,35–38]. Interestingly, single nucleotide polymorphisms (SNPs) found in other genes, for example *cytochrome c oxidase (COX)* and *arachidonate lipoxygenase (ALOX)*, may also influence levels of eicosanoids produced from EPA and AA [26,39]. *COX* and *ALOX* genes code for the cyclooxygenase and lipoxygenase enzymes, respectively, and are responsible for generating a range of eicosanoid mediators [16] (Figure 2). Consequently, both levels of dietary fatty acids and variation at the *FADS, COX* and *ALOX* loci may impact inflammatory processes and carcinogenesis.

There is increasing evidence to support the view that LCn-3 PUFA, specifically EPA and DHA, inhibit the growth of colorectal, breast and prostate cancer cell lines [27,40–42] and inhibit tumour growth in animal models [43–45]. Current evidence in humans is less clear and epidemiological data is largely inconsistent [9,27,28]. As inflammation is a predominant hallmark in many cancers, the relationship between inflammation and dietary LCn-3 PUFA is of high interest. Furthermore, the impact of genetic polymorphisms on the production of eicosanoids is important to consider. In this review, we discuss the interaction between LCn-3 PUFA and genotype, related to eicosanoid production, which may have an impact on the development and progression of cancers. The genes or family of genes under consideration include the *FADS* genes involved in the desaturation of LCn-3 PUFA [46], the *glutathione S-transferase (GST)* family of genes involved in oxidative stress and inflammation [47], and the *ALOX* and *COX* genes that generate pro- and anti-inflammatory mediators [48].

2. Methods

Articles utilised in this review were selected using the PubMed and Google Scholar databases. Key words used in the searches included: eicosanoid/s; polymorphism/s; cancer; dietary; polyunsaturated fatty acid; omega-3. One of these words must have also been present: prostate OR breast OR colorectal OR colon OR rectal AND FADS/fatty acid desaturase OR COX/cyclooxygenase OR ALOX/lipoxygenase OR GST/glutathione transferase. Included articles focused on human studies only. Exclusion criteria were: review articles; articles in any language other than English; articles older than 1990; articles focused on another disease other than breast, prostate or colorectal cancer; and articles lacking data on diet specific to PUFA or fish. Following searches of combinations of the above keywords, a total number of 417 articles were found. The titles of these 417 articles were read and after applying the exclusion criteria, 56 articles were selected for the next stage. Adjusting to the same exclusion criteria left a total number of 10 studies, which are summarised in Table 1.

Table 1. Polymorphisms associated with LCn-3 PUFA intake and cancer risk.

Reference	n	Subjects/methods	Exposure Measurement (PC; CC; CS)	Intervention (RCT)	Cancer type	Gene/s	Locus	Effect
Al-Hilal et al., 2013 [14]	367	6-month RCT/M + F, 45–70 year		EPA + DHA; 0.45, 0.9 or 1.9 g/day		FADS1 + FADS2	rs174537	↓D5D activity associated with T variant allele; ↑D5D activity in TG, TT with increasing doses; no association for D6D
Fradet et al., 2009 [12]	Control 478; case 466	CC/M, mean age 65 year	FFQ		Prostate	COX2	rs4648310	G allele correlated with aggressive PCa when n-3 FA intake was low, and low risk with high intake
Gago-Dominguez et al., 2004 [49]	Control 670; case 258	CC/F, 45–74 year	SQ FFQ		Breast	GSTM1, GSTT1, GSTP1	multiple	Lower activity genotypes associated with higher BCa protection with ↑intake of marine n-3 FA
Habermann et al., 2013 [11]	Control 912; case 712	CC/M + F, 30–79 year	CARDIA questionnaire		Rectal	ALOX12	rs11571339	G allele associated with ↓rectal cancer risk in those with low n-3 PUFA intake (NS)
Habermann et al., 2013 [11]	Control 1900; case 1543	CC/M + F, 30–79 year	CARDIA questionnaire		Colon	ALOX15	rs11568131	AA genotype have ↓risk of colon cancer with↑ intakes of n-3 PUFA (NS)
Habermann et al., 2013 [11]	Control 1900; case 1543	CC/M + F, 30–79 year	CARDIA questionnaire		Colon	COX1	rs10306110	Low EPA/DHA intake associated with higher colon cancer risk in variant allele carriers only
Hedelin et al., 2006 [50]	Control 1130; case1499	CC/M, 35–79 year	FFQ		Prostate	COX2	rs5275	C allele at locus rs5275 correlated with ↓risk of PCa with high intake of fatty fish
Hester et al., 2014 [13]	30	CS/Caucasian F, 21–65 year	Serum FA			FADS1	rs174537	T variant correlated with lower AA; GG genotype associated with ↑LTB$_4$ + 5-HETE
Hong et al., 2013 [37]	122	3 year PC/M, 35–59 year	Blood serum			FADS1, FADS2 + FADS3	rs174537 (FADS1); rs174575, rs2727270 (FADS2), rs1000778 (FADS3)	rs174537GG had ↑AA, AA/DGLA, DPA, LDL, oxLDL + ↓ETA. Rs17453 had↓AA, AA/DGLA, EPA, DPA, EPA/ALA + urinary PGF$_{2a}$
Poole et al., 2007 [51]	Control 626; case 716	CC/M + F, 30–74 year	FFQ		Colorectal	COX1	Phe17Leu	Modest↓risk of CRC for carriers of P17 with higher fish intake; L17 carriers have ↓risk of CRC with lower intake
Poole et al., 2010 [52]	Control 582; case 483	CC/M + F, 30–74 year	FFQ		Colorectal	PGES	rs7887087	Carriers of T allele have ↓risk of CRC with ↑fish intake
Poole et al., 2010 [52]	Control 582; case 483	CC/M + F, 30–74 year	FFQ		Colorectal	EP4	Val294Ile	Carriers of Ile variant showed correlation between ↑fish intake and ↑CRC risk
Porenta et al., 2013 [53]	108	6-month RCT/CRC at risk M + F	2 day FR + 24 h recall	Healthy People 2010 diet or Mediterranean diet	Colon	FADS cluster	rs174556 and rs174561 in FADS1, rs383445 in FADS2 and rs174537 of the FADS1/2 intragenic region	Wild-type alleles associated with lower AA in colonic mucosa in persons on Mediterranean Diet

PC: Prospective cohort; CC: Case-control; CS: Cross-sectional; RCT: Randomized controlled trial; M: Males; F: Females; EPA: Eicosapentaenoic acid; DHA: Docosahexaenoic acid; D5D: Delta-5 desaturase; D6D: Delta-6 desaturase; FA: Fatty acid; LTB: Leukotriene B$_4$; 5-HETE: 5-hydroxyeicosatetraenoic acid; CRC: Colorectal cancer; FR: Food recall; AA: Arachidonic acid; DGLA: Di-homo gamma linolenic acid; DPA: Docosapentaenoic acid; LDL: Low density lipoprotein; oxLDL: oxidized LDL; ETA: Eicosantetraenoic acid; ALA: Alpha-linolenic acid; PGF$_{2a}$: Prostaglandin F$_{2a}$; PUFA: Polyunsaturated fatty acid; NS: Non-significant; SQ: Semi-quantitative; FFQ: Food frequency questionnaire; BCa: Breast cancer; PCa: Prostate cancer.

3. The Role of Genetic Variation in Fatty Acid Desaturation

The *FADS* gene cluster is located on a highly polymorphic region of chromosome 11 and includes *FADS1* and *FADS2*, which encode delta 5 desaturase (D5D) and delta 6 desaturase (D6D), respectively [9]. These polymorphisms create a diverse set of haplotypes. The first demonstration of a relationship between *FADS* genotype and membrane-bound FAs was shown by Schaefer *et al.* (2006) [54] in serum phospholipids. Further evidence came from a study on infants, in which Danish infants carrying the *FADS* minor allele for locus rs1535 had a higher DHA level than those with the wild-type allele [55]. In contrast, those carrying the minor alleles of rs174448 (C) and rs174575 (G) had decreased DHA levels relative to wild-type [55]. Similarly, carriers of the T allele at rs174537 (in strong linkage disequilibrium with rs174546 and rs3834458) had lower levels of AA than the carriers of the G allele [37]. Additional examples have been presented by Al-Hilal *et al.* (2013) in which the minor allele of SNPs rs174537, rs174561 and rs3834458 correlate with higher amounts of ALA and lower levels of EPA, docosapentaenoic acid (DPA) and DHA, as well as lower activity of both D5D and D6D [14].

Of particular interest to the interplay with dietary LC*n*-3 PUFA, a 6-month intervention of an EPA/DHA supplement in individuals carrying a T allele at locus rs174537 showed rising activity of D5D with an increasing supplement dose [14]. Additionally, polymorphisms at *FADS* locus rs174546 correlated with serum triacylglycerides at baseline and 6 weeks following EPA/DHA supplementation [56]. At locus rs174537, the presence of a T-allele correlated with lower levels of AA, consistent with a similar study [37], and those carrying the GG genotype had higher levels of eicosanoids leukotriene B_4 (LTB$_4$) and 5-hydroxyeicosatetraenoic acid (5-HETE) [13]. LTB$_4$ and 5-HETE are pro-inflammatory compounds synthesized from AA by the leukotriene synthase and 5-LOX enzymes, respectively [39]. Therefore, it is possible that levels of circulating eicosanoids may be modulated by the interplay of diet and genotype. If these individuals are at particular risk for cancer, it would be advisable to increase the intake of LC*n*-3 PUFA.

Studies on colonic mucosal fatty acid compositions have revealed a diet-genotype effect. Lower concentrations of AA were observed in subjects carrying major alleles within the *FADS* gene cluster (rs174556 and rs174561 in *FADS1*, rs383445 in *FADS2* and rs174537 of the *FADS1/2* intragenic region) when consuming a Mediterranean diet compared to a Healthy Eating diet, due to increases in AA levels within the Healthy Eating group [53]. The Mediterranean diet has been extensively studied with regards to its effect on cancers. This diet is traditionally high in fat, but low in LC*n*-6 PUFA and *trans* fatty acids, and is typically high in olive oil, fresh fruit and vegetables [57,58]. The Mediterranean diet used in an intervention by Porenta *et al.* (2013) [53] was also high in fish and flaxseed. Additional studies are required to confirm these results, as diets were not strictly controlled and sample size was relatively small. A summary of the interaction between LC*n*-3 PUFA on prostate, breast and colorectal cancers as modified by *FADS* genotype, is provided in Table 1, alongside additionally discussed genotypes.

4. Genetic Polymorphisms Modulate Leukotriene Synthesis in Cancer

4.1. Lipoxygenases

Leukotrienes are eicosanoid inflammatory mediators produced by the oxidation of AA, and are implicated in inflammation and cancer [59]. Leukotriene synthesis begins with the formation of hydroperoxyeicosatetranoic acid (5-HPETE) and hydroperoxyeicosapentaenoic acid (5-HPEPE) from AA and EPA, respectively, by the lipoxygenases [16]. Although not statistically significant, a lower risk for colon cancer was demonstrated in wild-type homozygous individuals at locus rs11568131 of *ALOX15* when consuming high amounts of fish, an association that was absent in those carrying the variant allele [11]. Carriers of a G minor allele at locus rs11571339 of the *ALOX12* gene showed a lower risk for rectal cancer in those with low *n*-3 PUFA intake compared to higher intakes [11]. However, G allele carriers with high intakes showed no increased risk compared to the homozygous major allele reference group. Despite also demonstrating no statistical significance, this finding is particularly interesting, as a lower LCn-3 PUFA intake would generate fewer anti-inflammatory compounds than a higher intake. Furthermore, G allele carriers with lower intakes of LA and total PUFA showed a similar pattern. Studies investigating the differences in activity of 12-lipoxygenase due to this polymorphism could help to explain these findings.

A recent meta-analysis found that polymorphisms in the *ALOX12* gene at the Gln261Arg locus may influence cancer risk in Asian populations but not in Caucasians [60]. Furthermore, carriers of the variant in homozygous or heterozygous form had an increased risk for breast cancer, also demonstrating differences across ethnic populations [61]. The same polymorphism also showed an association with risk of colorectal adenomas [62]. To our knowledge, the interplay of this polymorphism with EPA/DHA intake has not been previously explored and is worthy of further investigation.

4.2. Glutathione S-Transferases

The glutathione S-transferase (GST) enzymes implicated in various types of cancer are important for the detoxification of environmental pollutants and chemical carcinogens, and modulate signaling of pathways associated with cell proliferation, cell differentiation and apoptosis [47]. In addition, GSTs are involved in the synthesis of leukotrienes from 5-HPETE. Finally, GSTs are also important for the detoxification of reactive oxygen species [63] and may help protect against DNA damage [64].

Raised levels of anti-oxidants can help activate *GST* genes and this in turn may help to reduce the increased levels of DNA damage that are associated with prostate cancer [36,64]. *GST* phenotype (e.g., *GSTT1* null genotype) is associated with risk of prostate cancer in Caucasians but this does not hold true for other races [47]. Unfortunately, no evidence appears to be available with respect to the modification of this effect by fatty acids in prostate cancer. However, van Hemelrijck *et al.* (2012) [65] identified an association between prostate cancer and the intake of heterocyclic aromatic amines (HCAs) that was modified by the genotype of HCA-metabolizing enzymes (e.g., *MnSOD* rs4880 and *GPX4* rs713041). HCAs are mutagenic and are generated by cooking meat at high temperatures [66]. Meat is a common source of animal fat and the effect of some monounsaturated fatty acids (e.g., palmitic and stearic acids) as well as n-6 PUFA (e.g., AA) on prostate cancer may be confounded by the presence of HCAs. For this reason, we propose that while the genotype of HCA-metabolizing enzymes may appear to interact with type of fatty acid intake and prostate cancer risk, in fact it is the presence of HCAs that is interacting with genotype to influence disease risk.

In contrast, a clear association has been shown between the polymorphic *GST* genes, breast cancer and marine FA intake [49]. Women carrying variants resulting in higher activity of the GST enzymes show a correlation with marine n-3 PUFA intake and risk of breast cancer, in which lower intake demonstrates a higher risk compared to those with higher intakes of the same genotypes. These associations were found in Chinese and Singaporean women [49].

5. Prostaglandin Synthesis

Cyclooxygenase enzymes, also known as prostaglandin endoperoxide synthases, catalyse the rate-limited formation of inflammatory prostaglandins. Two isozymes (*COX1* and *COX2*) exist, both of which are associated with injury and inflammation and demonstrate different tissue expression patterns [12]. Increased expression of *COX2* leads to hyperproliferation of colon epithelial cells, a process which was decreased following the presence of EPA [67]. Furthermore, the inhibitory effects of non-steroidal anti-inflammatory drugs (NSAIDs) associated with colorectal cancer are thought to relate to their inhibitory activity at both *COX1* and *COX2* [68].

In vitro studies have shown inhibitory actions of LCn-3 PUFA on prostate cancer cell growth. In different prostate cancer cell models, namely LNCaP and PacMetUT1, DHA appeared to sensitise the cells by attenuating the NF-κB survival pathway that promotes cancer cell survival, resulting in decreased cancer cell survival [69]. On the other hand, NF-κB does not appear to be involved in the induction of *COX2* expression in the prostate cancer cells, PC3, treated with DHA and EPA [70]. In regards to human studies, five of sixteen SNPs found within the *COX2* region were tested in a Swedish population with and without prostate cancer, identifying a relationship between two SNPs and the presence of prostate cancer [50,71]. Subsequently, the same authors demonstrated that the presence of a C allele at locus rs5275 was significantly associated with a decreased risk of prostate cancer in men with a high intake of fatty fish [50]. Similarly, Fradet *et al.* (2009) [12] assessed diet alongside nine *COX2* SNPs in men diagnosed with aggressive prostate cancer and found that LC*n*-3 PUFA intake was strongly associated with a decreased risk of aggressive prostate cancer. This effect was modified by the rs4648310 SNP, such that the increased risk of aggressive prostate cancer associated with a low intake of *n*-3 PUFA in those with the G allele (odds ratio = 5.49) could be reversed by increasing *n*-3 PUFA intake [12]. Therefore, it is reasonable to say that carriers of a G allele at the rs4648310 locus could benefit from increasing LC*n*-3 PUFA intake.

COX1 SNPs at the rs10306110 locus may modulate colon cancer risk. Habermann *et al.* (2013) [11] demonstrated an association between low LC*n*-3 PUFA intake and the variant allele, with an odds ratio of 1.56 and 1.62 for EPA and DHA, respectively. Total and monounsaturated fatty acid intake was associated with the variant allele at rs10306122 of *PTGS1*, the gene encoding *COX1*, and increased rectal cancer risk, although marine LC PUFA showed no effect [11].

The P17L polymorphism, leading to sequence changes within the signal peptide of *COX1*, was associated with risk of colorectal adenomas, in which higher fish intake in those homozygous for phenylalanine at position 17 had a modestly lower risk of adenomas with increasing fish intake [51]. Interestingly, those carrying at least one leucine at position 17 had a decreased risk of adenomas when consuming less fish per week [51]. Importantly, these individuals demonstrated a higher risk for colorectal cancer with increasing fish intake. This is a highly interesting finding which highlights the occurrence of inconsistencies in studies of cancer and LC*n*-3 PUFA and the importance of designing and performing studies that will provide clarity in this regard.

The same authors [51] then analysed the risk of colorectal adenomas between those in an assumed low risk group (high fish intake + NSAID use) and an assumed high risk group (low fish intake + no NSAID use) and variable intermediate groups, to assess the dual implications of both NSAID use and fish intake in the relationship between P17L polymorphisms and adenoma risk. PP homozygotes benefited from including more than 2 servings of fish per week as well as regular use of NSAIDs. However, those with PL and LL genotypes showed no statistically significant associations [51]. These findings are unexpected and it is necessary to replicate these investigations in larger studies with more detail on type of fish in the diet, as well as other dietary information.

Polymorphisms within the gene for *prostaglandin E$_2$ synthase-1 (PGES)* also correlate with colorectal adenoma risk. *PGES* catalyses the formation of PGE$_2$, a pro-inflammatory prostaglandin associated with increased cell proliferation [72,73]. Individuals carrying a T allele at rs7873087 had a lower risk for colorectal adenomas with increasing fish intake, whereas those homozygous for the A allele showed no significant association with fish intake [52]. Additional relationships were observed for polymorphisms within the *15-hydroxyprostaglandin dehydrogenase* gene and the *EP4 receptor* gene, which code for proteins responsible for the breakdown of PGE$_2$ and the corresponding PGE$_2$ receptor, respectively. These studies highlight the importance of inter individual differences in genes involved in the prostaglandin synthesis pathways from AA and EPA, and their complex association with colorectal cancer and fish intake. This relationship warrants further investigation.

Limitations in these studies include recall bias in the FFQ and diet diaries, which are commonly used in large studies such as cohorts or case-control designs due to lack of affordable and better alternatives. Furthermore, ethnicity must be adjusted for in studies, as ethnicity may influence the relationship between dietary *n*-3 PUFA, cancer risk and genotype, as highlighted earlier [60,61]. Additional factors potentially influencing the outcome of the studies reviewed herein, include the stage of the disease, as LC*n*-3 PUFA may interact differently with genotypes as the physiology of the tumour changes, and fish contaminants. Dioxins may increase cancer risk, which could generate substantial confounding [33]. In addition, it is important to note that this review highlights the current knowledge of the interplay between genes involved in eicosanoid synthesis only, and that there are a range of other genes that are likely to contribute to the relationship between cancer risk and LCn-3 PUFA intake, such as polymorphisms in DNA repair- and apoptosis-related genes [74].

6. Conclusions

The effects of LCn-3 PUFA on prostate, breast and colorectal cancer modified by genotype are presented in Table 1. It is clear that both dietary intake and polymorphisms of the *FADS* genes contribute to the concentrations of membrane-bound fatty acids such as EPA, DHA and AA. Although genetic variation within the *FADS* genes have not been directly associated with cancer, the effects on desaturase activity may influence the production of eicosanoids further downstream. Dietary LCn-3 PUFA (EPA, DPA and DHA) are inversely associated with aggressive prostate cancer [12] and prostate cancer risk. This protective effect can be modified by genotype including rs5275 [50] and rs4648310 [12] in *COX2*. On the other hand, the loss of expression of *FADS2*, in response to a mutation in *FAD2*, is associated with a more aggressive breast cancer tumour and reduced survival [9,75]. Breast cancer risk may also be modulated by dietary LCn-3 PUFA and activity of the GST enzymes [49]. Interestingly, an association between *ALOX12* polymorphisms and breast cancer, which was modified by ethnicity [60,61] could be further explored in regards to the relationship with LCn-3 PUFA intake. In regards to colon and rectal cancers, certain individuals may benefit largely from including LCn-3 PUFA in their diets while others do not, as demonstrated by polymorphisms in *ALOX12*, *ALOX15* and *PGES* genes [11,52]. Furthermore, there exists a positive association between increased risk of colorectal cancers and increased fish intake in some genotypes of the *COX1* gene, a relationship worthy of further investigation.

Compelling evidence from *in vivo* and *in vitro* studies has been presented on the inhibition of cancer progression. Here, evidence has been presented on the genotypic modification of response to LCn-3 PUFA and it is clear that we are on the brink of offering personalised nutritional advice with respect to these FAs. Such advice would ensure that people are correctly informed with respect to the types and amounts of LCn-3 PUFA they should consume in order to meet their specific requirements. In addition, further study could decipher the significance of the role of n-3 PUFA in cancer and inflammation, for example whether altered PUFA metabolism is a driver or a passenger in cancer [76].

Acknowledgments: The financial support of the Auckland Cancer Society Research Centre, Auckland, to KSB and LRF, is acknowledged.

Author Contributions: Georgia Lenihan-Geels and Karen S. Bishop conceived of the idea, conducted the literature search and wrote the article. Lynnette R. Ferguson edited the manuscript and provided guidance.

References

1. Ferlay, J.; Shin, H.-R.; Bray, F.; Forman, D.; Mathers, C.; Parkin, D.M. Estimates of worldwide burden of cancer in 2008: GLOBOCAN 2008. *Int. J. Cancer* **2010**, *127*, 2893–2917. [CrossRef] [PubMed]
2. Yu, Y.; Zheng, S.; Zhang, S.; Jin, W.; Liu, H.; Jin, M.; Chen, Z.; Ding, Z.; Wang, L.; Chen, K. Polymorphisms of inflammation-related genes and colorectal cancer risk: A population-based case-control study in China. *Int. J. Immunogenet.* **2014**, *41*, 289–297. [CrossRef] [PubMed]
3. De Marzo, A.M.; Platz, E.A.; Sutcliffe, S.; Xu, J.; Grönberg, H.; Drake, C.G.; Nakai, Y.; Isaacs, W.B.; Nelson, W.G. Inflammation in prostate carcinogenesis. *Nat. Rev. Cancer* **2007**, *7*, 256–269. [CrossRef] [PubMed]
4. Baena, R.; Salinas, P. Diet and colorectal cancer. *Maturitas* **2015**, *80*, 258–264. [CrossRef] [PubMed]
5. Shivappa, N.; Hébert, J.R.; Zucchetto, A.; Montella, M.; Serraino, D.; La Vecchia, C.; Rossi, M. Dietary inflammatory index and endometrial cancer risk in an Italian case-control study. *Br. J. Nutr.* **2015**, *115*, 138–146. [CrossRef] [PubMed]
6. Dasilva, G.; Pazos, M.; García-Egido, E.; Gallardo, J.M.; Rodríguez, I.; Cela, R.; Medina, I. Healthy effect of different proportions of marine ω-3 PUFAs EPA and DHA supplementation in Wistar rats: Lipidomic biomarkers of oxidative stress and inflammation. *J. Nutr. Biochem.* **2015**, *26*, 1385–1392. [CrossRef] [PubMed]

7.   Pelser, C.; Mondul, A.M.; Hollenbeck, A.R.; Park, Y. Dietary fat, fatty acids, and risk of prostate cancer in the NIH-AARP diet and health study. *Cancer Epidemiol. Biomark. Prev.* **2013**, *22*, 697–707. [CrossRef] [PubMed]

8.   Richman, E.L.; Kenfield, S.A.; Chavarro, J.E.; Stampfer, M.J.; Giovannucci, E.L.; Willett, W.C.; Chan, J.M. Fat intake after diagnosis and risk of lethal prostate cancer and all-cause mortality. *JAMA Intern. Med.* **2013**, *173*, 1318–1326. [CrossRef] [PubMed]

9.   Azrad, M.; Turgeon, C.; Demark-Wahnefried, W. Current evidence linking polyunsaturated Fatty acids with cancer risk and progression. *Front. Oncol.* **2013**, *3*, 224. [CrossRef] [PubMed]

10.   Burdge, G.C.; Calder, P.C. Conversion of alpha-linolenic acid to longer-chain polyunsaturated fatty acids in human adults. *Reprod. Nutr. Dev.* **2005**, *45*, 581–597. [CrossRef] [PubMed]

11.   Habermann, N.; Ulrich, C.M.; Lundgreen, A.; Makar, K.W.; Poole, E.M.; Caan, B.; Kulmacz, R.; Whitton, J.; Galbraith, R.; Potter, J.D.; *et al.* PTGS1, PTGS2, ALOX5, ALOX12, ALOX15, and FLAP SNPs: Interaction with fatty acids in colon cancer and rectal cancer. *Genes Nutr.* **2013**, *8*, 115–126. [CrossRef] [PubMed]

12.   Fradet, V.; Cheng, I.; Casey, G.; Witte, J.S. Dietary omega-3 fatty acids, cyclooxygenase-2 genetic variation, and aggressive prostate cancer risk. *Clin. Cancer Res.* **2009**, *15*, 2559–2566. [CrossRef] [PubMed]

13.   Hester, A.G.; Murphy, R.C.; Uhlson, C.J.; Ivester, P.; Lee, T.C.; Sergeant, S.; Miller, L.R.; Howard, T.D.; Mathias, R.A.; Chilton, F.H. Relationship between a common variant in the fatty acid desaturase (FADS) cluster and eicosanoid generation in humans. *J. Biol. Chem.* **2014**, *289*, 22482–22489. [CrossRef] [PubMed]

14.   Al-Hilal, M.; Alsaleh, A.; Maniou, Z.; Lewis, F.J.; Hall, W.L.; Sanders, T.A.B.; O'Dell, S.D. Genetic variation at the FADS1-FADS2 gene locus influences delta-5 desaturase activity and LC-PUFA proportions after fish oil supplement. *J. Lipid Res.* **2013**, *54*, 542–551. [CrossRef] [PubMed]

15.   Lenihan-Geels, G.; Bishop, K.S.; Ferguson, L.R. Alternative sources of omega-3 fats: Can we find a sustainable substitute for fish? *Nutrients* **2013**, *5*, 1301–1315. [CrossRef] [PubMed]

16.   Szefel, J.; Piotrowska, M.; Kruszewski, W.J.; Jankun, J.; Lysiak-Szydlowska, W.; Skrzypczak-Jankun, E. Eicosanoids in Prevention and Management of Diseases. *Curr. Mol. Med.* **2011**, *11*, 13–25. [CrossRef] [PubMed]

17.   Pischon, T.; Hankinson, S.E.; Hotamisligil, G.S.; Rifai, N.; Willett, W.C.; Rimm, E.B. Habitual dietary intake of *n*-3 and *n*-6 fatty acids in relation to inflammatory markers among US men and women. *Circulation* **2003**, *108*, 155–160. [CrossRef] [PubMed]

18.   Yli-Jama, P.; Seljeflot, I.; Meyer, H.E.; Hjerkinn, E.M.; Arnesen, H.; Pedersen, J.I. Serum non-esterified very long-chain PUFA are associated with markers of endothelial dysfunction. *Atherosclerosis* **2002**, *164*, 275–281. [CrossRef]

19.   Ferrucci, L.; Cherubini, A.; Bandinelli, S.; Bartali, B.; Corsi, A.; Lauretani, F.; Martin, A.; Andres-Lacueva, C.; Senin, U.; Guralnik, J.M. Relationship of Plasma Polyunsaturated Fatty Acids to Circulating Inflammatory Markers. *J. Clin. Endocrinol. Metable.* **2006**, *91*, 439–446. [CrossRef] [PubMed]

20.   Calder, P.C.; Ahluwalia, N.; Brouns, F.; Buetler, T.; Clement, K.; Cunningham, K.; Esposito, K.; Jönsson, L.S.; Kolb, H.; Lansink, M.; *et al.* Dietary factors and low-grade inflammation in relation to overweight and obesity. *Br. J. Nutr.* **2011**, *106*, S5–S78. [CrossRef] [PubMed]

21.   Tuncer, S.; Banerjee, S. Eicosanoid pathway in colorectal cancer: Recent updates. *World J. Gastroenterol.* **2015**, *21*, 11748–11766. [CrossRef] [PubMed]

22.   Wang, W.; Zhu, J.; Lyu, F.; Panigrahy, D.; Ferrara, K.W.; Hammock, B.; Zhang, G. ω-3 polyunsaturated fatty acids-derived lipid metabolites on angiogenesis, inflammation and cancer. *Prostaglandins Other Lipid Mediat.* **2014**, *113*, 13–20. [CrossRef] [PubMed]

23.   Hanahan, D.; Weinberg, R.A. Hallmarks of cancer: the next generation. *Cell* **2011**, *144*, 646–674. [CrossRef] [PubMed]

24.   Mazhar, D.; Ang, R.; Waxman, J. COX inhibitors and breast cancer. *Br. J. Cancer* **2006**, *94*, 346–350. [CrossRef] [PubMed]

25.   Eberhart, C.E.; Coffey, R.J.; Radhika, A.; Giardiello, F.M.; Ferrenbach, S.; DuBois, R.N. Up-regulation of cyclooxygenase 2 gene expression in human colorectal adenomas and adenocarcinomas. *Gastroenterology* **1994**, *107*, 1183–1188. [PubMed]

26.   Kleinstein, S.E.; Heath, L.; Makar, K.W.; Poole, E.M.; Seufert, B.L.; Slattery, M.L.; Xiao, L.; Duggan, D.J.; Hsu, L.; Curtin, K.; *et al.* Genetic variation in the lipoxygenase pathway and risk of colorectal neoplasia. *Genes. Chromosomes Cancer* **2013**, *52*, 437–449. [CrossRef] [PubMed]

27. Augustsson, K.; Michaud, D.S.; Rimm, E.B.; Leitzmann, M.F.; Stampfer, M.J.; Willett, W.C.; Giovannucci, E. A prospective study of intake of fish and marine fatty acids and prostate cancer. *Cancer Epidemiol. Biomark. Prev.* **2003**, *12*, 64–67.

28. Kantor, E.D.; Lampe, J.W.; Peters, U.; Vaughan, T.L.; White, E. Long-chain omega-3 polyunsaturated fatty acid intake and risk of colorectal cancer. *Nutr. Cancer* **2014**, *66*, 716–727. [CrossRef] [PubMed]

29. Catsburg, C.; Joshi, A.D.; Corral, R.; Lewinger, J.P.; Koo, J.; John, E.M.; Ingles, S.A.; Stern, M.C. Polymorphisms in carcinogen metabolism enzymes, fish intake, and risk of prostate cancer. *Carcinogenesis* **2012**, *33*, 1352–1359. [CrossRef] [PubMed]

30. Wallström, P.; Bjartell, A.; Gullberg, B.; Olsson, H.; Wirfält, E. A prospective study on dietary fat and incidence of prostate cancer (Malmö, Sweden). *Cancer Causes Control* **2007**, *18*, 1107–1121. [CrossRef] [PubMed]

31. Corella, D.; Ordovás, J.M. Interactions between dietary *n*-3 fatty acids and genetic variants and risk of disease. *Br. J. Nutr.* **2012**, *107*, S271–S283. [CrossRef] [PubMed]

32. Von Schacky, C. Omega-3 index and cardiovascular health. *Nutrients* **2014**, *6*, 799–814. [CrossRef] [PubMed]

33. World Health Organization. Exposure to Dioxins and Dioxin-like Substances: A Major Public Health Concern. Available online: http://www.who.int/ipcs/features/dioxins.pdf (accessed on 14 January 2016).

34. White, M.C.; Holman, D.M.; Boehm, J.E.; Peipins, L.A.; Grossman, M.; Jane Henley, S. Age and Cancer Risk. *Am. J. Prev. Med.* **2014**, *46*, S7–S15. [CrossRef] [PubMed]

35. Tintle, N.L.; Pottala, J.V.; Lacey, S.; Ramachandran, V.; Westra, J.; Rogers, A.; Clark, J.; Olthoff, B.; Larson, M.; Harris, W.; Shearer, G.C. A genome-wide association study of saturated, mono- and polyunsaturated red blood cell fatty acids in the Framingham Heart Offspring Study. *Prostaglandins Leukot. Essent. Fatty Acids* **2015**, *94*, 65–72. [CrossRef] [PubMed]

36. Bishop, K.S.; Erdrich, S.; Karunasinghe, N.; Han, D.Y.; Zhu, S.; Jesuthasan, A.; Ferguson, L.R. An investigation into the association between DNA damage and dietary fatty acid in men with prostate cancer. *Nutrients* **2015**, *7*, 405–422. [CrossRef] [PubMed]

37. Hong, S.H.; Kwak, J.H.; Paik, J.K.; Chae, J.S.; Lee, J.H. Association of polymorphisms in FADS gene with age-related changes in serum phospholipid polyunsaturated fatty acids and oxidative stress markers in middle-aged nonobese men. *Clin. Interv. Aging* **2013**, *8*, 585–596. [PubMed]

38. Chilton, F.H.; Murphy, R.C.; Wilson, B.A.; Sergeant, S.; Ainsworth, H.; Seeds, M.C.; Mathias, R.A. Diet-gene interactions and PUFA metabolism: A potential contributor to health disparities and human diseases. *Nutrients* **2014**, *6*, 1993–2022. [CrossRef] [PubMed]

39. Simopoulos, A.P. Genetic variants in the metabolism of omega-6 and omega-3 fatty acids: their role in the determination of nutritional requirements and chronic disease risk. *Exp. Biol. Med. (Maywood)* **2010**, *235*, 785–795. [CrossRef] [PubMed]

40. Zhang, C.; Yu, H.; Ni, X.; Shen, S.; Das, U.N. Growth inhibitory effect of polyunsaturated fatty acids (PUFAs) on colon cancer cells via their growth inhibitory metabolites and fatty acid composition changes. *PLoS ONE* **2015**, *10*, e0123256. [CrossRef] [PubMed]

41. Mansara, P.P.; Deshpande, R.A.; Vaidya, M.M.; Kaul-Ghanekar, R. Differential Ratios of Omega Fatty Acids (AA/EPA + DHA) Modulate Growth, Lipid Peroxidation and Expression of Tumor Regulatory MARBPs in Breast Cancer Cell Lines MCF7 and MDA-MB-231. *PLoS ONE* **2015**, *10*, e0136542. [CrossRef] [PubMed]

42. Rose, D.P.; Connolly, J.M. Effects of fatty acids and eicosanoid synthesis inhibitors on the growth of two human prostate cancer cell lines. *Prostate* **1991**, *18*, 243–254. [CrossRef] [PubMed]

43. Akinsete, J.A.; Ion, G.; Witte, T.R.; Hardman, W.E. Consumption of high ω-3 fatty acid diet suppressed prostate tumorigenesis in C3(1) Tag mice. *Carcinogenesis* **2012**, *33*, 140–148. [CrossRef] [PubMed]

44. Van Beelen, V.A.; Spenkelink, B.; Mooibroek, H.; Sijtsma, L.; Bosch, D.; Rietjens, I.M.; Alink, G.M. An *n*-3 PUFA-rich microalgal oil diet protects to a similar extent as a fish oil-rich diet against AOM-induced colonic aberrant crypt foci in F344 rats. *Food Chem. Toxicol.* **2009**, *47*, 316–320. [CrossRef] [PubMed]

45. Leslie, M.A.; Abdelmagid, S.A.; Perez, K.; Muller, W.J.; Ma, D.W. Mammary tumour development is dose-dependently inhibited by *n*-3 polyunsaturated fatty acids in the MMTV-neu(ndl)-YD5 transgenic mouse model. *Lipids Health Dis.* **2014**, *13*, 96. [CrossRef] [PubMed]

46. Glaser, C.; Rzehak, P.; Demmelmair, H.; Klopp, N.; Heinrich, J.; Koletzko, B. Influence of FADS polymorphisms on tracking of serum glycerophospholipid fatty acid concentrations and percentage composition in children. *PLoS ONE* **2011**, *6*, e21933. [CrossRef] [PubMed]

47. Zhou, T.-B.; Drummen, G.P.C.; Jiang, Z.-P.; Qin, Y.-H. GSTT1 polymorphism and the risk of developing prostate cancer. *Am. J. Epidemiol.* **2014**, *180*, 1–10. [CrossRef] [PubMed]

48. Chen, C. COX-2's new role in inflammation. *Nat. Chem. Biol.* **2010**, *6*, 401–402. [CrossRef] [PubMed]

49. Gago-Dominguez, M. Marine *n*-3 fatty acid intake, glutathione S-transferase polymorphisms and breast cancer risk in post-menopausal Chinese women in Singapore. *Carcinogenesis* **2004**, *25*, 2143–2147. [CrossRef] [PubMed]

50. Hedelin, M.; Chang, E.T.; Wiklund, F.; Bellocco, R.; Klint, A.; Adolfsson, J.; Shahedi, K.; Xu, J.; Adami, H.-O.; Grönberg, H.; Bälter, K.A. Association of frequent consumption of fatty fish with prostate cancer risk is modified by COX-2 polymorphism. *Int. J. Cancer* **2007**, *120*, 398–405. [CrossRef] [PubMed]

51. Poole, E.M.; Bigler, J.; Whitton, J.; Sibert, J.G.; Kulmacz, R.J.; Potter, J.D.; Ulrich, C.M. Genetic variability in prostaglandin synthesis, fish intake and risk of colorectal polyps. *Carcinogenesis* **2007**, *28*, 1259–1263. [CrossRef] [PubMed]

52. Poole, E.M.; Hsu, L.; Xiao, L.; Kulmacz, R.J.; Carlson, C.S.; Rabinovitch, P.S.; Makar, K.W.; Potter, J.D.; Ulrich, C.M. Genetic variation in prostaglandin E2 synthesis and signaling, prostaglandin dehydrogenase, and the risk of colorectal adenoma. *Cancer Epidemiol. Biomark. Prev.* **2010**, *19*, 547–557. [CrossRef] [PubMed]

53. Porenta, S.R.; Ko, Y.-A.; Gruber, S.B.; Mukherjee, B.; Baylin, A.; Ren, J.; Djuric, Z. Interaction of fatty acid genotype and diet on changes in colonic fatty acids in a Mediterranean diet intervention study. *Cancer Prev. Res. (Phila)* **2013**, *6*, 1212–1221. [CrossRef] [PubMed]

54. Schaeffer, L.; Gohlke, H.; Müller, M.; Heid, I.M.; Palmer, L.J.; Kompauer, I.; Demmelmair, H.; Illig, T.; Koletzko, B.; Heinrich, J. Common genetic variants of the FADS1 FADS2 gene cluster and their reconstructed haplotypes are associated with the fatty acid composition in phospholipids. *Hum. Mol. Genet.* **2006**, *15*, 1745–1756. [CrossRef] [PubMed]

55. Harsløf, L.B.S.; Larsen, L.H.; Ritz, C.; Hellgren, L.I.; Michaelsen, K.F.; Vogel, U.; Lauritzen, L. FADS genotype and diet are important determinants of DHA status: a cross-sectional study in Danish infants. *Am. J. Clin. Nutr.* **2013**, *97*, 1403–1410. [CrossRef] [PubMed]

56. Cormier, H.; Rudkowska, I.; Paradis, A.-M.; Thifault, E.; Garneau, V.; Lemieux, S.; Couture, P.; Vohl, M.-C. Association between polymorphisms in the fatty acid desaturase gene cluster and the plasma triacylglycerol response to an *n*-3 PUFA supplementation. *Nutrients* **2012**, *4*, 1026–1041. [CrossRef] [PubMed]

57. Davis, C.; Bryan, J.; Hodgson, J.; Murphy, K. Definition of the Mediterranean Diet; A Literature Review. *Nutrients* **2015**, *7*, 9139–9153. [CrossRef] [PubMed]

58. Trichopoulou, A.; Costacou, T.; Bamia, C.; Trichopoulos, D. Adherence to a Mediterranean diet and survival in a Greek population. *N. Engl. J. Med.* **2003**, *348*, 2599–2608. [CrossRef] [PubMed]

59. Wang, D.; Dubois, R.N. Eicosanoids and cancer. *Nat. Rev. Cancer* **2010**, *10*, 181–193. [CrossRef] [PubMed]

60. Shan, D.; Shen, K.; Zhu, J.; Feng, M.; Wu, Y.; Wan, C.; Shen, Y.; Xu, L. The polymorphism (Gln261Arg) of 12-lipoxygenase and cancer risk: A meta-analysis. *Int. J. Clin. Exp. Med.* **2015**, *8*, 488–495. [PubMed]

61. Prasad, V.V.; Kolli, P.; Moganti, D. Association of a functional polymorphism (Gln261Arg) in 12-lipoxygenase with breast cancer. *Exp. Ther. Med.* **2011**, *2*, 317–323. [CrossRef] [PubMed]

62. Gong, Z.; Hebert, J.R.; Bostick, R.M.; Deng, Z.; Hurley, T.G.; Dixon, D.A.; Nitcheva, D.; Xie, D. Common polymorphisms in 5-lipoxygenase and 12-lipoxygenase genes and the risk of incident, sporadic colorectal adenoma. *Cancer* **2007**, *109*, 849–857. [CrossRef] [PubMed]

63. Jin, Y.; Hao, Z. Polymorphisms of glutathione S-transferase M1 (GSTM1) and T1 (GSTT1) in ovarian cancer risk. *Tumour Biol.* **2014**, *35*, 5267–5272. [CrossRef] [PubMed]

64. Kanwal, R.; Pandey, M.; Bhaskaran, N.; Maclennan, G.T.; Fu, P.; Ponsky, L.E.; Gupta, S. Protection against oxidative DNA damage and stress in human prostate by glutathione S-transferase P1. *Mol. Carcinog.* **2014**, *53*, 8–18. [CrossRef] [PubMed]

65. Van Hemelrijck, M.; Rohrmann, S.; Steinbrecher, A.; Kaaks, R.; Teucher, B.; Linseisen, J. Heterocyclic aromatic amine [HCA] intake and prostate cancer risk: effect modification by genetic variants. *Nutr. Cancer* **2012**, *64*, 704–713. [CrossRef] [PubMed]

66. John, E.; Stern, M.; Sinha, R.; Koo, J. Meat Consumption, Cooking Practices, Meat Mutagens, and Risk of Prostate Cancer. *Nutr. Cancer* **2011**, *63*, 525–537. [CrossRef] [PubMed]

67. Yu, W.; Murray, N.R.; Weems, C.; Chen, L.; Guo, H.; Ethridge, R.; Ceci, J.D.; Evers, B.M.; Thompson, E.A.; Fields, A.P. Role of cyclooxygenase 2 in protein kinase C beta II-mediated colon carcinogenesis. *J. Biol. Chem.* **2003**, *278*, 11167–11174. [CrossRef] [PubMed]

68. Thun, M.J.; Henley, S.J.; Patrono, C. Nonsteroidal anti-inflammatory drugs as anticancer agents: Mechanistic, pharmacologic, and clinical issues. *J. Natl. Cancer Inst.* **2002**, *94*, 252–266. [CrossRef] [PubMed]

69. Cavazos, D.A.; Price, R.S.; Apte, S.S.; deGraffenried, L.A. Docosahexaenoic acid selectively induces human prostate cancer cell sensitivity to oxidative stress through modulation of NF-κB. *Prostate* **2011**, *71*, 1420–1428. [CrossRef] [PubMed]

70. Eser, P.O.; Vanden Heuvel, J.P.; Araujo, J.; Thompson, J.T. Marine- and plant-derived ω-3 fatty acids differentially regulate prostate cancer cell proliferation. *Mol. Clin. Oncol.* **2013**, *1*, 444–452. [PubMed]

71. Shahedi, K.; Lindström, S.; Zheng, S.L.; Wiklund, F.; Adolfsson, J.; Sun, J.; Augustsson-Bälter, K.; Chang, B.-L.; Adami, H.-O.; Liu, W.; Grönberg, H.; Xu, J. Genetic variation in the COX-2 gene and the association with prostate cancer risk. *Int. J. Cancer* **2006**, *119*, 668–672. [CrossRef] [PubMed]

72. Qiao, L.; Kozoni, V.; Tsioulias, G.J.; Koutsos, M.I.; Hanif, R.; Shiff, S.J.; Rigas, B. Selected eicosanoids increase the proliferation rate of human colon carcinoma cell lines and mouse colonocytes *in vivo*. *Biochim. Biophys. Acta* **1995**, *1258*, 215–223. [CrossRef]

73. Sheng, H.; Shao, J.; Washington, M.K.; DuBois, R.N. Prostaglandin E2 increases growth and motility of colorectal carcinoma cells. *J. Biol. Chem.* **2001**, *276*, 18075–18081. [CrossRef] [PubMed]

74. Stern, M.C.; Butler, L.M.; Corral, R.; Joshi, A.D.; Yuan, J.-M.; Koh, W.-P.; Yu, M.C. Polyunsaturated fatty acids, DNA repair single nucleotide polymorphisms and colorectal cancer in the Singapore Chinese Health Study. *J. Nutrigenet. Nutrigenom.* **2009**, *2*, 273–279. [CrossRef] [PubMed]

75. Lane, J.; Mansel, R.E.; Jiang, W.G. Expression of human delta-6-desaturase is associated with aggressiveness of human breast cancer. *Int. J. Mol. Med.* **2003**, *12*, 253–257. [CrossRef] [PubMed]

76. Azrad, M.; Zhang, K.; Vollmer, R.T.; Madden, J.; Polascik, T.J.; Snyder, D.C.; Ruffin, M.T.; Moul, J.W.; Brenner, D.; Hardy, R.W.; et al. Prostatic alpha-linolenic acid (ALA) is positively associated with aggressive prostate cancer: a relationship which may depend on genetic variation in ALA metabolism. *PLoS ONE* **2012**, *7*, e53104. [CrossRef] [PubMed]

6

Up-Regulation of Mitochondrial Antioxidant Superoxide Dismutase Underpins Persistent Cardiac Nutritional-Preconditioning by Long Chain *n*-3 Polyunsaturated Fatty Acids in the Rat

Grace G. Abdukeyum [1], Alice J. Owen [2], Theresa A. Larkin [3] and Peter L. McLennan [3,*]

[1] Division of Medical and Exercise Science, School of Medicine, Faculty of Science Medicine and Health, University of Wollongong, Wollongong NSW 2522, Australia; Grace.Abdukeyum@hnehealth.nsw.gov.au

[2] Centre of Cardiovascular Research & Education in Therapeutics, School of Public Health & Preventive Medicine, Monash University, Melbourne VIC 3004, Australia; alice.owen@monash.edu

[3] Centre for Human and Applied Physiology, Graduate School of Medicine, School of Medicine, Faculty of Science Medicine and Health, University of Wollongong, Wollongong NSW 2522, Australia; tlarkin@uow.edu.au

* Correspondence: petermcl@uow.edu.au

Academic Editors: Lindsay Brown, Bernhard Rauch and Hemant Poudyal

Abstract: Reactive oxygen species paradoxically underpin both ischaemia/reperfusion (I/R) damage and ischaemic preconditioning (IPC) cardioprotection. Long-chain omega-3 polyunsaturated fatty acids (LC*n*-3 PUFA) are highly susceptible to peroxidation, but are paradoxically cardioprotective. This study tested the hypothesis that LC*n*-3 PUFA cardioprotection is underpinned by peroxidation, upregulating antioxidant activity to reduce I/R-induced lipid oxidation, and the mechanisms of this nutritional preconditioning contrast to mechanisms of IPC. Rats were fed: fish oil (LC*n*-3 PUFA); sunflower seed oil (*n*-6 PUFA); or beef tallow (saturated fat, SF) enriched diets for six weeks. Isolated hearts were subject to: 180 min normoxic perfusion; a 30 min coronary occlusion ischaemia protocol then 120 min normoxic reperfusion; or a 3 × 5 min global IPC protocol, 30 min ischaemia, then reperfusion. Dietary LC*n*-3 PUFA raised basal: membrane docosahexaenoic acid (22:6*n*-3 DHA); fatty acid peroxidisability index; concentrations of lipid oxidation products; and superoxide dismutase (MnSOD) activity (but not CuZnSOD or glutathione peroxidase). Infarct size correlated inversely with basal MnSOD activity ($r^2 = 0.85$) in the ischaemia protocol and positively with I/R-induced lipid oxidation (lipid hydroperoxides (LPO), $r^2 = 0.475$; malondialdehyde (MDA), $r^2 = 0.583$) across ischaemia and IPC protocols. While both dietary fish oil and IPC infarct-reduction were associated with reduced I/R-induced lipid oxidation, fish oil produced nutritional preconditioning by prior LC*n*-3 PUFA incorporation and increased peroxidisability leading to up-regulated mitochondrial SOD antioxidant activity.

Keywords: fish oil; preconditioning; antioxidant; reactive oxygen species; ischaemia; reperfusion; *n*-3 PUFA; lipid oxidation; infarct

1. Introduction

Regular consumption of fish or fish oil reduces cardiovascular mortality [1], often without modifying classical risk factors. For example, sudden death is reduced in high-risk post-MI patients, without significant reductions in blood pressure, blood lipids or prevention of new cardiac events [2]. This cardioprotection, associated with omega-3 long-chain polyunsaturated fatty acid (LC*n*-3 PUFA) consumption, is observed independently of the prevention of ischaemic events [3], and therefore supports a cardiac origin related to incorporation of the fatty acids into myocardial membranes [4]. Ischaemic preconditioning (IPC) is a powerful cardioprotective process, wherein brief periods of ischaemia, insufficient to produce cellular damage, can protect the myocardium from the damaging effects of a subsequent more prolonged ischaemic insult. The protective envelope of IPC is twofold, categorised as: classical or early preconditioning, which provides cardioprotection for several hours after the IPC stimulus; with a second phase called late or delayed preconditioning which occurs 24–7 h after the stimulus. Experimentally, the LCn-3 PUFA confer their cardioprotection in part through nutritional preconditioning of the myocardium that in rat heart is at least as effective in reducing infarct size [5,6] and promoting post-ischaemic contractile recovery [5], and more effective in preventing ischaemia or reperfusion induced cardiac arrhythmias [5], as early ischaemic preconditioning (IPC). Classical, early IPC cardioprotection disappears within several hours of the initial preconditioning stimulus and repeated brief preconditioning episodes become ineffective in providing this early protection [7]. In contrast, the cardioprotection derived from dietary LCn-3 PUFA is obtained only after they are incorporated into and continuously present in the myocardium for at least seven days and it persists over weeks or months, for however long elevated membrane content is sustained [5,8,9]. There is no desensitisation apparent, with acute ischaemia or reperfusion arrhythmias prevented after five weeks [8] to 52 weeks [10] of continuous exposure to dietary LCn-3 PUFA. Therefore, the cardioprotective benefit of fish oil appears to mimic the more sustained, repeatable protection of late IPC and other persistent preconditioning stimuli [11–13]. Moreover, the LCn-3 PUFA [5] share with late IPC [14] the capacity to protect against both infarction and myocardial stunning.

Myocardial ischaemia and reperfusion (I/R) stimulates production of reactive oxygen species (ROS) and depletes antioxidants in the heart, creating oxidative stress, oxidation of biomolecules and cell damage. Paradoxically, these free radicals also act as triggers of IPC [15,16]. The highly unsaturated LCn-3 PUFA found in fish oil: 20:5n-3 eicosapentaenoic acid (EPA) and 22:6n-3 docosahexaenoic acid (DHA) with their numerous bisallylic carbon atoms, are more susceptible to peroxidation and generation of damaging reactive oxygen species than are shorter, less unsaturated fatty acids such as 18:2n-6 linoleic acid and 20:4n-6 arachidonic acid [17], which raises the prospect of adverse effects of fish oil supplementation. However, there is no clinical evidence to suggest that fish oil supplementation or high fish diets promote oxidative stress-related cardiovascular disease. In contrast, production of ROS is a mechanism invoked to explain the paradoxical effects of late IPC in the heart, which works by inducing upregulation of endogenous antioxidant protective mechanisms [16,18]. That protection occurs in lieu of the extreme oxidation of biomolecules and cell damage that usually occurs with I/R-induced oxidative stress and antioxidant depletion.

The current study tested the hypothesis that incorporation of LCn-3 PUFA into myocardial membranes increases their peroxidation potential and basal fatty acid oxidation, which by their constant presence, in turn increases endogenous antioxidant enzymes to confer physiological cardioprotective actions against I/R-stimulated oxidative stress. We propose that this will contrast to the mechanism of early IPC cardioprotection.

2. Experimental Section

2.1. Animals and Diets

Fifty-four male Wistar rats were randomly assigned to three experimental dietary groups. For six weeks they were fed one of three iso-energetic diets containing either predominantly saturated animal fat, n-6 PUFA or LCn-3 PUFA as the source of fat. The diets were based on the American Institute of Nutrition AIN93 rat diet, containing all essential vitamins and minerals with gelatine as a component of the protein source. The diet was prepared with 10% (dry wt) fat (23% metabolisable energy as fat) consisting of: 7% beef tallow plus 3% olive oil (SF diet); 5% sunflower seed oil plus 5% olive oil (n-6 PUFA diet); or 7% fish oil (Nu-Mega high DHA tuna fish oil) plus 3% olive oil (LCn-3 PUFA diet). In addition to delivering diets rich in saturated fat, n-6 PUFA or n-3 PUFA, the oil blends in the LCn-3 PUFA diet and the n-6 PUFA diet were designed to deliver similar total PUFA, and the oil blends in the LCn-3 PUFA diet and the SF diet were designed to deliver similar total n-6 PUFA, as previously described [5]. All diets contained sufficient PUFA to prevent essential fatty acid deficiency [5].

Animal care and experiments were conducted with the approval of the University of Wollongong, Animal Care and Ethics Committee according to the guidelines of the National Health and Medical Research Council, Australia, Australian Code of Practice for the Care and Use of Animals for Scientific Purposes [19].

2.2. Heart Preparation

After six weeks of feeding, rats were anaesthetised (pentobarbital sodium, 60 mg·kg^{-1} i.p.), the thorax was opened, the heart was rapidly excised, submerged in ice-cold perfusate to arrest beating, and immediately perfused by an aortic cannula in the Langendorff mode at a constant pressure of 75 mmHg delivering warm (37 °C) Krebs–Henseleit bicarbonate buffer gassed with 5% CO_2 in O_2 [5]. The left atrium was opened and a thin-walled balloon catheter was introduced into the left ventricle, with balloon volume adjusted to maintain end diastolic pressure of 6–8 mmHg. 6–0 silk suture was passed through the myocardium closely underlying the left anterior descending coronary artery near its origin.

2.3. Index Ischaemia and Ischaemic Preconditioning

Each dietary group ($n = 18$) was separated into groups of $n = 6$ and randomly assigned to one of three perfusion protocols for 180 min after initial 30 min equilibration perfusion (Figure 1).

1. Control normoxia protocol ($n = 6$ per diet): Hearts were perfused throughout with oxygenated Krebs–Henseleit solution.

2. Ischaemia protocol (n = 6 per diet): Hearts were normoxically perfused for 30 min followed by 30 min index-ischaemia and 120 min normoxic reperfusion. Index-ischaemia was induced by occluding the left anterior descending coronary artery.

3. Ischaemic preconditioning (IPC) protocol (n = 6 per diet): Hearts were subjected to three cycles of five minutes global ischaemia (zero perfusion), each followed by five minutes normoxic reperfusion, prior to the 30 min index-ischaemia then 120 min normoxic reperfusion [5].

On completion of 120 min reperfusion in the ischaemia and IPC protocols, the coronary artery was re-occluded to reveal the ischaemic zone at risk (I-z/r). Hearts were then cut into 2 mm slices. The central slice was incubated in a buffer containing triphenyl-tetrazolium chloride and sodium phosphate (pH 7.4), then stored in 10% formalin until photographed and analysed for infarct size. Infarct size was reported as a percentage of the zone at risk. The remaining slices were separated into non-ischaemic (non-I) and ischaemic (ISCH) segments (Figure 1). Samples of fresh ISCH and non-I tissue were used immediately for lipid hydroperoxide (LPO) analysis, with the remainder rapidly frozen and stored at −80 °C for analysis of other markers of oxidation and antioxidant status. Samples of control normoxic heart were always taken from the left ventricle anterior free wall, supplied by the left anterior descending coronary artery, that would have been subject to ischaemia in the other protocols. It represents the basal state of the ischaemic zone at risk.

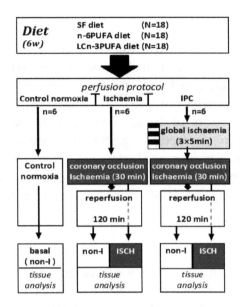

Figure 1. Flow chart illustrating the distribution of dietary groups into: Control normoxic; Ischaemia; and IPC perfusion protocols. In each protocol, isolated hearts were perfused for 180 min. Ischaemia protocol and IPC protocol hearts were dissected into non-ischaemic (non-I) and ischaemic (ISCH) tissue for biochemical analysis. IPC: ischaemic preconditioning.

2.4. Measurement of Oxidative Stress Biomarkers

Concentrations of LPO were measured by modification of the ferric thiocyanate assay using a colorimetric assay kit (Lipid Hydroperoxide Assay, Cayman Chemical Company, Ann Arbor, MI, USA) and were expressed per mg of protein. Concentrations of malondialdehyde (MDA) were measured in thawed tissue homogenates by reverse-phase HPLC with fluorescence detection [20].

2.5. Measurement of Antioxidants

Endogenous: Total superoxide dismutase (SOD) activity and CuZnSOD activity were measured in ventricle sections of: ISCH tissue; and non-I tissue using a BIOXYTECH®-SOD-525™ assay kit (Oxis Research™, Portland, OR, USA). The activity of mitochondrial SOD activated by manganese (MnSOD) was calculated as the difference between total SOD and CuZnSOD. The activity of SOD was expressed per mg of tissue protein. Glutathione peroxidase (GPX) activity was measured in ventricle sections of: ISCH; and non-I ventricle using BIOXYTECH®GPx-340TM assay kit (OxisResearch™, Portland OR, USA) and was expressed per mg of tissue protein. *Exogenous:* Myocardial vitamin E (alpha-tocopherol) was measured by HPLC with electrochemical detection, using a modification of the method described by Yang [21].

2.6. Myocardial Fatty Acid Analyses

Total lipids were extracted from 100 to 200 mg samples of ventricular myocardium using a modification of the Folch method [22]. Phospholipids were isolated from the total muscle lipid by solid phase extraction using silica Sep-pak™ cartridges (Waters, Rydalmere, NSW, Australia). Fatty acid methyl esters were prepared by direct transesterification of the phospholipid fraction [23] and analysed by gas chromatography using a Shimadzu GC-17A with flame ionization detection using a 30 m × 0.25 mm, 0.25 μm FAMEWAX column (J and W Scientific, Santa Clara CA, USA) with hydrogen as carrier gas and a step temperature program rising from 150 °C to 260 °C, over 27 min and held for 6 min. Individual fatty acids were identified by their retention times with reference to authentic fatty acid methyl ester standards (Sigma-Aldrich, Rydalmere, NSW, Australia) and expressed as a percentage of total phospholipid fatty acids.

2.7. Statistical Analyses

Results were expressed as mean $\pm$ SEM. Data were analysed by two-way analysis of variance (ANOVA) for diet and treatment main effects (normoxic perfusion, ischaemia, IPC + ischaemia) and by multi-way ANOVA for diet, treatment and ISCH *versus* non-I tissue main effects. Tukey's HSD test was used for *post-hoc* pairwise comparison of individual means and interactions. Within dietary groups, ISCH and non-I sections of the same hearts were compared using repeated measures ANOVA. Statistical analyses were performed using Statistix software, version 10 (Analytical Software, Tallahassee, FL, USA). Linear regression analysis with Pearson's correlation was performed to determine linear associations between lipid oxidation products, antioxidants and infarct size using Prism for Windows, version 6 (GraphPad Software, La Jolla, CA, USA). Statistical significance was accepted at $p < 0.05$.

3. Results

Neither the starting body weight, the final body weight nor the change in body weight over six weeks differed between dietary groups (Start: SF 348 $\pm$ 6 g; n-6 PUFA 351 $\pm$ 5 g; LCn-3 PUFA 352 $\pm$ 6 g. Six weeks: SF 460 $\pm$ 11 g; n-6 PUFA 457 $\pm$ 8 g; LCn-3 PUFA 480 $\pm$ 9 g. Change: SF 112 $\pm$ 7 g; n-6 PUFA 109 $\pm$ 9 g; LCn-3 PUFA 128 $\pm$ 7 g. n = 18 per diet).

3.1. Myocardial Membrane Phospholipid Fatty Acid Composition

The relative concentration of DHA (22:6n-3) was greater in phospholipid of LCn-3 PUFA hearts than in either n-6 PUFA or SF hearts ($p < 0.05$) (Table 1). The LCn-3 PUFA hearts contained significantly lower concentrations of linoleic (18:2n-6) and arachidonic acids (20:4n-6) compared with n-6 PUFA or SF hearts. Total n-3 PUFA was greater in LCn-3 PUFA hearts compared with either n-6 PUFA or SF hearts, and lower in n-6 PUFA than SF hearts ($p < 0.05$). The total concentration of n-6 PUFA was lower in LCn-3 PUFA hearts than in either n-6 PUFA or SF hearts and greater in n-6 PUFA than SF hearts ($p < 0.05$).

Table 1. Influence of dietary fat (six weeks) on phospholipid fatty acid composition as percentage of total phospholipid fatty acids of rat heart ventricle.

	DIET								
Fatty Acid	**SF**			**n-6 PUFA**			**LCn-3 PUFA**		
16:0	9.7	$\pm$	0.1	10.2	$\pm$	0.2	10.8	$\pm$	0.1
18:0	23.7	$\pm$	0.2	23.8	$\pm$	0.1	22.4	$\pm$	0.2
18:1n-9	[a] 9.5	$\pm$	0.1	[b] 5.4	$\pm$	0.1	[b] 4.3	$\pm$	0.3
18:1n-7	3.6	$\pm$	0.1	3.5	$\pm$	0.1	3.4	$\pm$	0.1
Total SFA	33.80	$\pm$	0.13	34.70	$\pm$	0.80	33.70	$\pm$	0.40
Total MUFA	[a] 13.50	$\pm$	0.12	[b] 8.95	$\pm$	0.30	[b] 7.75	$\pm$	1.10
18:2n-6 (LA)	[b] 17.50	$\pm$	0.20	[a] 18.7	$\pm$	0.40	[c] 5.60	$\pm$	0.03
20:4n-6 (AA)	[a] 23.30	$\pm$	0.30	[a] 23.5	$\pm$	0.20	[b] 13.30	$\pm$	0.15
22:5n-6	n.d			[a] 1.50	$\pm$	0.12	[a] 1.06	$\pm$	0.05
20:5n-3 (EPA)	n.d			n.d			1.30	$\pm$	0.01
22:5n-3 (DPA)	1.90	$\pm$	0.04	1.02	$\pm$	0.02	1.17	$\pm$	0.04
22:6n-3 (DHA)	[b] 12.20	$\pm$	0.04	[b] 10.02	$\pm$	0.20	[a] 28.30	$\pm$	0.04
Total (n-6) PUFA	[b] 40.80	$\pm$	0.20	[a] 43.80	$\pm$	0.60	[c] 20.00	$\pm$	0.16
Total (n-3) PUFA	[b] 14.10	$\pm$	0.06	[c] 11.00	$\pm$	0.20	[a] 30.70	$\pm$	0.08
Total PUFA	54.90	$\pm$	4.50	54.70	$\pm$	4.50	50.70	$\pm$	4.40
UI	[b] 215.40	$\pm$	1.20	[b] 215.10	$\pm$	0.50	[a] 260.58	$\pm$	1.20
Peroxidisability Index	[b] 156.20	$\pm$	1.20	[b] 149.50	$\pm$	1.60	[a] 201.10	$\pm$	0.70

SF: saturated fat enriched diet; n-6 PUFA: n-6 PUFA enriched diet; LCn-3 PUFA: n-3 PUFA enriched diet; SFA: saturated fatty acids; MUFA: monounsaturated fatty acids; PUFA: polyunsaturated fatty acids; LA: linoleic acid; AA: arachidonic acid; EPA: eicosapentaenoic acid; DPA: docosahexaenoic acid; DHA: docosahexaenoic acid. Unsaturation index (UI) was calculated according to the formula: UI = 1 $\times$ (% monoenoic acids) + 2 $\times$ (% dienoics) + 3 $\times$ (% trienoics) + 4 $\times$ (% tetraenoics) + 5 $\times$ (% pentaenoics) + 6 $\times$ (% hexaenoics) or sum (fatty acid percent) $\times$ (number of double bonds). Peroxidatisability index was calculated from the formula: (% dienoic acids $\times$ 1) + (% trienoics $\times$ 2) + (% tetraenoics $\times$ 3) + (% pentaenoics $\times$ 4) + (% hexaenoics $\times$ 5) [17]. n.d: not detected. n = 6 per dietary group. [a, b, c] Values not sharing a common letter superscript are significantly different (ANOVA, $p < 0.05$).

No significant dietary differences were observed in the membrane phospholipid total saturated fatty acids or total PUFA. The SF hearts had greater concentrations of total monounsaturated fatty acids (MUFA). Membrane unsaturation index (UI) and peroxidisability index (Figure 2A) were significantly greater in LCn-3 PUFA than in either n-6 PUFA or SF hearts ($p < 0.05$), which were not significantly different from each other.

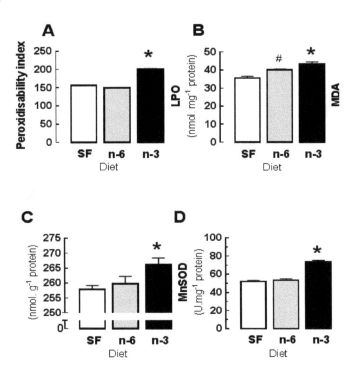

Figure 2. Influence of six weeks dietary fat feeding on basal: (**A**) membrane fatty acid peroxidisability index; and concentrations of (**B**) lipid hydroperoxides (LPO); (**C**) malondialdehyde (MDA); and (**D**) antioxidant superoxide dismutase (MnSOD) of basal or non-I regions of the heart after 180 min of isolated perfusion protocol. Open columns (SF): saturated fat diet; shaded columns (n-6): n-6 PUFA rich diet; filled columns (n-3): LCn-3 PUFA rich fish oil diet. Values are means $\pm$ SEM. $n = 18$ per dietary group except peroxidisability index: $n = 6$. * different from both other diet groups, $p < 0.05$. # different from SF group, $p < 0.05$.

3.2. Basal Properties: Effects of Diet on Oxidative Stress and Antioxidant Activity

The basal and non-I tissue derived from the three perfusion protocols exhibited no significant between protocol differences in tissue concentrations of lipid oxidation products LPO or MDA or anti-oxidants within any dietary group (pooled data shown in Figure 2). This establishes the non-I measures as representative of the basal state of the ISCH region.

The concentrations of LPO in basal and non-I tissue were significantly greater in LCn-3 PUFA than in either n-6 PUFA or SF hearts and greater in n-6 PUFA than SF hearts ($p < 0.05$) (Figure 3A). The concentrations of MDA in basal and non-I tissue were significantly greater in LCn-3 PUFA than in either n-6 PUFA or SF hearts ($p < 0.05$), which were not different from each other (Figure 3B).

The activity of MnSOD in basal and non-I tissue was significantly greater in LCn-3 PUFA hearts, than in SF or n-6 PUFA hearts (Figure 3C). In basal and non-I tissue there were no significant dietary differences in CuZnSOD activity (basal, non-I (U$\cdot$mg^{-1} protein): SF 15.3 ± 0.9; n-6 PUFA 16.9 ± 0.7; LCn-3 PUFA 17.4 ± 0.6 $n = 18$) ($p > 0.05$) or GPX (basal, non-I (mU$\cdot$mg^{-1} protein): SF 19.2 ± 1.5; n-6 PUFA 19.7 ± 1.5; LCn-3 PUFA 21 ± 1.2 $n = 15$). The concentration of α-tocopherol was significantly greater in n-6 PUFA hearts than in either LCn-3 PUFA or SF hearts ($p < 0.05$) (basal, non-I (μM): SF 6.1 ± 0.4; n-6 PUFA 6.9 ± 0.2; LCn-3 PUFA 5.9 ± 0.6 $n = 15$).

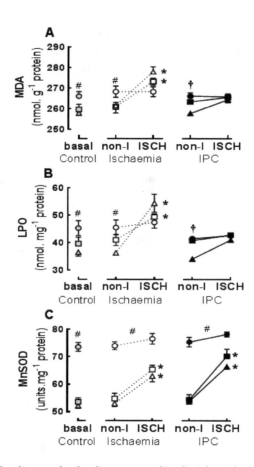

Figure 3. Influence of six weeks dietary fat feeding on cardiac lipid oxidation and antioxidant markers in ischaemic (ISCH) or non-ischaemic (non-I) regions after: Control normoxic perfusion (basal), Ischaemia perfusion, or ischaemic preconditioning (IPC) perfusion protocols: (**A**) lipid hydroperoxides (LPO); (**B**) malondialdehyde (MDA); and (**C**) superoxide dismutase (MnSOD). Data are from hearts that were normoxic throughout (basal), or the non-I and ISCH regions of hearts subjected to 30 min of regional ischaemia with or without prior IPC. Diet groups: ▲▲△—saturated fat (SF); ■■□—n-6 PUFA; ●●○—LCn-3 PUFA. Values are means ± SEM. n = 18 per diet, n = 6 per perfusion protocol. * ISCH different from non-I region within diet, $p < 0.05$; # n-3 PUFA different from SF $p < 0.05$; † LCn-3 PUFA and n-6 PUFA different from SF.

3.3. Ischaemic Responses: Effects of Diet and Ischaemic Preconditioning on Oxidative Stress and Antioxidant Capacity in Hearts Subjected to Regional I/R

Ischaemia: The concentrations of LPO (Figure 3A) and MDA (Figure 3B) were acutely increased in the ISCH compared to non-I region of n-6 PUFA and SF hearts ($p < 0.01$) but not in LCn-3 PUFA hearts. The concentrations of LPO and MDA in the ISCH region were significantly greater in SF hearts than in LCn-3 PUFA hearts (Figure 3A,B).

IPC: There were no significant acute changes in LPO or MDA in ISCH compared to non-I regions within any dietary group (Figure 3A,B), nor were there any significant between-diet differences within the ISCH regions of IPC + ischaemia hearts. Concentrations of LPO and MDA in ISCH regions were significantly lower in IPC + ischaemia hearts than in ischaemia only hearts ($p < 0.0001$). Pairwise comparison indicated that this IPC difference was evident in SF and n-6 PUFA diets only.

Myocardial MnSOD activity was significantly greater in ISCH compared to non-I regions of hearts from SF and n-6 PUFA fed rats but not significantly changed within LCn-3 PUFA hearts (Figure 3C). The perfusion protocol incorporating IPC + ischaemia had no different effect on MnSOD activity to ischaemia alone.

3.4. Infarct

In hearts subjected to the ischaemia perfusion protocol, infarct size was significantly smaller in LCn-3 PUFA hearts (ischaemia infarct size (% Iz/r): SF 50 $\pm$ 1 n = 6; n-6 PUFA 47 $\pm$ 1 n = 6; LCn-3 PUFA n = 6 11 $\pm$ 1 n = 6, ($p < 0.05$)). In hearts subjected to the IPC + ischaemia protocol, the infarct size was significantly smaller in the SF and n-6 PUFA hearts than in the corresponding ischaemia group ($p < 0.05$). There was no significant difference within the LCn-3 PUFA diet. (IPC + ischaemia infarct size (% Iz/r): SF 13 $\pm$ 1 n = 6; n-6 PUFA 12 $\pm$ 1 n = 6; LCn-3 PUFA 10 $\pm$ 1 n = 6).

3.5. Associations between Oxidation Biomarkers, Antioxidant and Infarct Size

Ischaemia protocol: Infarct size was positively associated with lipid oxidation biomarker production in the ISCH region, independent of diet (Table 2). The acute increases in LPO and MDA (ISCH compared to the non-I region) correlated better than the absolute ISCH concentrations of LPO and MDA. Lipid oxidation biomarkers LPO and MDA were correlated in the ISCH region. Ischaemic production of LPO and MDA and infarct size were inversely associated with the basal (non-I) MnSOD activity (Table 2). The strongest association was the inverse correlation between basal MnSOD and infarct size (Figure 4).

IPC: In hearts subjected to the IPC + ischaemia perfusion protocol, infarct size was not significantly correlated with LPO, MDA or MnSOD concentrations, and ischaemia-induced increase in MDA but not LPO was correlated with MnSOD activity. Lipid oxidation biomarkers LPO and MDA were correlated in the ISCH region (Table 2).

Pooled analysis of data from both perfusion protocols revealed significant correlations of infarct size with lipid oxidation markers and with MnSOD. Lipid oxidation biomarkers LPO and MDA were correlated in the ISCH region (Table 2).

Table 2. Correlations between lipid oxidation products, antioxidants and infarct size.

Dependent Variable	Independent Variable	Association	r^2	p for Slope
Ischaemia Protocol				
Infarct	LPO (ISCH)	positive	0.337 *	0.018
Infarct	LPO increase	positive	0.478 **	0.004
Infarct	MDA (ISCH)	positive	0.356 *	0.015
Infarct	MDA increase	positive	0.517 **	0.004
Infarct	MnSOD (basal)	negative	0.851 **	<0.0001
MDA (ISCH)	LPO (ISCH)	positive	0.481 **	0.006
LPO increase	MnSOD (basal)	negative	0.397 **	0.009
MDA increase	MnSOD (basal)	negative	0.617 **	0.001
IPC + Ischaemia Protocol				
Infarct	LPO (ISCH)	positive	0.039	0.483 n.s.
Infarct	LPO increase	positive	0.147	0.175 n.s.
Infarct	MDA (ISCH)	positive	0.175	0.150 n.s.
Infarct	MDA increase	positive	0.009	0.728 n.s.
Infarct	MnSOD (basal)	negative	0.058	0.335 n.s.
MDA (ISCH)	LPO (ISCH)	positive	0.764 **	<0.0001
LPO increase	MnSOD (basal)	negative	0.128	0.174 n.s.
MDA increase	MnSOD (basal)	negative	0.293 *	0.017
Overall				
Infarct	LPO increase	positive	0.583 **	<0.0001
Infarct	MDA increase	positive	0.475 **	<0.0001
Infarct	MnSOD (basal)	negative	0.270 *	0.0012
MDA (ISCH)	LPO (ISCH)	positive	0.760 **	<0.0001

LPO: lipid hydroperoxides. MDA: malondialdehyde. MnSOD: manganese superoxide dismutase. ISCH: ischaemic region. Basal: non-ischaemic region of ventricle wall. n.s.: not significant ($p > 0.05$); * $p < 0.05$; ** $p < 0.01$.

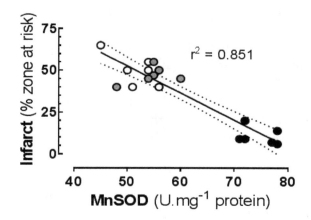

Figure 4. Correlation between: basal (non-I) concentration of superoxide dismutase; and infarct size in isolated rat hearts subjected to 30 min index ischaemia and 120 min reperfusion. Rats fed supplemented diets for six weeks—open symbols: saturated fat (SF) diet; shaded symbols: *n*-6 PUFA diet; closed symbols: LC*n*-3 PUFA fish oil diet.

4. Discussion

A diet rich in LC*n*-3 PUFA from fish oil modified the fatty acid profile of myocardial membrane phospholipids, increasing the percentage of fat as DHA and the peroxidisability index (predicting an increase in risk of oxidative damage), yet paradoxically reduced the measured oxidative damage following I/R. While the increased myocardial peroxidation potential was associated with an increase in basal fatty acid peroxidation, confirming effects of DHA feeding recorded in plasma and liver [24], it also induced a marked chronic increase in MnSOD (endogenous antioxidant) activity, and inhibited I/R-induced lipid oxidation and infarction. Reactive oxygen species act as both the agents of damage and of conservation in IPC, causing cellular damage yet triggering protective signalling processes [25]. In this respect, LC*n*-3 PUFA supplementation reflects both the low level generation of ROS through lipid peroxidation [26] and up-regulation of endogenous antioxidants that are implicated as triggers and mediators respectively of late phase IPC [27]. This aligns fish oil nutritional preconditioning [5] not only with this more persistent form of IPC (variously known as late, delayed or second window of IPC), but through LC*n*-3 PUFA continuous presence as a membrane component, it also provides a persistent tolerance to I/R injury. This persistent preconditioning is also observed with repeated stresses like exercise and heat exposure [12]. In contrast, early phase IPC did not acutely affect basal lipid oxidation or antioxidant activity during the 150 min post preconditioning time course of this study protocol. Moreover, IPC prevention of lipid oxidation and infarction during the index ischaemia was not additive to the effects of fish oil feeding. Admittedly the anti-infarct effects of both fish oil and IPC could be individually regarded as already maximal.

Fish oil-induced chronic increases in basal lipid oxidation directly correlated with basal MnSOD antioxidant activity in myocardium, which in turn was negatively correlated with the I/R-induced increase in lipid oxidation. This interdependence, which reflects the contrasting damaging influence and homeostatic signalling roles of ROS in ischaemia and IPC, can explain some of the lack of consistent correlation between oxidation products and anti-oxidants and sometime failure of oxidation markers to serve as clear criteria for defining oxidative stress [26]. The effects were consistent on LPO (an intermediate common to oxidation of all PUFA) and MDA (a stable end product of a single pathway also not specific for any PUFA family). Ultimately the infarct size was negatively correlated with MnSOD activity and directly correlated with the increase in lipid oxidation products in the ISCH region. Chronic elevation of plasma MnSOD has been previously observed during fish oil feeding [28], consistent with its persistent elevation over several days following multiple exposures to TNFα, exercise stress or heat stress [12].

Fish oil induced increases in antioxidant expression and reduced lipid peroxidation products were also reported in hepatic and renal tissue of immune suppressed mice [29,30] and hepatic tissue of hypertensive rats [31], conditions associated with heightened oxidative stress. In those studies, the fish oil diets were effective independently of varied provision of high or low concentrations of natural antioxidants in comparative n-6 PUFA or MUFA enriched diets. In the current study, the n-6 PUFA rich diet with its elevated vitamin E content did not change the membrane fatty acid composition sufficiently to modulate either membrane peroxidisability index or endogenous antioxidant enzyme activity relative to the low PUFA saturated fat enriched diet, and hearts from those diets were equally highly susceptible to oxidative damage. This is consistent with previous findings that both membrane effects and cardioprotective effects of n-6 PUFA are readily lost as the PUFA content is diluted by other fat sources [32,33]. This is not the case for LCn-3 PUFA, which sustain membrane composition [34,35], and cardiac [5,10,32,33,36] and other functional effects [35] to very low dietary concentrations. The ability of low (nutritionally relevant) intakes of fish oil to modify membrane composition and cardiac function, including prevention of I/R arrhythmias is important, since the provision of extremely high LCn-3 PUFA intakes can be pro-arrhythmic (fish oil concentrate 4 g/d/20 kg dog, equivalent to ⩾40/d standard fish oil capsules in an 80 kg man) [37], perhaps representing the harmful effects of excessive oxidation. Similarly, in a senescence-prone mouse model, high fish oil feeding in conjunction with high total PUFA enhances oxidative stress and decreases lifespan [38].

The present study suggests that LCn-3 PUFA exert protection from ischaemia by activating signalling pathways that resemble those involved in late IPC or exercise, and we describe this as "nutritional preconditioning". The current study used a LCn-3 PUFA intake equivalent to more than 30 g of fish oil per day in humans [34]. However, even very low doses in the range 0.16%–1.25% FO markedly increase myocardial DHA and peroxidation index (at 0.31% dietary fish oil equivalent to human 1–2 fish meals per week) DHA is increased from 7.7% to 14.9% of phospholipid fatty acids and PI is increased from 149 to 164 (calculated from Slee [34]). This is a dose that modulates skeletal muscle membrane fatty acids and muscle fatigue [35]. In skeletal muscle, reactive oxygen species capable of causing cellular damage when in physiological excess can at lower levels also act to optimise contractile performance and initiate long-term protective adaptations to the intermittent stress imposed by exercise training [39].

The present study deliberately used a high DHA fish oil, which does not reflect the composition of most nutritional supplement fish oils, but rather reflects the main LCn-3 PUFA derived from eating fish [4,40]. As the most abundant n-3 PUFA found in myocardium, DHA is also the main fatty acid underpinning the cardiac effects of fish and fish oil [4]. The use of two diets for comparison with fish oil allows specific attribution of the effects of fish oil feeding to its LCn-3 PUFA content, since similar total PUFA content was provided in the n-6 and LCn-3 PUFA diets; similar n-6 PUFA was provided in the SF and LCn-3 PUFA diets; and low saturated fat was provided in the n-6 PUFA diet, all without effect.

The increased expression of antioxidants within LCn-3 PUFA hearts was restricted to the mitochondrial form of SOD (MnSOD or SOD2) with CuZnSOD and GSx unchanged. This suggests localisation of the primarily influence of LCn-3 PUFA to the mitochondria. Increased MnSOD activity is similarly selectively implicated in the sustained cardioprotection elicited by heat stress and in late, delayed or second window of IPC [41], whereas over-expression of cardiac MnSOD in mice enhances contractile function, slows heart rate and increases efficiency of myocardial O_2 consumption [42], all properties shared by dietary fish oil [5,43,44]. Furthermore, the fish oil-reduced cardiac oxygen consumption and reduced susceptibility to I/R-damage and arrhythmias in rats is linked to mitochondrial Ca^{2+} handling [44]. In contrast, early IPC inhibited acute lipid oxidation and infarction did not involve upregulation of mitochondrial SOD, confirming its difference from late IPC [41] and highlighting a difference to the more persistent forms of preconditioning including exercise [45–47], late IPC [41] and now fish oil-induced nutritional preconditioning.

This study confirmed that increasing myocardial membrane percentage content of long chain n-3 highly polyunsaturated fatty acids by feeding fish oil, increased the basal peroxidation of cellular fatty acids, which in turn increased the activity of endogenous mitochondrial antioxidant superoxide dismutase. When these hearts were acutely subjected to regional I/R, the stimulated lipid oxidation and myocardial damage were reduced. The increase in peroxidation index of myocardial membranes through fatty acid compositional change and associated chronic mild elevation in lipid peroxidation products provokes a persistent physiological stress that might better be described as "oxidative shielding" [48], which if confirmed at lower fish oil intakes, could explain much of the cardioprotective effect of regular fish consumption. This readily available and safe nutritional approach appears to represent a natural form of late preconditioning, which, characterised by its persistence over time, would be particularly valuable in the clinical setting, where oxidative insults occur unexpectedly and preclude the use of planned preventative interventions [41]. The observation, however, also raises the possibility that like exercise training [45], effects of fish oil nutritional preconditioning may be blunted by concomitant antioxidant supplementation.

Acknowledgments: This research received no specific grant from any funding agency, commercial or not-for-profit sectors. The research was supported by the donation of high-DHA tuna fish oil from Clover Corporation and Nu-Mega Lipids (Altona North VIC, Australia).

Author Contributions: G.G.A., A.J.O. and P.L.M. conceived and designed the experiments; G.G.A., A.J.O. and T.A.L. performed the experiments and analysed the data; and G.G.A., A.J.O., T.A.L. and P.L.M. interpreted the data and provided important intellectual content for drafting the manuscript. P.L.M. had the primary responsibility for the final content.

References

1.   Trikalinos, T.A.; Lee, J.; Moorthy, D.; Yu, W.W.; Lau, J.; Lichtenstein, A.H.; Chung, M. Effects of eicosapentanoic acid and docosahexanoic acid on mortality across diverse settings: Systematic review and meta-analysis of randomized trials and prospective cohorts. Available online: http://www.ncbi.nlm. nih.gov/books/NBK91413/pdf/Bookshelf_NBK91413.pdf (accessed on 2 March 2016).

2.   Valagussa, F.; Franzosi, M.G.; Geraci, E.; Mininni, N.; Nicolosi, G.L.; Santini, M.; Tavazzi, L.; Vecchio, C.; Marchioli, R.; Bomba, E.; *et al.* Dietary supplementation with n-3 polyunsaturated fatty acids and vitamin E after myocardial infarction: Results of the GISSI-Prevenzione trial. *Lancet* **1999**, *354*, 447–455.

3.   Mozaffarian, D.; Rimm, E.B. Fish intake, contaminants, and human health—Evaluating the risks and the benefits. *JAMA* **2006**, *296*, 1885–1899. [CrossRef] [PubMed]

4.   McLennan, P.L. Cardiac physiology and clinical efficacy of dietary fish oil clarified through cellular mechanisms of omega-3 polyunsaturated fatty acids. *Eur. J. Appl. Physiol.* **2014**, *114*, 1333–1356. [CrossRef] [PubMed]

5.   Abdukeyum, G.G.; Owen, A.J.; McLennan, P.L. Dietary (n-3) long-chain polyunsaturated fatty acids inhibit ischemia and reperfusion arrhythmias and infarction in rat heart not enhanced by ischemic preconditioning. *J. Nutr.* **2008**, *138*, 1902–1909. [PubMed]

6.   Zeghichi-Hamri, S.; de Lorgeril, M.; Salen, P.; Chibane, M.; de Leiris, J.; Boucher, F.; Laporte, F. Protective effect of dietary n-3 polyunsaturated fatty acids on myocardial resistance to ischemia-reperfusion injury in rats. *Nutr. Res.* **2010**, *30*, 849–857. [CrossRef] [PubMed]

7.   Cohen, M.V.; Yang, X.M.; Downey, J.M. Conscious rabbits become tolerant to multiple episodes of ischemic preconditioning. *Circ. Res.* **1994**, *74*, 998–1004. [CrossRef] [PubMed]

8.   McLennan, P.L.; Abeywardena, M.Y.; Charnock, J.S. Dietary fish oil prevents ventricular fibrillation following coronary artery occlusion and reperfusion. *Am. Heart J.* **1988**, *116*, 709–717. [CrossRef]

9.   McLennan, P.L. Myocardial membrane fatty acids and the antiarrhythmic actions of dietary fish oil in animal models. *Lipids* **2001**, *36*, S111–S114. [CrossRef] [PubMed]

10.   McLennan, P.; Howe, P.; Abeywardena, M.; Muggli, R.; Raederstorff, D.; Mano, M.; Rayner, T.; Head, R. The cardiovascular protective role of docosahexaenoic acid. *Eur. J. Pharmacol.* **1996**, *300*, 83–89. [CrossRef]

11. Dana, A.; Baxter, G.F.; Walker, J.M.; Yellon, D.M. Prolonging the delayed phase of myocardial protection: Repetitive adenosine A(1) receptor activation maintains rabbit myocardium in a preconditioned state. *J. Am. Coll. Cardiol.* **1998**, *31*, 1142–1149. [CrossRef]

12. Hoshida, S.; Yamashita, N.; Otsu, K.; Hori, M. Repeated physiologic stresses provide persistent cardioprotection against ischemia-reperfusion injury in rats. *J. Am. Coll. Cardiol.* **2002**, *40*, 826–831. [CrossRef]

13. Marber, M.S.; Latchman, D.S.; Walker, J.M.; Yellon, D.M. Cardiac stress protein elevation 24 hours after brief ischemia or heat stress is associated with resistance to myocardial infarction. *Circulation* **1993**, *88*, 1264–1272. [CrossRef] [PubMed]

14. Bolli, R. The early and late phases of preconditioning against myocardial stunning and the essential role of oxyradicals in the late phase: An overview. *Basic Res. Cardiol.* **1996**, *91*, 57–63. [PubMed]

15. Baxter, G.F.; Ferdinandy, P. Delayed preconditioning of myocardium: Current perspectives. *Basic Res. Cardiol.* **2001**, *96*, 329–344. [CrossRef] [PubMed]

16. Zhou, X.B.; Zhai, X.L.; Ashraf, M. Direct evidence that initial oxidative stress triggered by preconditioning contributes to second window of protection by endogenous antioxidant enzyme in myocytes. *Circulation* **1996**, *93*, 1177–1184. [CrossRef] [PubMed]

17. Song, J.H.; Fujimoto, K.; Miyazawa, T. Polyunsaturated (*n*-3) fatty acids susceptible to peroxidation are increased in plasma and tissue lipids of rats fed docosahexaenoic acid-containing oils. *J. Nutr.* **2000**, *130*, 3028–3033. [PubMed]

18. Bolli, R.; Becker, L.; Gross, G.; Mentzer, R.; Balshaw, D.; Lathrop, D.A. Myocardial protection at a crossroads—The need for translation into clinical therapy. *Circ. Res.* **2004**, *95*, 125–134. [CrossRef] [PubMed]

19. National Health and Medical Research Council. *Australian Code of Practice for the Care and Use of Animals for Scientific Purposes*, 7th ed.; NHMRC: Canberra, Australia, 2004; p. 84.

20. Lepage, G.; Munoz, G.; Champagne, J.; Roy, C.C. Preparative steps necessary for the accurate measurement of malondialdehyde by high-performance liquid chromatography. *Anal. Biochem.* **1991**, *197*, 277–283. [CrossRef]

21. Yang, C.S.; Jung, L.M. Methodology of plasma retinol, tocopherol and carotenoid assays in cancer prevention studies. *J. Nutr. Growth Cancer* **1987**, *4*, 19–27.

22. Folch, J.; Lees, M.; Sloane-Stanley, G.H. A simple method for the isolation and purification of total lipids from animal tissues. *J. Biol. Chem.* **1957**, *226*, 497–509. [PubMed]

23. Lepage, G.; Roy, C. Direct transesterification of all classes of lipids in a one-step reaction. *J. Lipid Res.* **1986**, *27*, 114–121. [PubMed]

24. Song, J.H.; Miyazawa, T. Enhanced level of *n*-3 fatty acid in membrane phospholipids induces lipid peroxidation in rats fed dietary docosahexaenoic acid oil. *Atherosclerosis* **2001**, *155*, 9–18. [CrossRef]

25. Ray, P.D.; Huang, B.W.; Tsuji, Y. Reactive oxygen species (ROS) homeostasis and redox regulation in cellular signaling. *Cell. Signal.* **2012**, *24*, 981–990. [CrossRef] [PubMed]

26. Dotan, Y.; Lichtenberg, D.; Pinchuk, I. Lipid peroxidation cannot be used as a universal criterion of oxidative stress. *Prog. Lipid Res.* **2004**, *43*, 200–227. [CrossRef] [PubMed]

27. Stein, A.B.; Tang, X.L.; Guo, Y.; Xuan, Y.T.; Dawn, B.; Bolli, R. Delayed adaptation of the heart to stress—Late preconditioning. *Stroke* **2004**, *35*, 2676–2679. [CrossRef] [PubMed]

28. Erdogan, H.; Fadillioglu, E.; Ozgocmen, S.; Sogut, S.; Ozyurt, B.; Akyol, O.; Ardicoglu, O. Effect of fish oil supplementation on plasma oxidant/antioxidant status in rats. *Prostaglandins Leukot. Essent. Fatty Acids* **2004**, *71*, 149–152. [CrossRef] [PubMed]

29. Chandrasekar, B.; Fernandes, G. Decreased pro-inflammatory cytokines and increased antioxidant enzyme gene-expression by omega-3 lipids in murine lupus nephritis. *Biochem. Biophys. Res. Commun.* **1994**, *200*, 893–898. [CrossRef] [PubMed]

30. Venkatraman, J.T.; Chandrasekar, B.; Kim, J.D.; Fernandes, G. Effects of *n*-3 and *n*-6 fatty-acids on the activities and expression of hepatic antioxidant enzymes in autoimmune-prone NZBxNZW F1-mice. *Lipids* **1994**, *29*, 561–568. [CrossRef] [PubMed]

31. Ruiz-Gutierrez, V.; Vazquez, C.M.; Santa-Maria, C. Liver lipid composition and antioxidant enzyme activities of spontaneously hypertensive rats after ingestion of dietary fats (fish, olive and high-oleic sunflower oils). *Biosci. Rep.* **2001**, *21*, 271–285. [CrossRef] [PubMed]

32. McLennan, P.L.; Bridle, T.M.; Abeywardena, M.Y.; Charnock, J.S. Comparative efficacy of *n*-3 and *n*-6 polyunsaturated fatty acids in modulating ventricular fibrillation threshold in marmoset monkeys. *Am. J. Clin. Nutr.* **1993**, *58*, 666–669. [PubMed]

33. McLennan, P.L.; Abeywardena, M.Y. Membrane basis for fish oil effects on the heart: Linking natural hibernators to prevention of human sudden cardiac death. *J. Membr. Biol.* **2005**, *206*, 85–102. [CrossRef] [PubMed]

34. Slee, E.L.; McLennan, P.L.; Owen, A.J.; Theiss, M.L. Low dietary fish oil threshold for myocardial membrane *n*-3 PUFA enrichment independent of *n*-6 PUFA intake in rats. *J. Lipid Res.* **2010**, *51*, 1841–1848. [CrossRef] [PubMed]

35. Henry, R.; Peoples, G.E.; McLennan, P.L. Muscle fatigue resistance in the rat hindlimb *in vivo* from low dietary intakes of tuna fish oil that selectively increase phospholipid *n*-3 docosahexaenoic acid according to muscle fibre type. *Br. J. Nutr.* **2015**, *114*, 873–884. [CrossRef] [PubMed]

36. McLennan, P.L.; Owen, A.J.; Slee, E.L.; Theiss, M.L. Myocardial function, ischaemia and *n*-3 polyunsaturated fatty acids: A membrane basis. *J. Cardiovasc. Med.* **2007**, *8*, S15–S18. [CrossRef] [PubMed]

37. Billman, G.E.; Carnes, C.A.; Adamson, P.B.; Vanoli, E.; Schwartz, P.J. Dietary omega-3 fatty acids and susceptibility to ventricular fibrillation lack of protection and a proarrhythmic effect. *Circ. Arrhythm. Electrophysiol.* **2012**, *5*, 553–560. [CrossRef] [PubMed]

38. Tsuduki, T.; Honma, T.; Nakagawa, K.; Ikeda, I.; Miyazawa, T. Long-term intake of fish oil increases oxidative stress and decreases lifespan in senescence-accelerated mice. *Nutrition* **2011**, *27*, 334–337. [CrossRef] [PubMed]

39. Powers, S.K.; Jackson, M.J. Exercise-induced oxidative stress: Cellular mechanisms and impact on muscle force production. *Physiol. Rev.* **2008**, *88*, 1243–1276. [CrossRef] [PubMed]

40. McLennan, P.L.; Pepe, S. Weighing up fish and omega-3 PUFA advice with accurate, balanced scales: Stringent controls and measures required for clinical trials. *Heart Lung Circ.* **2015**, *24*, 740–743. [CrossRef] [PubMed]

41. Hausenloy, D.J.; Yellon, D.M. The Second Window of Preconditioning (SWOP) Where Are We Now? *Cardiovasc. Drugs Ther.* **2010**, *24*, 235–254. [CrossRef] [PubMed]

42. Kang, P.T.; Chen, C.-L.; Ohanyan, V.; Luther, D.J.; Meszaros, J.G.; Chilian, W.M.; Chen, Y.-R. Overexpressing superoxide dismutase 2 induces a supernormal cardiac function by enhancing redox-dependent mitochondrial function and metabolic dilation. *J. Mol. Cell. Cardiol.* **2015**, *88*, 14–28. [CrossRef] [PubMed]

43. Pepe, S.; McLennan, P.L. (*n*-3) long chain PUFA dose-dependently increase oxygen utilization efficiency and inhibit arrhythmias after saturated fat feeding in rats. *J. Nutr.* **2007**, *137*, 2377–2383. [PubMed]

44. Pepe, S.; McLennan, P.L. Cardiac membrane fatty acid composition modulates myocardial oxygen consumption and post-ischemic recovery of contractile function. *Circulation* **2002**, *105*, 2303–2308. [CrossRef] [PubMed]

45. Gomez-Cabrera, M.C.; Salvador-Pascual, A.; Cabo, H.; Ferrando, B.; Vina, J. Redox modulation of mitochondriogenesis in exercise. Does antioxidant supplementation blunt the benefits of exercise training? *Free Radic. Biol. Med.* **2015**, *86*, 37–46. [CrossRef] [PubMed]

46. Gomez-Cabrera, M.C.; Domenech, E.; Vina, J. Moderate exercise is an antioxidant: Upregulation of antioxidant genes by training. *Free Radic. Biol. Med.* **2008**, *44*, 126–131. [CrossRef] [PubMed]

47. Powers, S.K.; Smuder, A.J.; Kavazis, A.N.; Quindry, J.C. Mechanisms of Exercise-Induced Cardioprotection. *Physiology* **2014**, *29*, 27–38. [CrossRef] [PubMed]

48. Naviaux, R.K. Oxidative Shielding or Oxidative Stress? *J. Pharmacol. Exp. Ther.* **2012**, *342*, 608–618. [CrossRef] [PubMed]

7

Omega-3 Fatty Acids and Cancer Cell Cytotoxicity: Implications for Multi-Targeted Cancer Therapy

Donatella D'Eliseo [1,2] and Francesca Velotti [2,*]

[1]   Department of Molecular Medicine, Istituto Pasteur-Fondazione Cenci Bolognetti,
      Sapienza University of Rome, 00161 Rome, Italy; donatella.deliseo@uniroma1.it
[2]   Department of Ecological and Biological Sciences (DEB), La Tuscia University, Largo dell'Università,
      01100 Viterbo, Italy
*   Correspondence: velotti@unitus.it

Academic Editors: Lindsay Brown, Bernhard Rauch and Hemant Poudyal

Abstract: Cancer is a major disease worldwide. Despite progress in cancer therapy, conventional cytotoxic therapies lead to unsatisfactory long-term survival, mainly related to development of drug resistance by tumor cells and toxicity towards normal cells. n-3 polyunsaturated fatty acids (PUFAs), eicosapentaenoic acid (EPA) and docosahexaenoic acid (DHA), can exert anti-neoplastic activity by inducing apoptotic cell death in human cancer cells either alone or in combination with conventional therapies. Indeed, n-3 PUFAs potentially increase the sensitivity of tumor cells to conventional therapies, possibly improving their efficacy especially against cancers resistant to treatment. Moreover, in contrast to traditional therapies, n-3 PUFAs appear to cause selective cytotoxicity towards cancer cells with little or no toxicity on normal cells. This review focuses on studies investigating the cytotoxic activity of n-3 PUFAs against cancer cells via apoptosis, analyzing the molecular mechanisms underlying this effective and selective activity. Here, we highlight the multiple molecules potentially targeted by n-3 PUFAs to trigger cancer cell apoptosis. This analysis can allow a better comprehension of the potential cytotoxic therapeutic role of n-3 PUFAs against cancer, providing specific information and support to design future pre-clinical and clinical studies for a better use of n-3 PUFAs in cancer therapy, mainly combinational therapy.

Keywords: fatty acids (FAs); n-3 polyunsaturated fatty acids (PUFAs); docosahexaenoic acid (DHA); eicosapentaenoic acid (EPA); apoptosis; cytotoxicity; cancer therapy; combinational therapy; drug resistance; cancer stem cells

1. Introduction

Cancer is a major burden of disease worldwide and, in certain countries, it ranks the second most common cause of death following cardiovascular diseases [1]. Furthermore, as elderly people are most susceptible to cancer and population aging continues, cancer is projected to become the leading cause of death worldwide in many countries. Despite progress made in recent years in cancer therapy, traditional cytotoxic therapies such as chemo- and radio-therapy have multiple limitations, leading to treatment failure, cancer relapse and unsatisfactory long-term clinical results [2]. These limitations are mainly related to two important issues: (1) conventional therapies lead to development of drug resistance by tumor cells and/or fail to destroy cancer stem cells (CSCs) or tumor-initiating cells (TICs), a population of self-renewing and drug resistant cancer cells [3,4]; (2) conventional therapies can cause normal cells to die in massive number, leading to local and systemic toxicity. Since cancer cell survival is driven by complex molecular interactions between growth and death signals [5], most oncologists think that targeting a single molecular component may not be sufficient to disrupt this process and combinational therapies, targeting multiple molecules, pathways, or networks are needed to eradicate the tumor and increase patients' survival [6].

Omega-3 (ω-3 or n-3) fatty acids (FAs) are an important family of polyunsaturated fatty acids (PUFAs) and key nutrients, involved in normal growth and development of various human tissues [7–9]. Longer chain n-3 polyunsaturated fatty acids (PUFAs) are mainly composed of eicosapentaenoic acid (EPA) and docosahexaenoic acid (DHA). EPA has 20 carbon atoms and 5 double bonds (20:5n-3). DHA has a chain with 22 carbon atoms and 6 double bounds (22:6n-3), which makes it the longest chain and most unsaturated FA commonly found in biological systems. In the human body, DHA is either derived from β-oxidation of EPA or acquired from the diet. Cold-water oily fish are the main dietary source of essential n-3 PUFAs in humans, providing thus relatively large amount of EPA and DHA [10]. Beyond their role in physiological functions, n-3 PUFAs can affect some chronic diseases such as cancer [8,9,11–13]. Indeed, n-3 PUFAs or purified EPA and DHA can exert anti-neoplastic activity, playing a potential role either in cancer prevention or in cancer therapy [11–13].

Several decades ago, on the basis of human epidemiological studies, dietary oily fish and fish oil (FO) consumption have been associated with the protection against the development of some types of cancer, mainly colorectal, mammary and prostatic cancers [14,15]. Thereafter, most of the studies performed either in vitro or in vivo have demonstrated the protection by n-3 PUFAs against cancer risk. However, some reports question the effectiveness of these compounds in neoplastic prevention, and others argue that an increased n-3 PUFAs intake could induce some types of cancer [15–19]. Thus, the potential preventive role of n-3 PUFAs has become a subject of intense interest and debate. The biological effects of n-3 PUFAs on normal cells to prevent their transformation are not the topic of our dissertation, since exhaustive reviews have been written and have critically analyzed the data in the literature [15,16,20,21].

During recent years, extensive studies have also considered the potential therapeutic activity of n-3 PUFAs against established solid and hematological tumors [13,22]. A number of biological effects that could contribute to this activity have been suggested, including induced alteration by n-3 PUFAs of cancer cell invasion and metastasization, as well as proliferation and apoptosis [21–25]. The induction of tumor cell apoptosis plays an important role in cancer therapy and represents a prominent target of many treatment strategies. Several studies have demonstrated that n-3 PUFAs, EPA and DHA have inhibitory effects on tumor growth by inducing cancer cell death via apoptosis, either alone [22–25] or in combination with conventional anticancer therapies [26–31]. Although all these studies have proposed molecular mechanisms that account for the pro-apoptotic activity of n-3 PUFAs in cancer cells, the mechanisms are still not completely understood, and a large number of molecular targets of n-3 PUFAs have been identified and multiple mechanisms appear to underlie the induction of apoptosis by these FAs. However, notably, the cytotoxic activity exerted by n-3 PUFAs is very peculiar for two main reasons. First, it has the potential to increase the sensitivity of tumor cells to conventional cytotoxic therapies, possibly improving the efficacy of these therapies against some types of tumors, especially those otherwise resistant to treatments [26–35]. Second, it appears to be selective, in that n-3 PUFAs cause cytotoxicity against cancer cells with little or no toxicity on normal cells [28,36–45]. This is a very important point, since in order for a therapeutic agent to be truly effective, it should be toxic to cancer cells without harming normal cells; conversely, conventional chemotherapeutics kill cancer cells but also strike the healthy cells, causing adverse effects and severe morbidity. All the above considerations greatly support investigations carried out to assess the role of n-3 PUFAs as adjuvant, to improve the efficacy and tolerability of traditional anticancer therapies.

This review focuses on studies investigating the cytotoxic activity via apoptosis of n-3 PUFAs against cancer cells and analyzes the cellular and molecular mechanisms underlying this activity. In particular, it will be highlighted the wide range of molecules potentially targeted by n-3 PUFAs to induce cancer cell apoptosis. Firstly, in Section 2, it will be examined the pro-apoptotic activity exerted by n-3 PUFAs in different cancer models in vitro and in vivo, as well as the apoptotic pathways triggered by these FAs. Concerning this point, it will be also considered the important potential capability of

EPA and DHA of inducing cytotoxicity towards drug-resistant cancer cells such as CSCs or TICs. Next, in Section 3, it will be analyzed the molecular events upstream the triggering of apoptosis by n-3 PUFAs, highlighting the multiple potential molecular targets of these FAs. This review could allow a better comprehension of the potential cytotoxic therapeutic role of the principal long chain n-3 PUFAs EPA and DHA against cancer, providing specific information and support to design future pre-clinical and clinical studies, which lead to the development of a more proper and effective use of these FAs in human cancer therapy, mainly combinational therapy.

2. Induction of Cancer Cell Apoptosis by n-3 Polyunsaturated Fatty Acids (PUFAs) and Triggering of the Intrinsic and Extrinsic Apoptotic Pathways

Apoptosis is a programmed cell death process, occurring in physiological and pathological conditions [46]. Caspases are central to apoptosis mechanism, as they are both the initiators and executioners of this process. There are three pathways by which caspases can be activated. The two commonly described initiation pathways are the intrinsic (or mitochondrial) and the extrinsic (or death receptor) apoptotic pathways. Both pathways eventually lead to a common pathway or the execution phase of apoptosis mediated by the executioner caspase-3, -6 and -7. A third initiation pathway is the intrinsic endoplasmic reticulum (ER) pathway [46,47]. The intrinsic or mitochondrial pathway is activated by endogenous stress signals such as growth factor deprivation, DNA-damaging chemicals and reactive oxygen species (ROS), which increase mitochondrial membrane permeability by modifying the interplay between B cell lymphoma protein-2 (Bcl-2) family proteins, that interact with mitochondrial membrane voltage-dependent anion channels. Bcl-2 family proteins have either pro-apoptotic (e.g., Bak, Bax, or Bok) or anti-apoptotic (e.g., Bcl-2, Bcl-xL, or Mcl-1) roles; a Bcl-2 subfamily, the BH3-only protein family (e.g., Bad, Bid, Bim, Noxa or Puma) also modulate pro- and anti-apoptotic Bcl-2 protein interactions. Pro-apoptotic stimuli shift the balance towards apoptic proteins, promoting the mitochondrial outer membrane permeabilization (MOMP), the subsequent release of cytochrome C into the cytosol, followed by its complex formation with procaspase-9 and apoptotic protease-activating factor 1 (APAF1), leading to the activation of the initiator caspase-9; then, caspase-9 activates the executioner caspases. The extrinsic pathway of apoptosis is activated by signal originated by death receptors such as TNFα-receptors, CD95 (Fas) and TNF-related apoptosis-inducing ligand (TRAIL)-receptors, following their interaction with their corresponding ligands, TNFα, FasL and TRAIL. Receptor activation leads to recruitment, to receptor associated lipid rafts, of adaptor molecules to form death-inducing signaling complexes (DISCs), which contains TNF receptor-associated death domain (TRADD), Fas-associated death domain (FADD), procaspase-8/FLICE and receptor-interacting protein kinase 1 (RIPK1). This complex induces the activation of caspase-8 and -10, which activate the executioner caspases. In addition, caspase-8 can also truncate Bid (tBid), which can migrate to the mitochondria to associate with Bax, increasing membrane permeability and converging thus to the activation of the intrinsic apoptotic pathway. The intrinsic ER pathway of apoptosis is activated in response to diverse arrays of stress such as oxidative stress, calcium influx and ER stress. The ER has three main functions: (1) folding, glycosylation and sorting of proteins to their proper destination; (2) synthesizing cholesterol and other lipids; and (3) maintenance of Ca^{2+} homeostasis. Disruption of any of these processes causes ER stress and activates the unfolded protein response (UPR). However, following prolonged ER stress, imbalanced calcium storage will activate calpain, which can inactivate Bcl-Xl and also activate the executioner caspases, leading to apoptosis. Finally, the apoptotic cascade is regulated by regulatory proteins, such as FLICE-like inhibitory proteins (FLIPs), which inhibit the extrinsic apoptotic pathway by binding to FADD and causing dissociation of the FADD/caspase-8 complex. Additionally, families of inhibitor of apoptosis protein (IAP) (e.g., XIAP, cIAP, and survivin) bind to caspase-3 and -9, thereby inhibiting caspase activity. Moreover, XIAP associated factor 1 (XAF1) negatively regulates the antiapoptotic function of XIAP.

Evasion of apoptosis by tumor cells is a hallmark of cancer [5] and defects in cancer cell apoptosis have been described at any point along the apoptotic pathways, including impaired receptor signaling, disrupted balance of anti- and pro-apoptotic Bcl-2 family proteins, reduced expression of caspases and increased expression of regulatory proteins (e.g., IAPs).

2.1. In Vitro and in Vivo Induction of Cancer Cell Apoptosis by n-3 PUFAs

n-3 PUFAs, EPA and DHA can induce apoptosis in tumor cells *in vitro* and *in vivo*, in a dose- and time-dependent manner. They induce apoptosis *in vitro*, in tumor cell lines derived from a wide range of solid tumors including colorectal carcinoma [37,48–50], esophageal [51] and gastric cancers [52], hepatocellular carcinoma [53–55], pancreatic cancer [56–58], cholangiocarcinoma [59], breast [60,61], ovarian [62], prostate [63,64] and bladder [65] cancers, neuroblastoma [66] and glioma [67], lung cancer [68,69], squamous cell carcinoma (SCC) [42] and melanoma [70,71]. Apoptosis induced by n-3 PUFAs, EPA and DHA has been also described in cancer cell lines derived from hematological tumors such as myeloid and lymphoid leukemias and lymphomas [72–78], as well as multiple myeloma [44,79].

In addition, in these last years a great attention has been given to CSCs or TICs, a small population of cancer cells with self-renewal and drug resistance properties, involved in cancer initiation, maintenance, metastasis and recurrence [2–4,80]. Resistance of CSCs/TICs to standard anti-cancer therapies is responsible for ineffectiveness of these treatments, leading to tumor recurrence and metastasis [2–4]. Therefore, in order to establish efficient therapeutic strategies that can prevent tumor relapse and induce a long-lasting clinical response, it is important to develop drugs that can specifically target and eliminate CSCs/TICs. Remarkably, recent *in vitro* studies have indicated the capability of n-3 PUFAs to affect colorectal and breast CSCs [81–85]. Indeed, it was shown that both EPA and DHA (10–70 μM), separately, induced apoptosis in cancer stem-like cells derived from the SW620 colon cancer cell line, and the effect was markedly increased when they acted simultaneously. Moreover, both compounds enhanced the efficacy of chemotherapeutics agents such as 5-fluorouracil (5-FU) and mitomycin C against the same target cells [82]. Accordingly, it was observed that EPA alone and (with increased efficacy) in combination with 5-FU + oxaliplatin (OX) (FuOX) induced apoptosis in FuOX-resistant HT-29 and HCT116 colorectal carcinoma cells, highly enriched in CSCs [83]. In addition, de Carlo *et al.* [84] found that 25 μM EPA induced the differentiation of colon CSCs, by upregulating cytokeratin 20 and mucin 2 and downregulating CD133 expression; they hypothesized that the increased degree of colon CSC differentiation could be strictly related to the EPA-induced sensitization of CD133[+] cells to 5-FU. More recently, in human triple negative breast cancers, it has been shown that DHA inhibited mammosphere formation of TICs [85]. The capability of n-3 PUFAs to eliminate CSCs/TICs and/or increase their sensitivity to conventional antineoplastic drugs have a very important therapeutic potential, further supporting the anticancer use of these FAs as adjuvants in cancer therapies.

Suppression of tumor cell growth by n-3 PUFAs has been confirmed *in vivo*, in pre-clinical studies using cancer animal models mainly rapresented by transgenic "fat-1" mice (bearing the *Caenorhabditis elegans* "n-3 desaturase" gene able to convert n-6 to n-3 PUFAs, resulting thus in elevated n-3 PUFAs tissue content) and xenograft nude mice implanted with different tumor cell types [13,22,24,41,86–89]. However, it should be noted that most studies have been performed in experimental settings evaluating the suppression of tumor development and only few investigations have been realized in therapeutic settings, evaluating the capability of PUFAs to eradicate established tumors [24,41,86–89].

Encouraging results concerning the *in vivo* anti-neoplastic activity of n-3 PUFAs have been also obtained from clinical studies, even though they were mainly set-up to investigate cancer prevention and support, rather than cancer therapy [25,30,31,90–101]. Indeed, the outcomes mainly investigated included n-3 PUFAs membrane incorporation, immune and inflammatory responses, oxidative status, as well as body weight and composition or quality of life [31,96,97,99–101]. Few studies addressed n-3 PUFAs supplementation and decrease of tumor size or extension of patient survival [90–93,95,96,98,100] (Table 1).

Table 1. Overview of human studies investigating the clinical outcome or prognosis in cancer patients supplemented with *n*-3 polyunsaturated fatty acids (PUFAs).

Cancer Type	Study Type	Enrolled Subjects	Pts (n)	FA/Daily	Objectives	Outcomes	Ref.
CRC	Phase II double-blind RCT	Patients under-going liver resection surgery for CRCLM	43 (T) 45 (C)	EPA (2 g)	To evaluate: ki67 proliferation index; safety and tolerability; tumor FA content; CD31-positive vascularity.	No difference in Ki67 proliferation index. Treatment was safe and well tolerated. EPA was incorporated into CRC liver metastasis tissue. Treatment reduced vascularity of CRC liver metastases. In the first 18 months after CRCLM resection, EPA-treated patients obtained OS benefit compared with control, although early CRC recurrence rates were similar.	[95]
CRC	Systematic review and meta-analysis: 9 trials published until September 2014	Patients with CRC undergoing concomitant surgery (5 trials) or chemotherapy (3 trials)	242 (T) 233(C)	EPA + DHA (2.2 g; median daily dose (range 0.6-4.8)	To evaluate the effects of *n*-3 PUFAs on inflammatory mediators (cytokines and acute phase proteins): IL-6 and IL-1β, TNF, CRP and CRP/albumin ratio.	Benefits on some inflammatory mediators, but they are specific for some supplementation protocols (duration, dose, route) and concomitant anti-cancer treatment: reduction in IL-6 occurs in surgical patients that received 0.2 g/kg of FO parenterally at postoperative period ($p = 0.002$); increase in albumin occurs in surgical patients that received >2.5 g/d of EPA+DHA orally at preoperative period ($p = 0.038$); in patients undergoing chemo- therapy, the supplementation of 0.6 g/d of EPA+DHA during 9 week reduces CRP levels ($p = 0.017$), and CRP/albumin ratio ($p = 0.016$).	[101]
CRC	RCT with two arms, parallel groups, open label	Patients with advanced CRC never submitted to chemotherapy	17 (T) 13 (C)	FO (2 g); (0.6g/day EPA + DHA)	To evaluate clinical outcomes during and after chemotherapy in individuals with CRC who received FO in the first 9 week of treatment. Outcomes assessed were: number of chemotherapy cycles administered; days undergoing chemotherapy; number of delays and interruptions in the admi-nistration of chemotherapy; number of hospitalizations during chemothery; tumor progression; values of CEA; days until events (death and progression); and 3-year survival.	Time to tumor progression was significantly longer in treated (593 days ±211.5) *vs* control (330 days ±135.1) patients ($P = 0.04$); treated patients presented also lower CEA values after chemotherapy (however these differences were not statistically significant); other outcomes did not differ between groups.	[90]

Table 1. *Cont.*

Cancer Type	Study Type	Enrolled Subjects	Pts (n)	FA/Daily	Objectives	Outcomes	Ref.
Breast cancer	Open-label, one-arm phase II study	Metastatic breast cancer patients undergoing anthracycline-based chemotherapy (5-FU, epirubicin, cyclophosphamide) at first-line treatment for metastases	25 (T)	DHA (1.8 g)	To investigate the efficacy and safety of adding DHA to an oral supplement ROS generating chemotherapy treatment, by measuring response rate and OS.	No adverse effects. Higher plasma DHA concentrations were associated to greater median time to progression (8.7 months) and OS (34 months) compared to patients with low plasma DHA levels (3.5 and 18 months, respectively).	[91]
Breast cancer	A population-based follow-up study (using resources from the Long Island Breast Cancer Study Project)	Women newly diagnosed with first primary in situ (16%) or invasive (84%) breast cancer	1463	Variable dietary fish intake	To investigate whether dietary *n*-3 PUFA intake benefits survival after breast cancer.	All cause mortality was reduced by 16% to 34% among women with breast cancer who reported a high intake of fish and *n*-3 PUFAs.	[100]
NSCLC	Two-arm, non-randomized phase II study	Patients with advanced NSCLC undergoing platinum-based chemotherapy (carboplatin with vinorelbine or gemcitabine) as first-line treatment	15 (T) 31 (C)	EPA + DHA (2.5 g)	To evaluate whether the combination of FO and chemotherapy provided a benefit over standard of care on response rate and clinical benefit from chemotherapy.	Plasma EPA and DHA were higher in treated patients ($p < 0.001$ and $p = 0.004$, respectively). Treated patients had an increased response rate and greater clinical benefit compared with the control group (60.0% *vs* 25.8%, $p = 0.008$; 80.0% *vs* 41.9%, $p = 0.02$, respectively). The incidence of dose-limiting toxicity did not differ between groups ($p = 0.46$). One-year survival tended to be greater in treated patients (60.0% *vs* 38.7%; $p = 0.15$).	[93]
NSCLC	Prospective RCT	Adva-ced NSCLC receiving paclitaxel and cisplatin/carboplatin treatment	46 (T) 46 (C)	EPA (2 g)	To compare the effect of an oral EPA enriched supplement with an isocaloric diet on nutritional, clinical and inflammatory parameters and health-related quality of life. Response to chemotherapy and survival were also evaluated.	Improvement of energy and protein intake, body composition, and decreased fatigue, loss of appetite and neuropathy. There was no difference in response rate or OS between control and EPA group.	[96]
Pancreatic Cancer	A systematic evaluation of results of 11 prospective cohort RCTs	Unresectable pancreatic cancer patients	602 (T) 765 (C)	EPA (range 1-6 g) and/or DHA (range 0.96-1 g)	To systematically evaluate results of trials examining the effects of *n*-3 PUFA consumption on body weight, lean body mass, resting energy expenditure, and OS.	A significant increase in body weight ($p < 0.00001$) and lean body mass ($p < 0.00001$), a significant decrease in resting energy expenditure ($p = 0.03$), and an increase in OS (130–259 days *vs* 63–130 days) in patients who consumed an oral nutrition supplement enriched with *n*-3 PUFAs compared to those who consumed conventional nutrition.	[98]

Abbreviations: Pts (n), number of patients; FA, fatty acids; C, control; T, treated; CRC, colorectal; CRCLM, colorectal cancer liver metastases; OS, overall survival; RCT, randomized controlled trial; CEA, carcinoembryonic antigen; NSCLC, non-small-cell lung cancer; IL, interleukin; TNF, tumor necrosis factor ; CRP, C-reative protein; FO, fish oil; PUFAs, polyunsaturated fatty acids; DHA, docosaexaenoic acid; EPA, eicosapentaenoic acid; 5-FU, 5-fluorouracil; Ref, reference number.

Thus, although in these studies *n*-3 PUFAs supplementation was associated with improvement of clinical outcome and prognosis, the conclusion is limited because of the limited amount of data.

2.2. Triggering of the Intrinsic and Extrinsic Apoptotic Pathways by n-3 PUFAs

Many studies have reported that *n*-3 PUFAs induced apoptosis by triggering the intrinsic mitochondrial and ER pathways. In fact, EPA increased caspase-3 and -9, but not caspase-8, while inducing apoptosis in Ramos lymphoma cells [102]. Different studies in colon cancer (LS-174, HT-29, Caco-2 and COLO 201) cell lines showed that dietary FO [103] or DHA [104,105] modified the expression of Bcl-2 family proteins by increasing the levels of the pro-apoptotic proteins Bak and Bcl-xS and decreasing those of the anti-apoptotic proteins Bcl-2 and Bcl-xL. Similarly, Sun *et al.* [54] observed that DHA induced apoptosis in human Bel-7402 hepatocellular carcinoma cells, by up-regulating caspase-3 and Bax expression levels and downregulating the expression of Bcl-2 and Bim. Recently, Abdi *et al.* [44] demonstrated that EPA and DHA induced apoptosis in myeloma (L363, OPM-1, OPM-2 and U266) cells through mitochondrial perturbation and caspase-3 activation, whereas both compounds did not affect the viability of normal human peripheral blood mononuclear cells. Moreover, the analysis of gene modulation by *n*-3 PUFAs in myeloma cells revealed the modulation of several signal pathways, including nuclear factor (NF)-κB, Notch, Hedgehog, oxidative stress and Wnt, indicating the possible involvement of multiple molecular signals in the initiation of apoptosis by the intrinsic pathway. Finally, the activation of the intrinsic ER stress pathway has been also proposed underlying DHA-induced apoptosis in colon cancer cells. Indeed, Jackobsen *et al.* [106] showed that DHA, while inducing cell death in the aggressive SW620 colon cancer cell line, also induced extensive changes in gene expression patterns (mRNA) of ER stress; they also found abundant presence of phosphorylated eIF2α, increase in cytosolic Ca^{2+} and disturbances in lipid metabolism, suggesting that cytotoxic effects of DHA are associated with signaling pathways involving lipid metabolism and ER stress.

On the other hand, other studies have indicated the activation of the extrinsic pathway in the induction of apoptosis by *n*-3 PUFAs. Indeed, increased expression of both caspase-9 and caspase-8 was reported in EPA- [107] and DHA- [108] induced apoptosis in human HL-60 leukemia and Caco-2 colon cancer cells, respectively. In the case of colon cancer cell apoptosis, tBid expression was also enhanced, indicating a contribution of caspase-8 also to the activation of the mitochondrial pathway. Accordingly, in our laboratory we found the involvement of caspase-8 in DHA-mediated apoptosis in pancreatic and bladder cancer cell lines [65].

Finally, both DHA and EPA could exert an important pro-apoptotic effect in different colorectal cancer (Caco-2, HT-29, HCT116, LoVo, SW480) cells by the downregulation of two key regulatory elements of the extrinsic and intrinsic pathways, FLIP and XIAP, respectively; interestingly, DHA and EPA did not affect the viability of normal human colon mucosal epithelium (NCM460) cells [39].

3. Molecules, Signals and Networks Targeted by *n*-3 PUFAs: Upstream Events in the Triggering of the Apoptotic Pathways

Cancer is often described as a disorder of the balance between cell growth and death [5]. On the one hand, defects in signaling pathways promoting cell growth and survival occur in cancer cells and high constitutive levels of MEK/ERK, PI3K/Akt, JAK/STAT or IKK/IκB/NF-κB pathways are frequently observed in human cancers [5,109]. On the other hand, as already mentioned in Section 2, defects along the apoptotic pathways also occur in cancer cells, leading to resistance to apoptosis [5,110]. Therefore, all the molecules, signals and networks involved in cancer cell survival and death are potential targets for apoptosis-based cancer therapies.

The mechanisms by which *n*-3 PUFAs induce apoptosis in tumor cells are not fully determined in molecular terms; however, the proposed main routes of action of *n*-3 PUFAs are: (1) incorporation into cell membranes, leading to changes in the distribution and function of key survival and death signals; (2) generation of lethal levels of intracellular oxidative stress; (3) modulation of eicosanoid metabolites;

(4) binding to nuclear receptors, leading to changes in gene expression. These routes may underlie the pleiotropic and multifaceted effects of n-3 PUFAs, leading to the induction of apoptosis in cancer cells and/or to the sensibilization of tumor cells to traditional therapies. Therefore, in the context of these four routes of action of n-3 PUFAs, in this section we analyze studies investigating the mechanisms underlying the induction of apoptosis, highlighting the potential upstream molecular events targeted by n-3 PUFAs to trigger the apoptotic pathways in cancer cells.

3.1. Cell Membrane Enrichment in n-3 PUFAs and Changes in the Distribution and Function of Key Survival and Death Signals in Cancer Cells

Once ingested, n-3 PUFAs, EPA and DHA are uptaken and incorporated in tumor cell membranes by both passive or carrier-mediated transmembrane translocation [29]. The FA composition of membrane phospholipids can influence multiple cellular functions. It should be noted that DHA, for its high level of unsaturation and presence of several CH-CH$_2$-CH repeating units in its molecule, possesses an extremely flexible structure, more flexible than EPA, and it can rapidly isomerize through different conformational states [29]. Therefore, the enrichment of n-3 PUFAs in tumor cell membranes and the high molecular disorder originating from their (mainly DHA) incorporation into membrane phospholipids may affect physical-chemical properties of membranes, including their fluidity, permeability, deformability, as well as their lipid microdomain formation [29,111]. Plasma membrane is composed of microdomains of saturated lipids that segregate together to form "lipid rafts". Lipid rafts are enriched in glycosylphosphatidylinositol-linked proteins, contain several signaling proteins (e.g., epidermal growth factor receptor, EGFR) and play a key role in cell signal transduction, mainly by facilitating the association of signal molecules (e.g., those involved in cell survival). Cholesterol is a critical lipid component for lipid raft integrity and function, and DHA have poor affinity for cholesterol and influences lipid rafts, modifying their biochemical and biophysical features and changing their composition and/or the activity of raft-related signaling molecules. Therefore, concerning the regulation of apoptosis, n-3 PUFAs have the potential to modulate the function of death receptors, growth factor receptors, cytokines and hormones receptors, as well as oncogenes, tumor suppressor genes and signal transduction secondary messangers (e.g., adapter proteins, receptor-associated enzymes, protein kinases and phosphatases). As a consequence, n-3 PUFAs may alter the activation of transcription factors and expression of genes as well as the phenotype of tumor cells [111]. Thus, cell membrane enrichment in n-3 PUFAs can influence multiple cellular functions at multiple biological levels. Moreover, noteworthy, it has been reported that there are significant differences between tumor and normal cells in n-3 PUFAs uptake and membrane distribution, being tumor cells deficient in PUFAs (especially in arachidonic acid-ARA, EPA and DHA) as compared to normal cells, since they have decreased activity of Δ^5 and Δ^6 desaturases. Although the exact reason for the low activity of desaturases in cancer cells is not known, it has been proposed that it might be a defence mechanism adopted by tumor cells to protect themselves from toxic molecules such as free radicals derived from n-3 PUFAs peroxidation in cancer cells (see Section 3.2) [112,113]. Therefore, the specific enrichment of tumor cell membranes with n-3 PUFAs, EPA or DHA is one of the possible reasons underlying the capability of n-3 PUFAs to induce cytotoxicity in tumor cells, with no or little action on normal cells.

Discoveries over the last decade propose that n-3 PUFAs incorporation into cancer cell membranes is essential for apoptosis by n3-PUFAs in different cancer cell models [26,113–115]. However, currently, the precise mechanism of how a selective change in DHA and EPA content of membranes translates to a change in signaling events to induce apoptosis is not completely clear. Therefore, in the next sections (from Section 3.1.1 to 3.1.6), we analyze the studies investigating this issue. We take into consideration different possible actions by n-3 PUFAs, such as the displacement of lipid raft associated onco-proteins as well as the modulation of different survival signaling pathways in tumor cells, including Wnt/β-catenin, MAPK/Erk, PI3K/Akt/mTOR, JAK-STAT and NF-κB pathways.

3.1.1. Changes in Lipid Raft-Associated Onco-Proteins by n-3 PUFAs

The involvement of the modulation of EGFR and HER-2 signals in n-3 PUFAs-induced apoptosis has been reported by different studies, performed in different types of cancer (mainly breast cancer) cells. In 2007, Schley and coworkers [116] showed that apoptosis induced by a combination of EPA and DHA in MDA-MB-231 breast cancer cells was due to changes in lipid raft composition, leading to a decrease of EGFR levels as well as an increase of EGFR and p38 mitogen-activated protein kinase (MAPK) phosphorylation. Accordingly, in oral SCC cells, it was found that DHA- and EPA-induced apoptosis was mediated by amplification of the EGFR/ERK/p90RS kinase (K) pathway (i.e., EGFR autophosphorylation, sustained phosphorylation of ERK1/2 and of its downstream target p90RSK); to note, the viability of normal keratinocytes was not affected [42]. In contrast with these results, in three different (A549 lung, WiDr colon and MDA-MB-231 breast) cancer cell models it was found that DHA-induced apoptosis was caused by the exclusion of EGFR from caveolin-rich lipid raft fractions, resulting in a decreased association of Ras with Sos1 and the subsequent downregulation of Erk signaling; these data were confirmed in vivo, using xenograft athymic mice implanted with A549 cells [117]. Similarly, a reduction of EGFR activation was observed in EPA- or DHA-induced apoptosis in breast cancer (MDA-MB-231 and MCF-7) cells, associated to a reduction of Bcl2 and caspase-8 expression; moreover, DHA (probably related to its better capability to change lipid raft properties), but not EPA, also slightly reduced EGFR concentration [118]. More recently, in line with these results, it was found that DHA had the capability of decreasing cell surface levels of lipid rafts via their internalization and then fusion with lysosomes in MDA-MB-231 breast cancer cells. This implied that DHA displaced several raft-associated onco-proteins, including EGFR, Hsp90, Akt, and Src and also decreased total levels of those proteins via multiple pathways, including the proteasomal and lysosomal pathways, thereby decreasing their activities such as Hsp90 chaperone function [119]. Then, the therapeutic potential of DHA in the treatment of HER-2 positive breast cancers has been reported by two investigators. Ravacci [43], Mason [120] and coworkers showed that DHA induced apoptosis in transformed human mammary epithelial (HB4aC5.2) cells and in breast cancer (BT-474) cells, respectively, by the deplacement of HER-2 from lipid rafts and the decrease of Akt and ERK1/2 activation; no effects were observed in related untransformed (HB4a) cells.

New insight into the potential application of n-3 PUFAs in breast cancer treatment was also provided by a recent investigation in MCF-7 and T47D breast cancer cells, showing that DHA and EPA could shift the pro-survival estrogen signal to a pro-apoptotic effect by increasing the G protein coupled estrogen receptor 1-cyclic adenosine monophosphate-protein kinase A (GPER1-cAMP-PKA) signaling response, blunting EGFR, Erk 1/2 and AKT activity [121].

It is of interest that it has been also demonstrated that pre-treatment of estrogen receptor negative MDA-MB-231 cells with DHA increased the anti-cancer effects of doxorubicin, by increasing the plasma membrane raft content of CD95 and FADD. [122].

Finally, in prostate cancer (PC3 and LNCaP) cells, growth suppression by DHA was due to changes in cell plasma membrane phospholipid content, leading to the alteration of phosphatidylinositol phosphates (PIPs) content, $PI(3,4,5)P_3$ (PIP_3) and Akt localization, inhibition of Akt phosphorylation and thus of the AKT survival signaling pathway [123].

3.1.2. Inhibition of the Wnt/β-Catenin Pathway by n-3 PUFAs

Wnt functions causing an accumulation of β-catenin in the cytoplasm and its eventual translocation into the nucleus, to act as a transcriptional coactivator of transcription factors that belong to the T cell factor/lymphoid enhancer factor (TCF/LEF) family. Dysregulation of Wnt signaling and β-catenin expression is believed to be central in the regulation of tumor cell apoptosis [109].

In 2007, Calviello et al. [124] proposed that DHA exerted pro-apoptotic effects in colon cancer cells through proteasomal-dependent degradation of β-catenin, leading to down-regulation of the expression of TCF-β-catenin target genes such as survivin (a IAP family member). Then, Lim [53,59], Song [125] and coworkers showed that DHA- and EPA-induced apoptosis in human cholangiocarcinoma, hepatocellular and pancreatic carcinoma cells was caused by the inhibition of the β-catenin signaling pathway through two systems of β-catenin degradation, such as the activation (by dephosphorylation) of glycogen synthase kinase-3β (GSK-3β) and the induction of the formation of β-catenin/Axin/GSK-3β binding complex; similar results were obtained *in vivo*, in Fat-1 transgenic mice implanted with mouse pancreatic cancer (PANC02) cells [125]. More recently, the inhibition of the Wnt/β-catenin pathway was also found to be involved in growth suppression of breast MCF-7 cancer cells *in vitro* and in therapy experiments *in vivo*, performed in Babl/c mice bearing 4T1 mouse breast cancer and fed with a 5% FO diet [126].

3.1.3. Modulation of the Mitogen-Activated Protein Kinase (MAPK)/ERK (or Ras/Raf/MEK/ERK) Pathway by n-3 PUFAs

The MAPK/ERK pathway includes many MAPK proteins (originally called extracellular signal-regulated kinases, ERK), which function by adding phosphate groups to a neighboring protein, leading to change the expression of genes specific for molecules involved in cell cycle and apoptosis. This pathway represents a necessary step in the development and progression of many cancers. Although the activation of ERK is traditionally linked to cell survival and proliferation, recent studies have demonstrated that this is not always the case and ERK activation can also cause growth arrest or apoptosis [109]. Indeed, as reported below, both activation and inhibition of ERK have been associated with n-3 PUFAs-induced tumour cell apoptosis, suggesting that tissue- or cancer-specific mechanisms of n-3 PUFAs action might occur.

In 2008, Serini *et al.* [68] showed that DHA-induced apoptosis was due to decreased levels of phosphorylated MAPKs, especially ERK1/2 and p38 in lung cancer cells. Accordingly, n-3 PUFAs induced apoptosis in breast cancer cells *in vitro* and in a Fat-1 mice breast cancer model, by inhibition of the MEK/ERK/Bad signaling pathway; the inhibition was induced through the increased expression of the integral membrane protein syndecan-1 (SDC-1) [127]. On the other hand, in gastric cancer cells, DHA-induced apoptosis was caused by the activation of ERK and c-Jun N-terminal kinase (JNK), leading to the activation of AP-1 transcription factor, which induced the expression of apoptotic genes [52].

3.1.4. Inhibition of the PI3K/Akt/mTOR Pathway by n-3 PUFAs

PI3K (phosphatidylinositol-3-kinase) is one of the intracellular pathways responsible for the transmission of anti-apoptotic signals by cell survival factors. Phosphatase and tensin homologue deleted on chromosome ten (PTEN) is a lipid phosphatase, which catalyzes the dephosphorylation of PIP3 and thus serves as a major negative regulator of PI3K/Akt signaling; when it is phosphorylated, it becomes inactive. Akt (or protein kinase B, PKB) is a serine/threonine kinase, activated in response to cytokines and growth factors through its translocation to the plasma membrane and its phosphorylation at two key residues (Thr308 and Ser473). Akt activation promotes directly cell survival and protect cells from apoptosis by inactivating components of the cell death machinery (e.g., caspase-9, Bad); in addition, Akt promotes indirectly cell survival and protect cells from apoptosis by activating transcription factors such as NF-κB, that induces the transcription of pro-survival and anti-apoptotic genes. Mammalian target of rapamycin (mTOR) is a protein kinase that integrates both intracellular and extracellular signals, and serves as a central regulator of cell metabolism, growth and survival. It regulates the activity of p70S6K and eukaryotic initiation factor (eIF)4E binding protein-1 (4E-BP1). The mTOR pathway is deregulated and activated in several types of cancer, significantly contributing to the enhancement of proliferation and the inhibition of autophagy; overexpression of downstream mTOR effectors 4E-BP1, S6K and eIF4E4 leads to poor cancer prognosis. Therefore, inhibition of mTOR activity disrupts the balance between pro- and anti-apoptotic proteins, enhancing tumor cell death [109].

It was shown that EPA and DHA induced apoptosis in MDA-MB-231 breast cancer cells *in vitro* [128,129] and in a xenograft animal model [129] by the inhibition of the survival Akt/NF-κB signaling pathway, due to the inactivation of PI3K, through increased PTEN expression by *n*-3 PUFAs. On the other hand, DHA-mediated apoptosis in colon cancer (Caco-2) cells, was due to the inactivation of PI3K induced by reduced PTEN phosphorylation by *n*-3 PUFAs. This inactivation promoted inhibition of Akt/PKB and thus of Bad and forkhead transcription factor (FKHR); to note, the viability of normal colon (NCM460) cells was not compromised [40,130]. Then, the suppression of the activity of (3'-phosphoinositide-dependent kinase 1)-PDK1/Akt/Bad signaling was demonstrated underlying *n*-3 PUFA-induced apoptosis in prostate cancer (PC3, LNCaP and DU145) cells *in vitro* and *in vivo*; moreover, the suppression was dependent on the upregulation of SDC-1, and 15-LOX-1-mediated metabolism of DHA was required for SDC-1 upregulation [64].

From recent studies, it has emerged that DHA can also simultaneously induce apoptosis and autophagy in cancer cells, and this process involves mTOR repression [131,132]. Indeed, DHA treatment in human cervical cancer cells led to autophagy via p53-mediated (AMP-activated protein kinase)-AMPK/mTOR signaling (*i.e.*, mTOR inhibition and AMPK activation), and DHA-induced autophagy sensitized tumor cells to apoptosis [131]. Then, in non-small cell lung cancer cells, it was shown that DHA-induced apoptosis and autophagy were associated to mTOR suppression induced by both AMPK activation and PI3K/Akt inhibition; these data were confirmed in Fat-1 transgenic mice implanted with Lewis lung cancer cells [133].

3.1.5. Inhibition of the JAK-STAT Pathway by *n*-3 PUFAs

The JAK-STAT system consists of a receptor (activated by interferons, interleukins, growth factors, or other chemical messengers), the Janus kinase (JAK) and the signal transducer and activator of transcription (STAT) proteins. STAT proteins once activated translocate into the nucleus, where they bind to DNA, promoting the transcription of specific genes affecting basic cell functions such as cell growth and death. The activation of STAT3 pathway in tumor cells is mainly due to the effect of tumor released factors and plays a critical role in tumor cell-survival and chemo-resistance [109].

A very recent work by Rescigno *et al.* [134] demonstrated that DHA-induced apoptosis in aggressive SK-BR-3 breast cancer cells reduced both ERK1/2 and STAT3 phosphorylation; interestingly, DHA only arrested cell cycle progression of non-tumor MCF-10A breast cells, activating p21$^{Waf1/Cip1}$ and p53. Moreover, it was also shown that the elimination of aldehyde dehydrogenase positive cells and the inhibition of mammosphere formation of TICs in human triple negative breast cancer cells by DHA was due to the Src homology region 2 domain-containing protein tyrosine phosphatase-1 (SHP-1)-dependent suppression of STAT3 activation and of its downstream mediators c-Myc and cyclin D1 [85].

3.1.6. Inhibition of the NF-κB Pathway by *n*-3 PUFAs

NF-κB transcription factor plays a key role in many physiological processes, including inflammation, cell proliferation and death. The aberrant regulation of NF-kB and signaling pathways that control its activity are heavily implicated in promoting pro-survival signaling and may be critical for resistance to chronic oxidative stress (*i.e.*, drug resistance) [2].

In prostate cancer (LNCaP, DU145, PC3) cells, it was shown that DHA synergistically enhanced the cytotoxic effect of docetaxel, through increased apoptosis by suppression of genes involved in the NF-κB pathway [135]. Then, always in prostate cancer (LNCaP and PacMetUT1) cells, it was reported that exposure of cells to DHA attenuated H_2O_2-induced NF-κB transcriptional activity and diminished the expression of the downstream anti-apoptotic target survivin; this activity was specific, since it was not observed in normal human prostate (PrEC) cells [136].

3.2. Cell Membrane Enrichment in n-3 PUFAs and Increased Oxidative Stress in Tumor Cells

One of the main characteristics of *n*-3 PUFAs is the fact that they are optimal substrates for oxidants inside the cell, undergoing thus nonenzymatic lipid peroxidation into cell membranes; moreover, nonenzymatic lipid peroxidation triggers a further increase of the formation of oxygen radicals and

ROS [29]. Tumor cells contain higher levels of ROS compared to normal cells, principally due to their accelerated metabolism needed to maintain their high proliferation rate. Thus, ROS in tumor cells can react with intracellular n-3 PUFAs giving rise to nonenzymatic lipid peroxidation products that are highly toxic [38]. The methylene group, located between two double bonds ($-$CH=CH$-$CH$_2$$-$CH=CH$-$), is particularly vulnerable to radical attack by reactive species, thus entailing the abstraction of hydrogen [29]. Moreover, DHA, possessing an additional double bond with respect to EPA, is more susceptible to nonenzymatic lipid peroxidation, providing a variety of lipid hydroxiperoxides and aldehydic breakdown products such as malonaldehyde (MDA; a marker for lipid peroxidation) with toxic as well as prooxidant properties [13,24]. Indeed, the nonenzymatic lipid peroxidation triggers a further increase of the generation of intracellular radical species; the further increase of intracellular ROS levels and oxidative stress in tumor cells by n-3 PUFAs (EPA > DHA) causes the disruption of the mitochondrial membrane potential, the release of cytochrome C and thus the triggering of the intrinsic apoptotic pathway (see Section 2). Moreover, DHA can be readily incorporated in mitochondrial membranes, altering their permeability and decreasing the mitochondrial membrane potential [29]. It has been also reported that DHA is mostly present in the mitochondrion in association with cardiolipins; cardiolipin-DHA molecules are under attack of radical species, with the consequent decrease of their binding affinity for cytochrome C, enhancement of its release and the release of other pro-apoptotic factors (e.g., Smac/Diablo) from mitochondria to cytosol, and the triggering of the intrinsic apoptotic pathway [29]. In addition, it is known that ROS can also oxidize and inhibit key signaling pathways involved in cell proliferation, survival and apoptosis, such as MAPK and NF-κB pathways [55,137]. Therefore, all these considerations indicate that lipid peroxidation and increased ROS levels play a key role in the induction of tumor cell apoptosis by n-3 PUFAs. Interestingly, it has been reported that there are significant differences in tumor vs normal cells not only in the uptake and distribution of n-3 PUFAs, but also in the ability to generate reactive species and oxidative stress from intracellular n-3 PUFAs. Indeed, as mentioned, tumor cells contain higher levels of oxygen radicals compared to normal cells and in presence of DHA they increase the production of cytotoxic lipid hydroperoxydes and other peroxides, undergoing apoptosis. In contrast to tumor cells, normal cells can use DHA to protect themselves from oxidative stress-induced apoptosis through a certain number of mechanisms, including the activation of the survival PI3K/Akt pathway as well as the increased production of cytoprotective molecules such as resolvins and protectins (see also Section 3.3) [138–140]. As reported in the next section, several investigators have shown that, as exogenous n-3 PUFAs are provided to cancer cells, these FAs can induce apoptosis by augmenting free radical generation and lipid peroxidation, whereas normal cells are not influenced [36,130,138].

Since ROS have been proposed as common mediators of apoptosis, the majority of cytotoxic anticancer agents (including ionizing radiations, most chemotherapeutic agents and some targeted therapies) work through ROS generation [29]. However, although they initially generate ROS production, most cancer cells following prolonged treatment with these drugs develop the capability to reduce ROS levels, resulting in drug-resistance. Evidence exists on the capability of n-3 PUFAs to increase both the efficacy of conventional anticancer therapies towards drug resistance and their tolerability towards normal cell damage. Indeed, n-3 PUFAs can increase the susceptibility of tumor cells to oxidative stress induced by conventional therapies, by maintaining high ROS levels in cancer cells, thereby precluding drug resistance [27,29]. Moreover, n-3 PUFAs can increase the tolerability to conventional therapies, by promoting both the selective induction of letal levels of oxidative stress in tumor cells and the selective production of protective lipid mediators in normal cells. Both activities have important therapeutic potential, further supporting the use of n-3 PUFAs as adjuvant in conventional cancer therapies.

Increased Oxidative Stress in Cancer Cells by n-3 PUFAs and Induction of Apoptosis

Early $in\ vitro$ studies performed in breast [60] and pancreatic [56] cancer cells proposed the involvement of oxidative mechanisms in the induction of cancer cell apoptosis by EPA and n-3 PUFAs, respectively; interestingly, increased oxidative stress and apoptosis were not observed in human normal cells, such as fibroblasts [60]. Further studies have shown that oxidative stress in cancer cells was generated by n-3 PUFAs through both generating lethal ROS levels and decreasing anti-oxidant activities in tumor cells [38].

In our laboratory, we showed that DHA promoted apoptosis in the human PaCa-44 pancreatic cell line through the induction of an active extrusion process of intracellular reduced glutathione (GSH), depleting tumor cells of one of the endogenous antioxidant defences, and increasing thus tumor cell sensibility to lipid peroxidation and oxidative stress [57]. This data has important implications for cancer therapy, since elevated GSH levels in tumors have been associated with resistance to apoptosis and chemotherapy [29]. Similarly, Ding and co-workers [141] found downregulation of the antioxidant enzyme superoxide dismutase 1 (SOD1) expression in the DHL-4 lymphoid cell line undergoing apoptotsis by DHA. Then, in the same laboratory, it was shown that DHA-mediated cytotoxicity in human ovarian cancer cell lines was associated to a reduction of glutathione peroxidase (GPx)-4 protein expression and that DHA-mediated cytotoxicity was reversed by vitamin E, suggesting that GPx-4 downregulation was due to oxidative stress [142]. Moreover, it was reported that the *in vitro* and *in vivo* sensitization of MDA-MB-231 breast cancer cells to anthracyclines (doxorubicin) by DHA was caused by a decrease of cytosolic GPx-1 activity and a concomitant increase of ROS levels [143].

On the other hand, n-3 PUFAs can also promote apoptosis by increasing lipid peroxidation and intracellular oxidative stress. It has been shown that DHA enhanced arsenic-trioxide-induced apoptosis in arsenic-trioxide resistant HL-60 (myeloid leukemia), SH-1 (hairy cell-leukemia), and Daudi (Burkitt lymphoma) cell lines by an increase of lipid peroxidation and a reduction of the mitochondrial membrane potential; these effects were reversed by the addition of the antioxidant vitamin E [144]. Similarly, Lindskog *et al.* [66] showed that DHA-mediated neuroblastoma cell death was associated with production of ROS and depolarization of the mitochondrial membrane potential, whereas vitamin E inhibited both mitochondrial depolarization and cell death; of note, nontransformed fibroblasts were not substantially affected by DHA. Moreover, DHA also significantly enhanced the cytotoxicity of arsenic trioxide, nonsteroidal antiinflammatory drug (diclofenac) and conventional chemotherapeutic agents (cisplatin, doxorubicin and irinotecan) both in chemosensitive and in multidrug-resistant neuroblastoma cells. More recently, similar effects were found in human HT-29 colorectal adenocarcinoma cells treated with DHA-combined treatment with 5-FU, OX and irinotecan (IRI); the anticancer action of DHA, observed in presence of low doses of chemotherapeutic drugs (1 μM 5-FU, 1 μM OX and 10 μM IRI), was carried out by loss of mitochondrial membrane potential and caspase-9 activation [145]. Increased lipid peroxidation associated to the activation of the intrinsic apoptotic pathway was confirmed by other investigators as mechanism underlying DHA- or EPA-mediated apoptosis, in different human cancer colon (HT-29 and Caco-2) [146] and gastric (MGC and SGC) [147] cell lines. In addition, in DHA-induced apoptotic human papillomavirus (HPV)-infected cancer cells, it was reported that the overproduction of mitochondrial ROS by DHA promoted the activation of the cellular ubiquitin-proteasome system, which leads to the degradation of E6/E7 oncoproteins, essential in the maintenance of HPV-associated malignancies [148].

Furthermore, it has been found that oxidative stress could induce apoptosis by triggering not only the intrinsic pathway, but also by the extrinsic pathway. Indeed, Kang *et al.* [149] found that DHA promoted apoptosis in MCF-7 breast cancer cells *in vitro* and *in vivo* via both ROS formation and caspase-8 activation, in that antioxidants or knockdown of caspase-8 each effectively abrogated cytotoxicity by DHA. To explain caspase-8 activation, the authors have hypothesized that ROS accumulation in plasma membrane lipid rafts might induce the assembly of DISC, triggering thus the extrinsic pathway. Then, the same investigators [58] also showed the induction of both ROS accumulation and caspase-8-dependent cell death by EPA and DHA, in human pancreatic cancer (MIA-PaCa-2 and Capan-2) cells *in vitro* and in xenografts athymic nude mice fed with 5% FO.

Recently, Jeong *et al.* [137] reported that the activation of MAPKs such as ERK/JNK/p38 was involved in DHA-induced apoptosis and that this activation was associated with mitochondrial ROS overproduction. Accordingly, Zhang *et al.* [55] showed that EPA caused apoptosis in HepG2 cells by evoking ROS formation, leading to both [Ca2+] accumulation and increased activation of JNK; both events promoted MOMP, the release of cytochrome C from mitochondria, and the activation of caspase-9 and caspase-3; to notice, EPA had no significant effect on the viability of normal liver (L-02) cells.

Finally, while it is well established that excessive ROS can instigate apoptosis, emerging data have also revealed a signaling role for ROS in the activation of autophagy. In PC3 and DU145 prostate cancer cells, with mutant p53 and exposed to DHA, it was found that ROS-mediated apoptosis and autophagy were caused by the inhibition of Akt-mTOR signaling [132]. According to these results, Zajdel *et al.* [150] showed that oxidative stress induced in human A549 lung cancer cells by EPA and DHA influenced apoptosis as well as tumor cell autophagy; the inhibition of the autophagic process suppressed cell death and decreased activation of caspase-3/7, indicating that EPA- and DHA-mediated autophagy could amplify cancer cell apoptosis.

3.3. Cell Membrane Enrichment in n-3 PUFAs and Changes in the Level and Quality of Eicosanoid Metabolites

Eicosanoids are generally considered as oxidized derivatives of 20-carbon FAs in the cell membrane, such as ARA (20:4n-6) and EPA. They include prostaglandins (PGs), thromboxanes (TXs), leukotrienes (LXs) and lipoxins (LXs). The major n-6 PUFA ARA, because of its prevalence in the phospholipids of cell membranes, is generally the major substrate for eicosanoid synthesis. Once released from membrane phospholipids, free ARA acts as a substrate for cyclooxygenases (COXs), lipoxygenases (LOXs) and cytochrome P450 enzymes; COX enzymes lead to 2-series PGs (e.g., PGE2) and TXs, and LOX enzymes to 4-series LTs and LXs, known as pro-inflammatory and pro-tumorigenic mediators. In fact, inflammation confers to tumor survival and drug resistance. On the other hand, EPA is also a substrate for COXs, LOXs and cytochrome P450 enzymes, giving rise to 3-series PGs (e.g., PGE3) and TXs and to 5-series LTs, known as anti-inflammatory and anti-tumorigenic mediators. These bioproducts bind specific receptors, usually G protein-coupled receptors, leading to the activation of signaling pathways involved in the regulation of cancer cell growth and death [9,13]. In addition, EPA and DHA give rise to anti-inflammatory and inflammation resolving metabolites, including resolvins produced from EPA (E-series) and DHA (D-series) and protectins and maresins produced from DHA [113,139,140,151,152]. Anti-inflammatory LXs, resolvins and protectins inhibit the expression of pro-inflammatory cytokines and adhesion molecules, thereby inhibiting tumor cell growth and invasion. Moreover, as mentioned in Section 3.2, it has been proposed that they behave as endogenous cytoprotective molecules for normal cells against lipid peroxidation-mediated damage by n-3 PUFAs. Indeed, enrichment of normal cell membranes in EPA and DHA, both *in vitro* and *in vivo*, may allow normal cells to produce enhanced amounts of resolvins and protectins, protecting themselves against toxic chemicals such as anti-cancer drugs [81]. Tumor cell membrane enrichment in n-3 PUFAs can induce changes in the level and quality of eicosanoid products by two main ways: (1) directly, by increasing specific metabolites derived from their metabolic conversion (e.g., PGE3); (2) indirectly, by inhibiting the conversion of ARA to pro-tumorigenic n-6 series eicosanoids (e.g., PGE-2). This second way might be pursued by displacing ARA from cell membranes (*i.e.*, n-3 PUFAs membrane incorporation partially replace ARA, reducing its availability), by competing with ARA for enzymes (e.g., EPA can act as an alternative substrate for COX-2, leading to a reduction in PGE2 in favour of PGE3), or by inhibiting NF-κB activation, thus decreasing COX-2 enzyme expression [9,29]. Moreover, DHA can inhibit COX-2 activity by binding the substrate channel of COX-2 [9].

COX-2 is overexpressed in many types of cancer leading to the formation of excess of PGE2 [153], and the autocrine COX-2/PGE2 pathway can confer tumor cell resistance to apoptosis by different ways, including the up-regulation of the β-catenin and Ras/Raf/MEK/ERK signaling pathways [154].

Modulation of Eicosanoid Bioproducts by *n*-3 PUFAs and Induction of Cancer Cell Apoptosis

Several studies have indicated that the modulation of eicosanoid production by *n*-3 PUFAs (mainly EPA) may contribute to the induction of apoptosis in cancer cells.

Some investigations have demonstrated that *n*-3 PUFAs can inhibit the autocrine anti-apoptotic COX-2/PGE2 pathway in tumor cells, leading thus to cancer cell apoptosis. Early *in vitro* and *in vivo* studies reported that decreased PGE2 production was associated with decreased growth of prostate [155,156] and breast [157] cancer cells. Furthermore, *n*-3 PUFAs inhibited tumor cell growth in a xenograft prostate cancer model by decreasing PGE2 as well as COX-2 levels [158]. Later, Funahashi *et al.* [159] showed that EPA decreased the growth of COX-2-positive and COX-2-negative PaCa pancreatic cancer cells and the COX-2-dependent mechanism was mediated by the binding of PGE3 to EP2 and EP4 receptors. Accordingly, dietary intake of *n*-3 PUFAs decreased the pancreatic cancer cell growth in a xenograft model through increasing PGE3 and decreasing PGE2 in tumor tissues. The down-regulation of COX-2 by *n*-3 PUFAs might be a crucial mechanism underlying their apoptotic effect in other types of tumors, including colon cancer [160,161]. In colorectal cancer cells, it was shown that EPA not only decreased COX-2 expression and PGE2 formation, but also increased the COX-dependent formation of EPA-derived metabolites [153]. All these results suggest that EPA may act as a "natural COX inhibitor". Very recently, Zhang C. *et al.* [113] found that the tumoricidal action of *n*-3 PUFAs on LoVo and RKO colorectal cancer cells *in vitro* was associated not only with the decreased production of pro-inflammatory PGE2 and LTB4, COX-2, arachidonate 5-LOX and microsomal PGE synthase expression, but also with the increased formation of anti-inflammtory LXA4, supporting the hypothesis that LXs, resolvins and protectins have a direct growth inhibitory action on tumor cells; in contrast, 5-FU produced opposite effects on these indices. On the other hand, concerning DHA metabolites, Gleissman *et al.* [138] showed that the cytotoxic action exerted by DHA in neuroblastoma cells was related to its conversion by 15-LOX and, at much lower degree by autoxidation, to 17-hydroxydocosahexaenoic acid (17-HDHA), via 17-hydroxyperoxydocosahexaenoic acid (17-HPDHA), a compound with significant cytotoxicity potency compared to DHA. In normal nervous tissue, DHA was converted by 5-LOX to anti-inflammatory and cytoprotective resolvins and protectins. In contrast, although neuroblastoma cells contained both 15-LOX and 5-LOX enzymes, the complete conversion of DHA into resolvins and protectins did not take place in cancer cells; thus, 17-HPDHA accumulated and exerted high cytotoxicity. Moreover, DHA, similarly to EPA, inhibited the secretion of PGE2 and augmented the cytotoxic potency of the COX-2-inhibitor celecoxib, by competing with ARA metabolites and by binding to catalytic sites of elongases, desaturases, and COX-2.

3.4. Binding of Nuclear Receptors by n-3 PUFAs and Changes in Gene Expression

Once released from the cell membrane, *n*-3 PUFAs can bind nuclear receptors such as peroxisome proliferator activating receptors (PPARs) in tumor cells [26], which, as ligand-activated transcription factors, regulate the expression of specific/target genes involved in several biological processes, including lipid metabolism and cell death. However, many of nuclear receptor-mediated effects of EPA and DHA are still unexplored.

It was shown that DHA-induced apoptosis in Reh and Ramos cells was mediated by PPARγ, which in turn up-regulated the p53 protein, leading to the activation of caspase-9 and caspase-3 [77]. Moreover, *in vitro* treatment of breast [162] and prostate [163] cancer cells with DHA activated PPARγ, which in turn up-regulated SDC-1 expression, inducing thus apoptosis. According to these results, O'Flaherty [164], Hu [165] and coworkers showed that 15-LOX metabolites of DHA, such as 17-HPDHA, 17-HDHA, 10,17-dihydroxy- and 7,17-dihydroxy-DHA, while exerting a more potent cytotoxicity on prostate PC3 cancer cells than DHA, like DHA induced apoptotic PC3 cells to activate a PPARγ reporter, which up-regulated SDC-1 expression; apoptosis was reduced by pharmacological inhibition or knockdown of PPARγ or SDC-1. In addition, 15-LOX-1-mediated metabolism of DHA was required to upregulate SDC-1 and to regulate the PDK/Akt signaling pathway that elicited prostate cancer cell apoptosis.

Table 2. Overview of studies investigating the apoptotic targets of *n*-3 PUFAs in human tumor cell lines *in vitro*.

Cell Lines	Cancer Type	Fatty Acid	Anti-Cancer Drug	Molecular Targets	Ref.
Caco-2, HT-29	Colorectal	FO	-	↓COX-2 signaling; ↓Bcl-2 expression	[103]
COLO 201	Colorectal	DHA	-	Bcl-2 family proteins: ↑Bak and Bcl-xS; ↓Bcl-xL and Bcl-2	[104]
LS-174, Colo 320 (p53-wild-type), HT-29 and Colo 205 (p53-mutant)	Colorectal	DHA	↑Susceptibility to 5-FU	Bcl-2 family proteins: ↓Bcl-xL and Bcl-2	[105]
SW620	Colorectal	DHA	-	↑ER stress genes (ERK-ATF4-CHOP pathway); ↑eIF2α, ↑cytosolic Ca^{2+}; Bcl-2 family proteins: ↑Bid; ↓Bad and Bik	[106]
Caco-2	Colorectal	DHA	-	Modulation of apoptotic genes: caspase-9 and -8 activation; pro-apoptotic Bcl-2 family, PG family, LOX, PPARα and γ	[108]
Caco-2, HT-29, HCT116, LoVo, SW480	Colorectal	DHA, EPA	-	↓FLIP, ↓XIAP	[39]
SW480, HCT116	Colorectal	DHA	-	↑Proteosomal degradation of β-catenin: ↓TCF-β-catenin target genes expression (survivin)	[124]
Caco-2	Colorectal	DHA	↑ Susceptibility to 5-FU, OX and irinotecan	↓PI3K and↓p38 MAPK/Akt pathway	[130], [40]
HT-29	Colorectal	DHA	-	Caspase-9 activation	[145]
HT-29, Caco-2	Colorectal	EPA, DHA	-	↑Lipid peroxidation, ↓Bcl-2 levels	[146]
HCA-7	Colorectal	EPA	-	↑COX-2-dependent PGE$_2$/PGE$_3$ switch	[153]
LoVo	Colorectal	EPA$^{(1)}$, DHA$^{(2)}$	-	$^{(1)}$↑PGE2, LTB4, COX-2, ALOX and mPGEs; $^{(2)}$↑LXA4, ↓LTB4, COX-2, ALOX5 and mPGES; ↑PGE2 and LXA4	[113]
MDA-MB-231	Breast	n-3 PUFAs	-	Lipid raft composition: ↑EGFR onco-protein; ↑EGFR and p38 MAPK signaling	[116]
A549, WiDr, MDA-MB-231	Lung, Colorectal, Breast	DHA	-	Lipid raft composition: ↓EGFR onco-protein; ↓EGFR and ERK signaling	[117]
MDA-MB-231, MCF-7	Breast	EPA, DHA	-	↓EGFR signaling; ↓Bcl-2; caspase-8 activation	[118]
MDA-MB-231	Breast	DHA	-	Lipid raft internalization: ↓lipid-raft-associated onco-proteins (EGFR, Hsp90, Akt, Src)	[119]
HB4aC5.2	Breast	EPA	-	Lipid raft disruption : ↓HER-2 onco-protein-mediated Akt and ERK1/2 signaling	[43]
BT-474	Breast	DHA	-	↓HER-2 onco-protein-mediated Akt and ERK1/2 signaling	[120]
MCF-7, T47D	Breast	DHA, EPA	-	↑Estrogen-mediated GPER1-cAMP-PKA signaling	[121]
MDA-MB-231	Breast	DHA	-	↑CD95-induced apoptosis	[122]
MCF-7	Breast	DHA	-	↓Wnt/β-catenin pathway	[126]
MCF-7, SK-BR-3	Breast	DHA	↑Susceptibility to doxorubicin	↑SDC-1 expression: ↓MEK/ERK/ Bad signaling	[127]
MDA-MB-231	Breast	n-3 PUFAs	-	↓PIK3/Akt/NF-κB signaling	[128]
MDA-MB-231	Breast	DHA, EPA	-	↑PTEN: ↓PIK3/Akt/NF-κB signaling and ↓transcription of Bcl-2 and Bcl-XL genes	[129]
SK-BR-3	Breast	DHA	-	↓ERK1/2 and STAT3 signaling	[134]
TIC	Breast	DHA	-	↑SHP-1: ↓STAT3 phosphorylation	[85]
MDA-MB-231	Breast	DHA	↑Susceptibility to doxorubicin	↓GPx-1	[143]
MCF-7	Breast	DHA	-	↑ROS production and caspase-8 activation	[149]
MCF-7	Breast	DHA	-	PPARγ activation: ↑SDC-1 expression	[162]
PC3, LNCaP	Prostate	DHA	-	↓PIP3 and Akt localization: ↓Akt signaling	[123]
PC3, LNCaP, DU145	Prostate	DHA	-	↑SDC-1 expression: ↓PDK1/Akt/Bad signaling	[64]
PC3, DU145	Prostate	DHA	-	↓Mitochondrial ROS: ↓Akt-mTOR signaling	[132]
LNCaP, DU145, PC3	Prostate	DHA	-	↓NF-κB pathway	[135]
LNCaP, PacMetUT1	Prostate	DHA	↑Susceptibility to docetaxel	↓NF-κB pathway: ↓survivin and ↑oxidative stress	[136]
PC3	Prostate	DHA	-	↑DHA oxidation and 17-HPDHA: binds PPARγ and ↑SDC-1 expression	[163], [164], [165]
A549, BEN	Lung	DHA	-	↑MPK-1: ↓ERK1/2 and p38 MAPK phosphorylation	[68]
A549, H1299	Lung	DHA	-	↑AMPK and ↓PI3K/Akt signaling; ↓mTOR	[133]
A549	Lung	DHA, EPA	-	↓Oxidative stress: ↑autophagy	[150]

Table 2. *Cont.*

Cell Lines	Cancer Type	Fatty Acid	Anti-Cancer Drug	Molecular Targets	Ref.
AGS	Gastric	DHA	-	↑ERK and JNK signaling; ↑AP-1, which induces apoptotic genes expression	[52]
MGC, SGC	Gastric	EPA, DHA	-	↑Lipid peroxidation	[147]
PaCa-44, MIA-PaCa-2, Capan-2	Pancreatic	DHA	-	↑GSH extrusion	[57]
MIA-PaCa-2, Capan-2	Pancreatic	EPA	-	↑ROS production and caspase-8 activation; ↑autophagy	[58]
SW1990, PANC-1	Pancreatic	DHA, EPA	-	↑β-catenin/Axin/GSK-3β complex-mediated β-catenin degradation	[125]
PaCa-44, EJ	Pancreatic, Bladder	DHA	-	Caspase-8 activation	[65]
Hep3B, Huh-7, HepG2	Hepatic	DHA, EPADHA	-	↑GSK-3β-mediated β-catenin degradation; ↓COX-2/PGE2 signaling	[53]
Bel-7402	Hepatic	DHA	-	Bcl-2 family proteins: ↓Bcl-2 and Bim;↑Bax; caspase-3 activation	[54]
HepG2	Hepatic	EPA	-	↑ROS-Ca²⁺-JNK mitochondrial pathway	[55]
SCC-13, SCC-25	Oral squamous cell	EPA	-	↑EGFR/ERK/p90RSK signaling	[42]
CCLP1, HuCCT1, SG231	Cholangiocarcinoma	DHA, EPA	-	↓Wnt/β-catenin; ↓COX-2 signaling	[59]
SK-N-DZ, SH-SY5Y (chemo-sensitive), SK-N-BE(2) (multi-drug resistant), SK-N-AS, IMR-32	Neuroblastoma	DHA	↑Susceptibility to cisplatin, doxorubicin and irinotecan	↑ROS production and depolarization of mitochondrial membrane potential	[66]
SK-N-BE(2) (multi-drug resistant), SH-SY5Y	Neuroblastoma	DHA	↑Susceptibility to celecoxib	DHA oxidation by 15-LOX to 17-HPDHA; no DHA oxidation by 5-LOX into resolvins and protectins; ↓COX-2/PGE2 signaling	[138]
HeLa (expressing HPV-18), SiHa	Cervical	DHA	-	↑Mitochondrial ROS: ubiquitin-proteasome system activation, leading to E6/E7 onco-proteins degradation	[148]
HL-60	Myeloid leukemia	EPA	-	Caspase-9 and -8 activation	[107]
HL-60 (arsenic trioxide resistant), SH-1, Daudi	Myeloid leukemia, Hairy cell leukemia, Burkitt lymphoma	DHA	↑Susceptibility to arsenic-trioxide	↑Lipid peroxidation	[144]
Ramos	Burkitt's lymphoma	EPA	-	Caspase-9 and -3 (but not caspase-8) activation	[102]
DHL-4	B cell lymphoma	DHA	-	↓SOD1 expression	[141]
Reh	Acute lymphocytic leukemia	DHA	-	PPARγ activation: ↑p53 protein, activating caspase-9 and -3	[77]
L363, OPM-1, OPM-2, U266	Multiple myeloma	EPA, DHA	↑Susceptibility to bortezomib	↓NF-κB: ↑mytocondrial oxidative stress and caspase-3 activation	[44]
SiHa, A549, MCF-7	Cervical, Lung, Breast	DHA	-	↓p53/AMPK/mTOR signaling; ↑autophagy	[131]
A2780, A2780/CP70, HL-60, Raji, CEM, MCF-7, MM1.S, MM1.R, C8161, HT29, Panc-1	Ovarian, Leukemia, Breast, Multiple myeloma, Colorectal, Pancreatic	DHA	-	↓GPx-4	[142]
PA-1, H1299, SiHa, D54MG	Ovarian, Lung, Cervical, Glioblastoma	DHA	-	↑Mitochondrial ROS: ↑ERK/JNK/p38 signaling	[137]

Abbreviations: EPA, eicosapentaenoic acid; DHA, docosahexaenoic acid; FO, fish oil; PUFAs, polyunsatured fatty acids; 5-FU, 5-fluorouracil; OX, oxaliplatin; COX-2, cyclooxygenase-2; Bcl, B-cell lymphoma; ATF, activating transcription factor; eIF, eukaryotic initiation factor; MAPK, mitogen-activated protein kinase; PG, prostaglandins; PPAR, peroxisome proliferator-activated receptor; LOX, lipoxygenase; ALOX, arachidonate-lipoxygenase; mPGES, microsomal PG synthase; FLIP, FLICE-like inhibitory protein; XIAP, X-linked inhibitor of apoptosis protein; TCF, T-cell factor; PI3K, phosphoinositide 3-kinase; LTB4, leukotriene B4; LX, lipoxin; EGFR, epidermal growth factor receptor; HSP, heat shock protein; GPER, G protein-coupled estrogen receptor; cAMP, cyclic adenosine monophosphate; PKA, protein kinase A; STAT, signal transducer and activator of transcription; PIP3, phosphatidylinositol (3,4,5)-trisphosphate; SDC-1, syndecan-1; MEK, mitogen/extracellular signal-regulated kinase; NF-κB, nuclear factor-κB; PTEN, phosphatase and tensin homolog deleted on chromosome ten; mTOR, mammalian target of rapamycin; JNK, Jun N-terminal kinase; GSH, glutathione; ROS, reactive oxygen species; PDK, phosphoinositide-dependent kinase; ERK, extracellular-signal-regulated kinase; GSK-3β, glycogen synthase kinase-3β; p90RSK, 90 kDa ribosomal protein S6 kinase ; SOD-1, superoxide dismutase-1; 17 HPDHA, 17-hydroxyperoxydocosahexaenoic acid; AMPK, AMP-activated protein kinase; GPx, glutathione peroxidase; Ref, reference number.

Table 3. Overview of studies investigating apoptotic targets involved in the suppression of tumor growth by *n*-3 PUFAs in animal models.

Animal Model	Cancer Type	Diet Fatty Acid	Anti-Cancer Drug	Molecular Targets	Ref.
Athymic nude mice implanted with human tumor xenograft HCT-15	Colorectal	FO	-	↓COX2, HIF-1α/VEGF-A and MMPs signal pathways	[166]
Babl/c mice bearing 4T1 mouse breast cancer	Breast	FO	-	↓Wnt/β-catenin pathway ↑PTEN expression:	[126]
Athymic nude mice implanted with human tumor xenograft MDA-MB-231	Breast	FO	-	↓PIK3/Akt/NF-κB signaling, ↓transcription of Bcl-2 and Bcl-XL genes, ↑caspase-3 activation	[129]
Spontaneous NMU-induced rat mammary tumor	Breast	FO	↑Susceptibi-lity to epirubicin	↑GPx-1 response	[143]
Athymic nude mice implanted with human tumor xenograft MCF-7	Breast	FO	-	↑ROS production and caspase-8 activation	[149]
Athymic nude mice implanted with human tumor xenograft MDA-MB-231	Breast	EPA or DHA ethyl esters	-	↓PGE2 production	[157]
Athymic nude mice implanted with human tumor xenograft DU145	Prostate	FO	-	↓PGE2 production	[156]
SCID mice implanted with human tumor xenograft LAPC4	Prostate	FO	-	↓COX-2/PGE2 pathway	[158]
Athymic nude mice implanted with human tumor xenograft A549	Lung	DHA	-	↓EGFR onco-protein; ↓EGFR and ERK signaling	[117]
Fat-1 transgenic mice implanted with Lewis	Lung	-	-	↓AMK and PI3K/Akt singnaling: ↑autophagy and apoptosis	[133]
Athymic nude mice implanted with human tumor xenograft MIA-PaCa-2	Pancreatic	FO	-	↑ROS production; ↑autophagosome formation	[58]
Fat-1 transgenic mice implanted with PANC02	Pancreatic	-	-	↓Wnt/β-catenin signaling	[125]
Athymic nude mice implanted with human tumor xenograft COX-2 negative and positive BxPC-3	Pancreatic	FO	-	↓COX-2/PGE2 pathway, ↑PGE3	[159]
Athymic nude rats implanted with human tumor xenograft multi-drug resistant SK-N-BE(2)	Neuroblastoma	DHA	-	↑lipid peroxidation	[41]

Abbreviations: EPA, eicosapentaenoic acid; DHA, docosahexaenoic acid; FO, fish oil; PUFAs, polyunsatured fatty acids; HIF-1α, hypoxia-inducible factor 1-α; VEGF, vascular endothelial growth factor; MMPs, matrix metalloproteinases; COX, cyclooxygenase; Bcl, B-cell lymphoma; PI3K, phosphoinositide 3-kinase; NF-κB, nuclear factor-κB; PTEN, phosphatase and tensin homolog deleted on chromosome ten; ERK, extracellular signal-regulated kinase; EGFR, epidermal growth factor receptor; ROS, reactive oxygen species; PG, prostaglandin, GPx, glutathione peroxidase; AMK, adenosine monophosphate kinase; SCID, severe combined immunodeficiency; Ref., reference number.

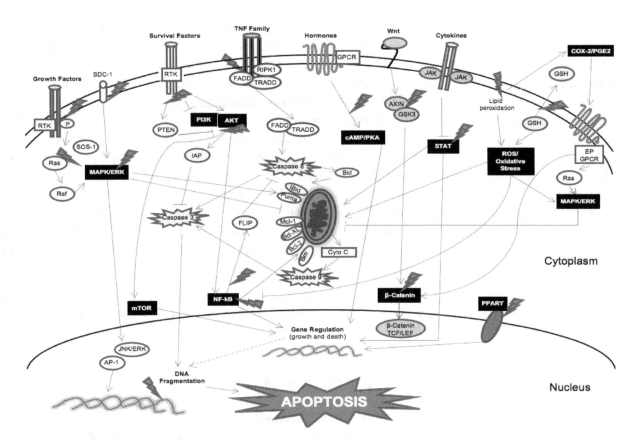

Figure 1. Multiple apoptotic molecular signals targeted by *n*-3 PUFAs in cancer cells. Abbreviations: RTK, protein tyrosine kinase; SOS-1, son of sevenless-1; Erk, extracellular-signal-regulated kinase; MAPK, mitoge*n*-activated protein kinase; JNK, Jun *N*-terminal kinase; AP-1, activator protei*n*-1; SDC-1, syndeca*n*-1; PTEN, phosphatase and tensin homolog deleted on chromosome ten; PI3K, phosphatidylinositol-3-kinase; mTOR, mammalian target of rapamycin; IAP, inhibitor of apoptosis; NF-κB, nuclear factor-κB; FLIP, FLICE-like inhibitory protein; RIPK-1, receptor-like protein kinase-1; FADD, Fas-associated death domain; TRADD, TNF receptor-associated death domain; Bcl-2, B-cell lymphoma protei*n*-2; Bim, Cyto C, cytochrome C; GPCR, G-protein coupled receptor; cAMP, cyclic adenosine monophosphate; PKA, protein kinase A; GSK, glycogen synthase kinase; TCF, T-cell factor; LEF, lymphoid enhancer-binding factor; JAK, Janus kinase; STAT, signal transducer and activator of transcription; ROS, reactive oxygen species; GSH, glutathione; COX-2, cyclooxygenase-2; PGE2, prostaglandin E2; PPAR-γ, peroxisome proliferator-activated receptor γ. arrows, activation; ⊥, inhibition; dashed arrows, indirect action; red/blue flash, targeted by *n*-3 PUFAs.

4. Conclusions

The targeting of tumor cell apoptosis has important therapeutic potential. It is known that essentially all chemotherapeutic drugs and radiotherapy regimens that are in clinical use induce apoptosis of malignant cells when they work properly. However, the resistance to therapy, due to the modulation of the expression of multiple genes and gene products involved in cell death and survival, prompt oncologists to believe that, for a more effective apoptosis-based treatment, combinational therapies are needed to target multitude molecular signals involved in cancer cell death. Several studies have proposed the potential cability of *n*-3 PUFAs DHA and EPA to enhance the efficacy as well as the tolerability of conventional anticancer therapies. Taken together, the data presented in this review, showing the ability of *n*-3 PUFAs, DHA and EPA to induce cytotoxicity via apoptosis in different tumor cell types *in vitro* (Table 2) and *in vivo* (Table 3), indicate that these FAs potentially target multiple molecular signals involved in tumor cell death (Figure 1).

The use of multiple different pathways by *n*-3 PUFAs to trigger apoptosis in tumor cells may be partly related to the diverse activities possibly exerted in diverse cellular cancer models, but also to the different *n*-3 PUFAs used (EPA, DHA or FO), as well as to the different ways of administration, such as doses and kinetics. The context is complex and it might be even more complex if we consider that most of the molecular signals converge into the nucleus, altering gene expression. The pleiotropic nature of transcriptional changes induced by *n*-3 PUFAs have been recently illustrated by studies where global gene expression patterns were determined by microarray analysis *in vitro* and *in vivo* [44,166,167]. Several genes, potentially involved directly or indirectly in cancer cell apoptosis, appear to be regulated by *n*-3 PUFAs, underlining the complexity of the mechanisms involved in the induction of cancer cell apoptosis by these FAs. Therefore, further basic research is needed to show which pathways are crucial for the control of tumor cell apoptosis by *n*-3 PUFAs. Moreover, a clear need appears for further clinical studies, evaluating the potential role of DHA and EPA supplementation, mainly in combination with chemo- and radio-therapeutic anticancer regimens, in the improvement of patients' clinical outcome and survival.

Acknowledgments: This work has been funded by the" bando FILAS Regione Lazio Lr 13/2008" (Project "Innovazioni tecnologiche per migliorare i processi produttivi e le qualità nutraceutiche e salutistiche dei prodotti di specie vegetali del territorio laziale").

References

1.   Ma, X.; Yu, H. Global burden of cancer. *J. Biol. Med.* **2006**, *79*, 85–94.
2.   Basile, K.J.; Aplin, A.E. Resistance to chemotherapy: Short-term drug tolerance and stem cell-like subpopulations. *Adv. Pharmacol.* **2012**, *65*, 315–334. [PubMed]
3.   Reya, T.; Morrison, S.J.; Clarke, M.F.; Weissman, I.L. Stem cells, cancer, and cancer stem cells. *Nature* **2001**, *414*, 105–111. [CrossRef] [PubMed]
4.   Maugeri-Saccà, M.; Vigneri, P.; de Maria, R. Cancer stem cells and chemosensitivity. *Clin. Cancer Res.* **2011**, *17*, 4942–4947. [CrossRef] [PubMed]
5.   Hanahan, D.; Weinberg, R.A. Hallmarks of cancer: The next generation. *Cell* **2011**, *144*, 646–674. [CrossRef] [PubMed]
6.   Pritchard, J.R.; Bruno, P.M.; Gilbert, L.A.; Capron, K.L.; Lauffenburger, D.A.; Hemann, M.T. Defining principles of combination drug mechanisms of action. *Proc. Natl. Acad. Sci. USA* **2013**, *110*, E170–E179. [CrossRef] [PubMed]
7.   Burlingame, B.; Nishida, C.; Uauy, R.; Weisell, R. Fats and fatty acids in human nutrition: Introduction. *Ann. Nutr. Metable* **2009**, *55*, 5–7. [CrossRef] [PubMed]
8.   Riediger, N.D.; Othman, R.A.; Suh, M.; Moghadasian, M.H. A systemic review of the roles of *n*-3 fatty acids in health and disease. *J. Am. Diet. Assoc.* **2009**, *109*, 668–679. [CrossRef] [PubMed]
9.   Calder, P.C. Marine ω-3 Fatty acids and inflammatory processes: Effects, mechanisms and clinical relevance. *Biochim. Biophys. Acta* **2015**, *1851*, 469–484. [CrossRef] [PubMed]
10. Gil, A.; Gil, F. Fish, a Mediterranean source of *n*-3 PUFA: Benefits do not justify limiting consumption. *Br. J. Nutr.* **2015**, *113*, S58–S67. [CrossRef] [PubMed]
11. Laviano, A.; Rianda, S.; Molfino, A.; Rossi Fanelli, F. ω-3 Fatty acids in cancer. *Curr. Opin. Clin. Nutr. Metab. Care* **2013**, *16*, 156–161. [CrossRef] [PubMed]
12. Bhagat, U.; Das, U.N. Potential role of dietary lipids in the prophylaxis of some clinical conditions. *Arch. Med. Sci.* **2015**, *11*, 807–818. [CrossRef] [PubMed]
13. Murray, M.; Hraiki, A.; Bebawy, M.; Pazderka, C.; Rawling, T. Anti-tumor activities of lipids and lipid analogues and their development as potential anticancer drugs. *Pharmacol. Ther.* **2015**, *150*, 109–128. [CrossRef] [PubMed]
14. Bang, H.O.; Dyerberg, J.; Nielsen, A.B. Plasma lipid and lipoprotein pattern in Greenlandic West-coast Eskimos. *Lancet* **1971**, *1*, 1143–1145. [CrossRef]
15. Gu, Z.; Shan, K.; Chen, H.; Chen, Y.Q. *n*-3 Polyunsaturated fatty acids and their role in cancer chemoprevention. *Curr. Pharmacol. Rep.* **2015**, *5*, 283–294. [CrossRef] [PubMed]

16. Serini, S.; Fasano, E.; Piccioni, E.; Cittadini, A.R.; Calviello, G. Dietary *n*-3 polyunsaturated fatty acids and the paradox of their health benefits and potential harmful effects. *Chem. Res. Toxicol.* **2011**, *24*, 2093–2105. [CrossRef] [PubMed]

17. Chapkin, R.S.; DeClercq, V.; Kim, E.; Fuentes, N.R.; Fan, Y.Y. Mechanisms by which pleiotropic amphiphilic *n*-3 PUFA reduce colon cancer risk. *Curr. Colorectal Cancer Rep.* **2014**, *10*, 442–452. [CrossRef] [PubMed]

18. Kiyabu, G.Y.; Inoue, M.; Saito, E.; Abe, S.K.; Sawada, N.; Ishihara, J.; Iwasaki, M.; Yamaji, T.; Shimazu, T.; *et al.* JPHC Study Group. Fish, *n*-3 polyunsaturated fatty acids and *n*-6 polyunsaturated fatty acids intake and breast cancer risk: The Japan Public Health Center-based prospective study. *Int. J. Cancer.* **2015**, *137*, 2915–2926. [CrossRef] [PubMed]

19. Brasky, T.M.; Darke, A.K.; Song, X.; Tangen, C.M.; Goodman, P.J.; Thompson, I.M.; Meyskens, F.L., Jr.; Goodman, G.E.; Minasian, L.M.; *et al.* Plasma phospholipid fatty acids and prostate cancer risk in the SELECT trial. *J. Natl. Cancer Inst.* **2013**, *105*, 1132–1141. [CrossRef] [PubMed]

20. Calder, P.C.; Deckelbaum, R.J. Dietary fatty acids in health and disease: Greater controversy, greater interest. *Curr. Opin. Clin. Nutr. Metab. Care* **2014**, *17*, 111–115. [CrossRef] [PubMed]

21. Weylandt, K.H.; Serini, S.; Chen, Y.Q.; Su, H.M.; Lim, K.; Cittadini, A.; Calviello, G. ω-3 Polyunsaturated fatty acids: The way forward in times of mixed evidence. *Biomed. Res. Int.* **2015**, *2015*, 143109. [CrossRef] [PubMed]

22. Berquin, I.M.; Edwards, I.J.; Chen, Y.Q. Multi-targeted therapy of cancer by ω-3 Fatty acids. *Cancer Lett.* **2008**, *269*, 363–377. [CrossRef] [PubMed]

23. Serini, S.; Piccioni, E.; Merendino, N.; Calviello, G. Dietary polyunsaturated fatty acids as inducers of apoptosis: Implications for cancer. *Apoptosis* **2009**, *14*, 132–152. [CrossRef] [PubMed]

24. Gleissman, H.; Johnsen, J.I.; Kogner, P. ω-3 Fatty acids in cancer, the protectors of good and the killers of evil? *Exp. Cell Res.* **2010**, *316*, 1365–1373. [CrossRef] [PubMed]

25. Vaughan, V.C.; Hassing, M.R.; Lewandowski, P.A. Marine polyunsaturated fatty acids and cancer therapy. *Br. J. Cancer* **2013**, *108*, 486–492. [CrossRef] [PubMed]

26. Biondo, P.D.; Brindley, D.N.; Sawyer, M.B.; Field, C.J. The potential for treatment with dietary long-chain polyunsaturated *n*-3 fatty acids during chemotherapy. *J. Nutr. Biochem.* **2008**, *19*, 787–796. [CrossRef] [PubMed]

27. Siddiqui, R.A.; Harvey, K.A.; Xu, Z.; Bammerlin, E.M.; Walker, C.; Altenburg, J.D. Docosahexaenoic acid: A natural powerful adjuvant that improves efficacy for anticancer treatment with no adverse effects. *Biofactors* **2011**, *37*, 399–412. [CrossRef] [PubMed]

28. Wang, J.; Luo, T.; Li, S.; Zhao, J. The powerful applications of polyunsaturated fatty acids in improving the therapeutic efficacy of anticancer drugs. *Expert Opin. Drug Deliv.* **2012**, *9*, 1–7. [CrossRef] [PubMed]

29. Merendino, N.; Costantini, L.; Manzi, L.; Molinari, R.; D'Eliseo, D.; Velotti, F. Dietary ω-3 polyunsaturated fatty acid DHA: A potential adjuvant in the treatment of cancer. *Biomed. Res. Int.* **2013**, *2013*, 310186. [CrossRef] [PubMed]

30. Hajjaji, N.; Bougnoux, P. Selective sensitization of tumors to chemotherapy by marine-derived lipids: A review. *Cancer Treat. Rev.* **2013**, *39*, 473–488. [CrossRef] [PubMed]

31. de Aguiar Pastore Silva, J.; Emilia de Souza Fabre, M.; Waitzberg, D.L. ω-3 Supplements for patients in chemotherapy and/or radiotherapy: A systematic review. *Clin. Nutr.* **2015**, *34*, 359–366. [CrossRef] [PubMed]

32. Das, U.N.; Madhavi, N.; Sravan Kumar, G.; Padma, M.; Sangeetha, P. Can tumour cell drug resistance be reversed by essential fatty acids and their metabolites? *Prostaglandins Leukot. Essent. Fatty Acids* **1998**, *58*, 39–54. [CrossRef]

33. Slagsvold, J.E.; Pettersen, C.H.; Størvold, G.L.; Follestad, T.; Krokan, H.E.; Schønberg, S.A. DHA alters expression of target proteins of cancer therapy in chemotherapy resistant SW620 colon cancer cells. *Nutr. Cancer* **2010**, *62*, 611–621. [CrossRef] [PubMed]

34. Kuan, C.Y.; Walker, T.H.; Luo, P.G.; Chen, C.F. Long-chain polyunsaturated fatty acids promote paclitaxel cytotoxicity via inhibition of the MDR1 gene in the human colon cancer Caco-2 cell line. *J. Am. Coll. Nutr.* **2011**, *30*, 265–273. [CrossRef] [PubMed]

35. Gelsomino, G.; Corsetto, P.A.; Campia, I.; Montorfano, G.; Kopecka, J.; Castella, B.; Gazzano, E.; Ghigo, D.; Rizzo, A.M.; Riganti, C. ω3 Fatty acids chemosensitize multidrug resistant colon cancer cells by down-regulating cholesterol synthesis and altering detergent resistant membranes composition. *Mol. Cancer* **2013**, *12*, 137. [CrossRef] [PubMed]

36. Das, U.N.; Begin, M.E.; Ells, G.; Huang, Y.S.; Horrobin, D.F. Polyunsaturated fatty acids augment free radical generation in tumor cells *in vitro*. *Biochem. Biophys. Res. Commun.* **1987**, *145*, 15–24. [CrossRef]

37. Tsai, W.S.; Nagawa, H.; Kaizaki, S.; Tsuruo, T.; Muto, T. Inhibitory effects of *n*--3 polyunsaturated fatty acids on sigmoid colon cancer transformants. *J. Gastroenterol.* **1998**, *33*, 206–212. [CrossRef] [PubMed]

38. Siddiqui, R.A.; Harvey, K.; Stillwell, W. Anticancer properties of oxidation products of docosahexaenoic acid. *Chem. Phys. Lipids* **2008**, *153*, 47–56. [CrossRef] [PubMed]

39. Giros, A.; Grzybowski, M.; Sohn, V.R.; Pons, E.; Fernandez-Morales, J.; Xicola, R.M.; Sethi, P.; Grzybowski, J.; Goel, A.; *et al.* Regulation of colorectal cancer cell apoptosis by the *n*-3 polyunsaturated fatty acids Docosahexaenoic and Eicosapentaenoic. *Cancer Prev. Res.* **2009**, *2*, 732–742. [CrossRef] [PubMed]

40. Toit-Kohn, J.L.; Louw, L.; Engelbrecht, A.M. Docosahexaenoic acid induces apoptosis in colorectal carcinoma cells by modulating the PI3 kinase and p38 MAPK pathways. *J. Nutr. Biochem.* **2009**, *20*, 106–114. [CrossRef] [PubMed]

41. Gleissman, H.; Segerström, L.; Hamberg, M.; Ponthan, F.; Lindskog, M.; Johnsen, J.I.; Kogner, P. ω-3 Fatty acid supplementation delays the progression of neuroblastoma *in vivo*. *Int. J. Cancer* **2011**, *128*, 1703–1711. [CrossRef] [PubMed]

42. Nikolakopoulou, Z.; Nteliopoulos, G.; Michael-Titus, A.T.; Parkinson, E.K. ω-3 Polyunsaturated fatty acids selectively inhibit growth in neoplastic oral keratinocytes by differentially activating ERK1/2. *Carcinogenesis* **2013**, *34*, 2716–2725. [CrossRef] [PubMed]

43. Ravacci, G.R.; Brentani, M.M.; Tortelli, T.Jr.; Torrinhas, R.S.; Saldanha, T.; Torres, E.A.; Waitzberg, D.L. Lipid raft disruption by docosahexaenoic acid induces apoptosis in transformed human mammary luminal epithelial cells harboring HER-2 overexpression. *J. Nutr. Biochem.* **2013**, *24*, 505–515. [CrossRef] [PubMed]

44. Abdi, J.; Garssen, J.; Faber, J.; Redegeld, F.A. ω-3 Fatty acids, EPA and DHA induce apoptosis and enhance drug sensitivity in multiple myeloma cells but not in normal peripheral mononuclear cells. *J. Nutr. Biochem.* **2014**, *25*, 1254–1262. [CrossRef] [PubMed]

45. Berstad, P.; Thiis-Evensen, E.; Vatn, M.H.; Almendingen, K. Fatty acids in habitual diet, plasma phospholipids, and tumour and normal colonic biopsies in young colorectal cancer patients. *J. Oncol.* **2012**, *2012*, 254801. [CrossRef] [PubMed]

46. Thomas, G.C. Apoptosis and cancer: The genesis of a research field. *Nature Rev. Cancer* **2009**, *9*, 501–507.

47. Logue, S.E.; Gorman, A.M.; Cleary, P.; Keogh, N.; Samali, A. Current concepts in ER stress-induced apoptosis. *J. Carcinogene Mutagene* **2013**. [CrossRef]

48. Mengeaud, V.; Nano, J.L.; Fournel, S.; Rampal, P. Effects of eicosapentaenoic acid, γ-linolenic acid and prostaglandin E1 on three human colon carcinoma cell lines. *Prostaglandins Leukot. Essent. Fatty Acids* **1992**, *47*, 313–319. [CrossRef]

49. Clarke, R.G.; Lund, E.K.; Latham, P.; Pinder, A.C.; Johnson, I.T. Effect of eicosapentaenoic acid on the proliferation and incidence of apoptosis in the colorectal cell line HT29. *Lipids* **1999**, *34*, 1287–1295. [CrossRef] [PubMed]

50. Chen, Z.Y.; Istfan, N.W. Docosahexaenoic acid is a potent inducer of apoptosis in HT-29 colon cancer cells. *Prostaglandins Leukot. Essent. Fatty Acids* **2000**, *63*, 301–308. [CrossRef] [PubMed]

51. Kubota, H.; Matsumoto, H.; Higashida, M.; Murakami, H.; Nakashima, H.; Oka, Y.; Okumura, H.; Yamamura, M.; Nakamura, M.; Hirai, T. Eicosapentaenoic acid modifies cytokine activity and inhibits cell proliferation in an oesophageal cancer cell line. *Anticancer Res.* **2013**, *33*, 4319–4324. [PubMed]

52. Lee, S.E.; Lim, J.W.; Kim, H. Activator protein-1 mediates docosahexaenoic acid-induced apoptosis of human gastric cancer cells. *Ann. N. Y. Acad. Sci.* **2009**, *1171*, 163–169. [CrossRef] [PubMed]

53. Lim, K.; Han, C.; Dai, Y.; Shenm, M.; Wu, T. ω-3 Polyunsaturated fatty acids inhibit hepatocellular carcinoma cell growth through blocking β-catenin and cyclooxygenase-2. *Mol. Cancer Ther.* **2009**, *8*, 3046–3055. [CrossRef] [PubMed]

54. Sun, S.N.; Jia, W.D.; Chen, H.; Ma, J.L.; Ge, Y.S.; Yu, J.H.; Li, J.S. Docosahexaenoic acid (DHA) induces apoptosis in human hepatocellular carcinoma cells. *Int. J. of Clin. Exp. Pathol.* **2013**, *6*, 281–289.

55. Zhang, Y.; Han, L.; Qi, W.; Cheng, D.; Ma, X.; Hou, L.; Cao, X.; Wang, C. Eicosapentaenoic acid (EPA) induced apoptosis in HepG2 cells through ROS-Ca^{2+}-JNK mitochondrial pathways. *Biochem. Biophys. Res. Commun.* **2015**, *456*, 926–932. [CrossRef] [PubMed]

56.   Hawkins, R.A.; Sangster, K.; Arends, M.J. Apoptotic death of pancreatic cancer cells induced by polyunsaturated fatty acids varies with double bond number and involves an oxidative mechanism. *J. Pathol.* **1998**, *185*, 61–70. [CrossRef]

57.   Merendino, N.; Loppi, B.; D'Aquino, M.; Molinari, R.; Pessina, G.; Romano, C.; Velotti, F. Docosahexaenoic acid induces apoptosis in the human PaCa-44 pancreatic cancer cell line by active reduced glutathione extrusion and lipid peroxidation. *Nutr. Cancer* **2005**, *52*, 225–233. [CrossRef] [PubMed]

58.   Fukui, M.; Kang, K.S.; Okada, K.; Zhu, B.T. EPA, an ω-3 Fatty acid, induces apoptosis in human pancreatic cancer cells: Role of ROS accumulation, caspase-8 activation, and autophagy induction. *J. Cell. Biochem.* **2013**, *114*, 192–203. [CrossRef] [PubMed]

59.   Lim, K.; Han, C.; Xu, L.; Isse, K.; Demetris, A.J.; Wu, T. Cyclooxygenase-2-derived prostaglandin E2 activates β-catenin in human cholangiocarcinoma cells: Evidence for inhibition of these signaling pathways by ω 3 polyunsaturated fatty acids. *Cancer Res.* **2008**, *68*, 553–560. [CrossRef] [PubMed]

60.   Rose, D.P.; Connolly, J.M. Effects of fatty acids and inhibitors of eicosanoid synthesis on the growth of a human breast cancer cell line in culture. *Cancer Res.* **1990**, *50*, 7139–7144. [PubMed]

61.   Chamras, H.; Ardashian, A.; Heber, D.; Glaspy, J.A. Fatty acid modulation of MCF-7 human breast cancer cell proliferation, apoptosis and differentiation. *J. Nutr. Biochem.* **2002**, *13*, 711–716. [CrossRef]

62.   Sharma, A.; Belna, J.; Logan, J.; Espat, J.; Hurteau, J.A. The effects of ω-3 fatty acids on growth regulation of epithelial ovarian cancer cell lines. *Gynecol. Oncol.* **2005**, *99*, 58–64. [CrossRef] [PubMed]

63.   Narayanan, N.K.; Narayanan, B.A.; Reddy, B.S. A combination of docosahexaenoic acid and celecoxib prevents prostate cancer cell growth *in vitro* and is associated with modulation of nuclear factor-κB, and steroid hormone receptors. *Int. J. Oncol.* **2005**, *26*, 785–792. [CrossRef] [PubMed]

64.   Hu, Y.; Sun, H.; Owens, R.T.; Gu, Z.; Wu, J.; Chen, Y.Q.; O'Flaherty, J.T.; Edwards, I.J. Syndecan-1-dependent suppression of PDK1/Akt/bad signaling by docosahexaenoic acid induces apoptosis in prostate cancer. *Neoplasia* **2010**, *12*, 826–836. [CrossRef] [PubMed]

65.   Molinari, R.; D'Eliseo, D.; Manzi, L.; Zolla, L.; Velotti, F.; Merendino, N. The n3-polyunsaturated fatty acid docosahexaenoic acid induces immunogenic cell death in human cancer cell lines via pre-apoptotic calreticulin exposure. *Cancer Immunol. Immunother.* **2011**, *60*, 1503–1507. [CrossRef] [PubMed]

66.   Lindskog, M.; Gleissman, H.; Ponthan, F.; Castro, J.; Kogner, P.; Johnsen, J.I. Neuroblastoma cell death in response to docosahexaenoic acid: Sensitization to chemotherapy and arsenic induced oxidative stress. *Int. J. Cancer* **2006**, *118*, 2584–2593. [CrossRef] [PubMed]

67.   Faragó, N.; Fehér, L.Z.; Kitajka, K.; Das, U.N.; Puskás, L.G. MicroRNA profile of polyunsaturated fatty acid treated glioma cells reveal apoptosis-specific expression changes. *Lipids Health Dis.* **2011**, *10*, 173. [CrossRef] [PubMed]

68.   Serini, S.; Trombino, S.; Oliva, F.; Piccioni, E.; Monego, G.; Resci, F.; Boninsegna, A.; Picci, N.; Ranelletti, F.O.; Calviello, G. Docosahexaenoic acid induces apoptosis in lung cancer cells by increasing MKP-1 and down-regulating p-ERK1/2 and p-p38 expression. *Apoptosis* **2008**, *13*, 1172–1183. [CrossRef] [PubMed]

69.   Yao, Q.H.; Zhang, X.C.; Fu, T.; Gu, J.Z.; Wang, L.; Wang, Y.; Lai, Y.B.; Wang, Y.Q.; Guo, Y. ω-3 polyunsaturated fatty acids inhibit the proliferation of the lung adenocarcinoma cell line A549 *in vitro*. *Mol. Med. Rep.* **2014**, *9*, 401–406. [PubMed]

70.   Albino, A.P.; Juan, G.; Traganos, F.; Reinhart, L.; Connolly, J.; Rose, D.P.; Darzynkiewicz, Z. Cell cycle arrest and apoptosis of melanoma cells by docosahexaenoic acid: Association with decreased pRb phosphorylation. *Cancer Res.* **2000**, *60*, 4139–4145. [PubMed]

71.   Denkins, Y.; Kempf, D.; Ferniz, M.; Nileshwar, S.; Marchetti, D. Role of ω-3 polyunsaturated fatty acids on cyclooxygenase-2 metabolism in brain-metastatic melanoma. *J. Lipid Res.* **2005**, *46*, 1278–1284. [CrossRef] [PubMed]

72.   Finstad, H.S.; Myhrstad, M.C.; Heimli, H.; Lømo, J.; Blomhoff, H.K.; Kolset, S.O.; Drevon, C.A. Multiplication and death-type of leukemia cell lines exposed to very long-chain polyunsaturated fatty acids. *Leukemia* **1998**, *12*, 921–929. [CrossRef] [PubMed]

73.   Finstad, H.S.; Drevon, C.A.; Kulseth, M.A.; Synstad, A.V.; Knudsen, E.; Kolset, S.O. Cell proliferation, apoptosis and accumulation of lipid droplets in U937-1 cells incubated with eicosapentaenoic acid. *Biochem. J.* **1998**, *336*, 451–459. [CrossRef] [PubMed]

74.   Chiu, L.C.M.; Wan, J.M.F. Induction of apoptosis in HL-60 cells by eicosapentaenoic acid (EPA) is associated with downregulation of BCL-2 expression. *Cancer Letters* **1999**, *145*, 17–27. [CrossRef]

75. Chiu, L.C.; Wong, E.Y.; Ooi, V.E. Docosahexaenoic acid modulates different genes in cell cycle and apoptosis to control growth of human leukemia HL-60 cells. *Int J Oncol.* **2004**, *25*, 737–744. [CrossRef] [PubMed]

76. Siddiqui, R.A.; Jenski, L.J.; Neff, K.; Harvey, K.; Kovacs, R.J.; Stillwell, W. Docosahexaenoic acid induces apoptosis in Jurkat cells by a protein phosphatase-mediated process. *Biochim. Biophys. Acta* **2001**, *1499*, 265–275. [CrossRef]

77. Zand, H.; Rhimipour, A.; Bakhshayesh, M.; Shafiee, M.; Nour Mohammadi, I.; Salimi, S. Involvement of PPAR-γ and p53 in DHA-induced apoptosis in Reh cells. *Mol. Cell. Biochem.* **2007**, *304*, 71–77. [CrossRef] [PubMed]

78. Yamagami, T.; Porada, C.D.; Pardini, R.S.; Zanjani, E.D.; Almeida-Porada, G. Docosahexaenoic acid induces dose dependent cell death in an early undifferentiated subtype of acute myeloid leukemia cell line. *Cancer Biol. Ther.* **2009**, *8*, 331–337. [CrossRef] [PubMed]

79. Sravan Kumar, G.; Das, U.N. Cytotoxic action of α-linolenic and eicosapentaenoic acids on myeloma cells *in vitro*. *Prostaglandins Leukot. Essent. Fatty Acids* **1997**, *56*, 285–293. [CrossRef]

80. Ricci-Vitiani, L.; Lombardi, D.G.; Pilozzi, E.; Biffoni, M.; Todaro, M.; Peschle, C.; de Maria, R. Identification and expansion of human colon-cancer-initiating cells. *Nature* **2007**, *445*, 111–115. [CrossRef] [PubMed]

81. Das, U.N. Essential fatty acids and their metabolites as modulators of stem cell biology with reference to inflammation, cancer, and metastasis. *Cancer Metastasis Rev.* **2011**, *30*, 311–324. [CrossRef] [PubMed]

82. Yang, T.; Fang, S.; Zhang, H.X.; Xu, L.X.; Zhang, Z.Q.; Yuan, K.T.; Xue, C.L.; Yu, H.L.; Zhang, S.; Li, Y.F.; *et al.* n-3 PUFA shave antiproliferative and apoptotic effects on human colorectal cancer stemlike cells *in vitro*. *J. Nutr. Biochem.* **2013**, *24*, 744–753. [CrossRef] [PubMed]

83. Vasudevan, A.; Yu, Y.; Banerjee, S.; Woods, J.; Farhana, L.; Rajendra, S.G.; Patel, A.; Dyson, G.; Levi, E.; Maddipati, K.R.; *et al.* ω-3 Fatty acid is a potential preventive agent for recurrent colon cancer. *Cancer Prev. Res.* **2014**, *7*, 1138–1148. [CrossRef] [PubMed]

84. De Carlo, F.; Witte, T.R.; Hardman, W.E.; Claudio, P.P. ω-3 Eicosapentaenoic acid decreases CD133 colon cancer stem-like cell marker expression while increasing sensitivity to chemotherapy. *PLoS ONE* **2013**, *8*, e69760.

85. Xiong, A.; Yu, W.; Liu, Y.; Sanders, B.G.; Kline, K. Elimination of ALDH+ breast tumor initiating cells by docosahexanoic acid and/or γ tocotrienol through SHP-1 inhibition of Stat3 signaling. *Mol. Carcinog.* **2015**. [CrossRef] [PubMed]

86. Rose, D.P.; Connolly, J.M.; Rayburn, J.; Coleman, M. Influence of diets containing eicosapentaenoic or docosahexaenoic acid on growth and metastasis of breast cancer cells in nude mice. *J. Natl. Cancer Inst.* **1995**, *87*, 587–592. [CrossRef] [PubMed]

87. Yam, D.; Peled, A.; Huszar, M.; Shinitzky, M. Dietary fish oil suppresses tumor growth and metastasis of Lewis lung carcinoma in mice. *J. Nutr. Biochem.* **1997**, *8*, 619–622. [CrossRef]

88. Boudreau, M.D.; Sohn, K.H.; Rhee, S.H.; Lee, S.W.; Hunt, J.D.; Hwang, D.H. Suppression of tumor cell growth both in nude mice and in culture by n-3 polyunsaturated fatty acids: Mediation through cyclooxygenase-independent pathways. *Cancer Res.* **2001**, *61*, 1386–1391. [PubMed]

89. Kato, T.; Hancock, R.L.; Mohammadpour, H.; McGregor, B.; Manalo, P.; Khaiboullina, S.; Hall, M.R.; Pardini, L.; Pardini, R.S. Influence of ω-3 fatty acids on the growth of human colon carcinoma in nude mice. *Cancer Lett.* **2002**, *187*, 169–177. [CrossRef]

90. Camargo, C.Q.; Mocellin, M.C.; Pastore Silva, J.A.; de Souza Fabre, M.E.; Nunes, E.A.; de Moraes Trinidade, E.B. Fish oil supplementation during chemotherapy increases posterior time to tumor progression in colorectal cancer. *Nutr. Cancer*, (in press). Available online: http://.doi.org/10.1080/01635581.2016.1115097 (accessed on 19 January 2016).

91. Bougnoux, P.; Hajjaji, N.; Ferrasson, M.N.; Giraudeau, B.; Couet, C.; le Floch, O. Improving outcome of chemotherapy of metastatic breast cancer by docosahexaenoic acid: A phase II trial. *Br. J. Cancer* **2009**, *1011978–1011985*. [CrossRef] [PubMed]

92. Cockbain, J.; Toogood, G.J.; Hull, M.A. ω-3 Polyunsaturated fatty acids for the treatment and prevention of colorectal cancer. *Gut* **2012**, *61*, 135–149. [CrossRef] [PubMed]

93. Murphy, R.A.; Mourtzakis, M.; Chu, Q.S.; Baracos, V.E.; Reiman, T.; Mazurak, V.C. Supplementation with fish oil increases first-line chemotherapy efficacy in patients with advanced non-small cell lung cancer. *Cancer* **2011**, *117*, 3774–3780. [CrossRef] [PubMed]

94. Patterson, R.E.; Flatt, S.W.; Newman, V.A.; Natarajan, L.; Rock, C.L.; Thomson, C.A.; Caan, B.J.; Parker, B.A.; Pierce, J.P. Marine fatty acid intake is associated with breast cancer prognosis. *J. Nutr.* **2011**, *141*, 201–206. [CrossRef] [PubMed]

95. Cockbain, A.J.; Volpato, M.; Race, A.D.; Munarini, A.; Fazio, C.; Belluzzi, A.; Loadman, P.M.; Toogood, G.J.; Hull, M.A. Anticolorectal cancer activity of the ω-3 polyunsaturated fatty acid eicosapentaenoic acid. *Gut* **2014**, *63*, 1760–1768. [CrossRef] [PubMed]

96. Sánchez-Lara, K.; Turcott, J.G.; Juárez-Hernández, E.; Nuñez-Valencia, C.; Villanueva, G.; Guevara, P.; de la Torre-Vallejo, M.; Mohar, A.; Arrieta, O. Effects of an oral nutritional supplement containing eicosapentaenoic acid on nutritional and clinical outcomes in patients with advanced non-small cell lung cancer: Randomised trial. *Clin. Nutr.* **2014**, *33*, 1017–1023. [CrossRef] [PubMed]

97. Arshad, A.; Chung, W.Y.; Isherwood, J.; Mann, C.D.; Al-Leswas, D.; Steward, W.P.; Metcalfe, M.S.; Dennison, A.R. Cellular and plasma uptake of parenteral ω-3 rich lipid emulsion fatty acids in patients with advanced pancreatic cancer. *Clin. Nutr.* **2014**, *33*, 895–899. [CrossRef] [PubMed]

98. Ma, Y.J.; Yu, J.; Xiao, J.; Cao, B.W. The consumption of ω-3 polyunsaturated fatty acids improves clinical outcomes and prognosis in pancreatic cancer patients: A systematic evaluation. *Nutr. Cancer* **2015**, *67*, 112–118. [CrossRef] [PubMed]

99. Nabavi, S.F.; Bilottom, S.; Russom, G.L.; Orhan, I.E.; Habtemariam, S.; Daglia, M.; Devi, K.P.; Loizzo, M.R.; Tundis, R.; Nabavi, S.M. ω-3 polyunsaturated fatty acids and cancer: Lessons learned from clinical trials. *Cancer Metastasis Rev.* **2015**, *34*, 359–380. [CrossRef] [PubMed]

100. Khankari, N.K.; Bradshaw, P.T.; Steck, S.E.; He, K.; Olshan, A.F.; Shen, J.; Ahn, J.; Chen, Y.; Ahsan, H.; Terry, M.B.; *et al.* Dietary intake of fish, polyunsaturated fatty acids, and survival after breast cancer: A population-based follow-up study on Long Island, New York. *Cancer* **2015**. [CrossRef] [PubMed]

101. Mocellin, M.C.; Camargo, C.Q.; Nunes, E.A.; Fiates, G.M.; Trindade, E.B. A systematic review and meta-analysis of the *n*-3 polyunsaturated fatty acids effects on inflammatory markers in colorectal cancer. *Clin. Nutr.* **2015**. [CrossRef] [PubMed]

102. Heimli, H.; Giske, C.; Naderi, S.; Drevon, C.A.; Hollung, K. Eicosapentaenoic acid promotes apoptosis in Ramos cells via activation of caspase-3 and -9. *Lipids* **2002**, *37*, 797–802. [CrossRef] [PubMed]

103. Llor, X.; Pons, E.; Roca, A.; Alvarez, M.; Mañé, J.; Fernández-Bañares, F.; Gassull, M.A. The effects of fish oil, olive oil, oleic acid and linoleic acid on colorectal neoplastic processes. *Clin. Nutr.* **2003**, *22*, 71–79. [CrossRef] [PubMed]

104. Danbara, N.; Yuri, T.; Tsujita-Kyutoku, M.; Sato, M.; Senzaki, H.; Takada, H.; Hada, T.; Miyazawa, T.; Okazaki, K.; Tsubura, A. Conjugated docosahexaenoic acid is a potent inducer of cell cycle arrest and apoptosis and inhibits growth of colo 201 human colon cancer cells. *Nutr. Cancer* **2004**, *50*, 71–79. [CrossRef] [PubMed]

105. Calviello, G.; Di Nicuolo, F.; Serini, S.; Piccioni, E.; Boninsegna, A.; Maggiano, N.; Ranelletti, F.O.; Palozza, P. Docosahexaenoic acid enhances the susceptibility of human colorectal cancer cells to 5-fluorouracil. *Cancer Chemother. Pharmacol.* **2005**, *55*, 12–20. [CrossRef] [PubMed]

106. Jakobsen, C.H.; Størvold, G.L.; Bremseth, H.; Follestad, T.; Sand, K.; Mack, M.; Olsen, K.S.; Lundemo, A.G.; Iversen, J.G.; Krokan, H.E.; *et al.* DHA induces ER stress and growth arrest in human colon cancer cells: Associations with cholesterol and calcium homeostasis. *J. Lipid. Res.* **2008**, *49*, 2089–2100. [CrossRef] [PubMed]

107. Arita, K.; Kobuchi, H.; Utsumi, T.; Takehara, Y.; Akiyama, J.; Horton, A.A.; Utsumi, K. Mechanism of apoptosis in HL-60 cells induced by *n*-3 and *n*-6 polyunsaturated fatty acids. *Biochem. Pharmacol.* **2001**, *62*, 821–828. [CrossRef]

108. Narayanan, B.A.; Narayanan, N.K.; Reddy, B.S. Docosahexaenoic acid regulated genes and transcription factors inducing apoptosis in human colon cancer cells. *Int. J. Oncol.* **2001**, *19*, 1255–1262. [CrossRef] [PubMed]

109. Kolch, W.; Halasz, M.; Granovskaya, M.; Kholodenko, B.N. The dynamic control of signal transduction networks in cancer cells. *Nat. Rev. Cancer* **2015**, *15*, 515–527. [CrossRef] [PubMed]

110. Huang, C.Y.; Yu, L.C. Pathophysiological mechanisms of death resistance in colorectal carcinoma. *World J. Gastroenterol.* **2015**, *21*, 11777–11792. [CrossRef] [PubMed]

111. Glatz, J.F.; Luiken, J.J.; van Nieuwenhoven, F.A.; van der Vusse, G.J. Molecular mechanism of cellular uptake and intracellular translocation of fatty acids. *Prostaglandins Leukot. Essent. Fatty Acids* **1997**, *57*, 3–9. [CrossRef]

112. Wassall, S.R.; Stillwell, W. Polyunsaturated fatty acid-cholesterol interactions: Domain formation in membranes. *Biochim. Biophys. Acta* **2009**, *1788*, 24–32. [CrossRef] [PubMed]

113. Zhang, C.; Yu, H.; Ni, X.; Shen, S.; Das, U.N. Growth inhibitory effect of polyunsaturated fatty acids (PUFAs) on colon cancer cells via their growth inhibitory metabolites and fatty acid composition changes. *PLoS ONE* **2015**, *10*, e0123256.

114. Ibarguren, M.; López, D.J.; Escribá, P.V. The effect of natural and synthetic fatty acids on membrane structure, microdomain organization, cellular functions and human health. *Biochim. Biophys. Acta* **2014**, *1838*, 1518–1528. [CrossRef] [PubMed]

115. Corsetto, P.A.; Cremona, A.; Montorfano, G.; Jovenitti, I.E.; Orsini, F.; Arosio, P.; Rizzo, A.M. Chemical-physical changes in cell membrane microdomains of breast cancer cells after ω-3 PUFA incorporation. *Cell Biochem. Biophys.* **2012**, *64*, 45–59. [CrossRef] [PubMed]

116. Schley, P.D.; Brindley, D.N.; Field, C.J. (*n*-3) PUFA alter raft lipid composition and decrease epidermal growth factor receptor levels in lipid rafts of human breast cancer cells. *J. Nutr.* **2007**, *137*, 548–553. [PubMed]

117. Rogers, K.R.; Kikawa, K.D.; Mouradian, M.; Hernandez, K.; McKinnon, K.M.; Ahwah, S.M.; Pardini, R.S. Docosahexaenoic acid alters epidermal growth factor receptor-related signaling by disrupting its lipid raft association. *Carcinogenesis* **2010**, *31*, 1523–1530. [CrossRef] [PubMed]

118. Corsetto, P.A.; Montorfano, G.; Zava, S.; Jovenitti, I.E.; Cremona, A.; Berra, B.; Rizzo, A.M. Effects of *n*-3 PUFAs on breast cancer cells through their incorporation in plasma membrane. *Lipids Health Dis.* **2011**, *10*, 73. [CrossRef] [PubMed]

119. Lee, E.J.; Yun, U.J.; Koo, K.H.; Sung, J.Y.; Shim, J.; Ye, S.K.; Hong, K.M.; Kim, Y.N. Down-regulation of lipid raft-associated onco-proteins via cholesterol-dependent lipid raft internalization in docosahexaenoic acid-induced apoptosis. *Biochim. Biophys. Acta* **2014**, *1841*, 190–203. [CrossRef] [PubMed]

120. Mason, J.K.; Klaire, S.; Kharotia, S.; Wiggins, A.K.; Thompson, L.U. α-linolenic acid and docosahexaenoic acid, alone and combined with trastuzumab, reduce HER2-overexpressing breast cancer cell growth but differentially regulate HER2 signaling pathways. *Lipids Health Dis.* **2015**, *14*, 91. [CrossRef] [PubMed]

121. Cao, W.; Ma, Z.; Rasenick, M.M.; Yeh, S.; Yu, J. *n*-3 poly-unsaturated fatty acids shift estrogen signaling to inhibit human breast cancer cell growth. *PLoS ONE* **2012**, *7*, e52838. [CrossRef] [PubMed]

122. Ewaschuk, J.B.; Newell, M.; Field, C.J. Docosahexanoic acid improves chemotherapy efficacy by inducing CD95 translocation to lipid rafts in ER⁻ breast cancer cells. *Lipids* **2012**, *47*, 1019–1030. [CrossRef] [PubMed]

123. Gu, Z.; Wu, J.; Wang, S.; Suburu, J.; Chen, H.; Thomas, M.J.; Shi, L.; Edwards, I.J.; Berquin, I.M.; Chen, Y.Q. Polyunsaturated fatty acids affect the localization and signaling of PIP3/AKT in prostate cancer cells. *Carcinogenesis* **2013**, *34*, 1968–1975. [CrossRef] [PubMed]

124. Calviello, G.; Resci, F.; Serini, S.; Piccioni, E.; Toesca, A.; Boninsegna, A.; Monego, G.; Ranelletti, F.O.; Palozza, P. Docosahexaenoic acid induces proteasome-dependent degradation of β-catenin, down-regulation of survivin and apoptosis in human colorectal cancer cells not expressing COX-2. *Carcinogenesis* **2007**, *28*, 1202–1209. [CrossRef] [PubMed]

125. Song, K.S.; Jing, K.; Kim, J.S.; Yun, E.J.; Shin, S.; Seo, K.S.; Park, J.H.; Heo, J.Y.; Kang, J.X.; Suh, K.S.; et al. ω-3-Polyunsaturated fatty acids suppress pancreatic cancer cell growth *in vitro* and *in vivo* via downregulation of Wnt/β-catenin signaling. *Pancreatology* **2011**, *11*, 574–584. [CrossRef] [PubMed]

126. Xue, M.; Wang, Q.; Zhao, J.; Dong, L.; Ge, Y.; Hou, L.; Liu, Y.; Zheng, Z. Docosahexaenoic acid inhibited the Wnt/β-catenin pathway and suppressed breast cancer cells *in vitro* and *in vivo*. *J. Nutr. Biochem.* **2014**, *25*, 104–110. [CrossRef] [PubMed]

127. Sun, H.; Hu, Y.; Gu, Z.; Owens, R.T.; Chen, Y.Q.; Edwards, I.J. ω-3 Fatty acids induce apoptosis in human breast cancer cells and mouse mammary tissue through syndecan-1 inhibition of the MEK-Erk pathway. *Carcinogenesis* **2011**, *32*, 1518–1524. [CrossRef] [PubMed]

128. Schley, P.D.; Jijon, H.B.; Robinson, L.E.; Field, C.J. Mechanisms of ω-3 fatty acid-induced growth inhibition in MDAMB-231 human breast cancer cells. *Breast Cancer Res. Treat.* **2005**, *92*, 187–195. [CrossRef] [PubMed]

129. Ghosh-Choudhury, T.; Mandal, C.C.; Woodruff, K.; St Clair, P.; Fernandes, G.; Choudhury, G.G.; Ghosh-Choudhury, N. Fish oil targets PTEN to regulate NFκB for downregulation of anti-apoptotic genes in breast tumor growth. *Breast Cancer Res. Treat.* **2009**, *118*, 213–228. [CrossRef] [PubMed]

130. Engelbrecht, A.M.; Toit-Kohn, J.L.; Ellis, B.; Thomas, M.; Nell, T.; Smith, R. Differential induction of apoptosis and inhibition of the PI3-kinase pathway by saturated, monounsaturated and polyunsaturated fatty acids in a colon cancer cell model. *Apoptosis* **2008**, *13*, 1368–1377. [CrossRef] [PubMed]

131. Jing, K.; Song, K.S.; Shin, S.; Kim, N.; Jeong, S.; Oh, H.R.; Park, J.H.; Seo, K.S.; Heo, J.Y.; Han, J.; *et al.* Docosahexaenoic acid induces autophagy through p53/AMPK/mTOR signaling and promotes apoptosis in human cancer cells harboring wild-type p53. *Autophagy* **2011**, *7*, 1348–1358. [CrossRef] [PubMed]

132. Shin, S.; Jing, K.; Jeong, S.; Kim, N.; Song, K.S.; Heo, J.Y.; Park, J.H.; Seo, K.S.; Han, J.; Park, J.I.; *et al.* The ω-3 polyunsaturated fatty acid DHA induces simultaneous apoptosis and autophagy via mitochondrial ROS-mediated Akt-mTOR signaling in prostate cancer cells expressing mutant p53. *Biomed. Res. Int.* **2013**, *2013*, 568671. [CrossRef] [PubMed]

133. Kim, N.; Jeong, S.; Jing, K.; Shin, S.; Kim, S.; Heo, J.Y.; Kweon, G.R.; Park, S.K.; Wu, T.; Park, J.I.; *et al.* Docosahexaenoic acid induces cell death in human non-small cell Lung cancer cells by repressing mTOR via AMPK activation and PI3K/Akt inhibition. *Biomed. Res. Int.* **2015**, *2015*, 239764. [CrossRef] [PubMed]

134. Rescigno, T.; Capasso, A.; Tecce, M.F. Effect of Docosahexaenoic acid on cell cycle pathways in Breast cell lines with different transformation degree. *J. Cell. Physiol.* **2015**. [CrossRef] [PubMed]

135. Shaikh, I.A.; Brown, I.; Schofield, A.C.; Wahle, K.W.; Heys, S.D. Docosahexaenoic acid enhances the efficacy of docetaxel in prostate cancer cells by modulation of apoptosis: The role of genes associated with the NF-κB pathway. *Prostate* **2008**, *68*, 1635–1646. [CrossRef] [PubMed]

136. Cavazos, D.A.; Price, R.S.; Apte, S.S.; de Graffenried, L.A. Docosahexaenoic acid selectively induces human prostate cancer cell sensitivity to oxidative stress through modulation of NF-κB. *Prostate* **2011**, *71*, 1420–1428. [CrossRef] [PubMed]

137. Jeong, S.; Jing, K.; Kim, N.; Shin, S.; Kim, S.; Song, K.S.; Heo, J.Y.; Park, J.H.; Seo, K.S.; Han, J.; *et al.* Docosahexaenoic acid-induced apoptosis is mediated by activation of mitogen-activated protein kinases in human cancer cells. *BMC Cancer* **2014**, *14*, 481. [CrossRef] [PubMed]

138. Gleissman, H.; Yang, R.; Martinod, K.; Lindskog, M.; Serhan, C.N.; Johnsen, J.I.; Kogner, P. Docosahexaenoic acid metabolome in neural tumors: Identification of cytotoxic intermediates. *FASEB J.* **2010**, *24*, 906–915. [CrossRef] [PubMed]

139. Serhan, C.N.; Arita, M.; Hong, S.; Gotlinger, K. Resolvins, docosatrienes, and neuroprotectins, novel ω-3-derived mediators, and their endogenous aspirin-triggered epimers. *Lipids* **2004**, *39*, 1125–1132. [CrossRef] [PubMed]

140. Hong, S.; Lu, Y.; Yang, R.; Gotlinger, K.H.; Petasis, N.A.; Serhan, C.N. Resolvin D1, protectin D1, and related docosahexaenoic acid-derived products: Analysis via electrospray/low energy tandem mass spectrometry based on spectra and fragmentation mechanisms. *J. Am. Soc. Mass Spectrom.* **2007**, *18*, 128–144. [CrossRef] [PubMed]

141. Ding, W.Q.; Vaught, J.L.; Yamauchi, H.; Lind, S.E. Differential sensitivity of cancer cells to docosahexaenoic acid-induced cytotoxicity: The potential importance of down-regulation of superoxide dismutase 1 expression. *Mol. Cancer Ther.* **2004**, *3*, 1109–1117. [PubMed]

142. Ding, W.Q.; Lind, S.E. Phospholipid hydroperoxide glutathione peroxidase plays a role in protecting cancer cells from docosahexaenoic acid-induced cytotoxicity. *Mol. Cancer Ther.* **2007**, *6*, 1467–1474. [CrossRef] [PubMed]

143. Vibet, S.; Goupille, C.; Bougnoux, P.; Steghens, J.P.; Goré, J.; Mahéo, K. Sensitization by docosahexaenoic acid (DHA) of breast cancer cells to anthracyclines through loss of glutathione peroxidase (GPx1) response. *Free Radic. Biol. Med.* **2008**, *44*, 1483–1491. [CrossRef] [PubMed]

144. Sturlan, S.; Baumgartner, M.; Roth, E.; Bachleitner-Hofmann, T. Docosahexaenoic acid enhances arsenic trioxidemediated apoptosis in arsenic trioxide-resistant HL-60 cells. *Blood* **2003**, *101*, 4990–4997. [CrossRef] [PubMed]

145. Granci, V.; Cai, F.; Lecumberri, E.; Clerc, A.; Dupertuis, Y.M.; Pichar, C. Colon cancer cell chemosensitisation by fish oil emulsion involves apoptotic mitochondria pathway. *Br. J. Nutr.* **2013**, *109*, 1188–1195. [CrossRef] [PubMed]

146. Hossain, Z.; Hosokawa, M.; Takahashi, K. Growth inhibition and induction of apoptosis of colon cancer cell lines by applying marine phospholipid. *Nutrition and Cancer* **2009**, *61*, 123–130. [CrossRef] [PubMed]

147. Dai, J.; Shen, J.; Pan, W.; Shen, S.; Das, U.N. Effects of polyunsaturated fatty acids on the growth of gastric cancer cells *in vitro*. *Lipids Health Dis.* **2013**, *12*, 71. [CrossRef] [PubMed]

148. Jing, K.; Shin, S.; Jeong, S.; Kim, S.; Song, K.S.; Park, J.H.; Heo, J.Y.; Seo, K.S.; Park, S.K.; Kweon, G.R.; et al. Docosahexaenoic acid induces the degradation of HPV E6/E7 oncoproteins by activating the ubiquitin-proteasome system. *Cell Death Dis.* **2014**, *5*, e1524. [CrossRef] [PubMed]

149. Kang, K.S.; Wang, P.; Yamabe, N.; Fukui, M.; Jay, T.; Zhu, B.T. Docosahexaenoic acid induces apoptosis in MCF-7 cells *in vitro* and *in vivo* via reactive oxygen species formation and caspase 8 activation. *PLoS ONE* **2010**, *5*, e10296. [CrossRef] [PubMed]

150. Zajdel, A.; Wilczok, A.; Tarkowski, M. Toxic effects of *n*-3 polyunsaturated fatty acids in human lung A549 cells. *Toxicol. Vitro* **2015**. [CrossRef] [PubMed]

151. Serhan, C.N.; Hong, S.; Gronert, K.; Colgan, S.P.; Devchand, P.R.; Mirick, G.; Moussignac, R.L. Resolvins: A family of bioactive products of ω-3 fatty acid transformation circuits initiated by aspirin treatment that counter proinflammation signals. *J. Exp. Med.* **2002**, *196*, 1025–1037. [CrossRef] [PubMed]

152. Wang, Q.; Hu, M.; Xu, H.; Yang, X. Anti-inflammatory and Pro-resolving effects of *n*-3 PUFA in Cancers: Structures and Mechanisms. *Curr. Top Med. Chem.* **2016**, *16*, 888–894. [CrossRef] [PubMed]

153. Hawcroft, G.; Loadman, P.M.; Belluzzi, A.; Hull, M.A. Effect of eicosapentaenoic acid on E-type prostaglandin synthesis and EP4 receptor signaling in human colorectal cancer cells. *Neoplasia* **2010**, *12*, 618–627. [CrossRef] [PubMed]

154. Poorani, R.; Bhatt, A.N.; Dwarakanath, B.S.; Das, U.N. COX-2, aspirin and metabolism of arachidonic, eicosapentaenoic and docosahexaenoic acids and their physiological and clinical significance. *Eur. J. Pharmacol.* **2015**. [CrossRef] [PubMed]

155. Karmali, R.A.; Reichel, P.; Cohen, L.A.; Terano, T.; Hirai, A.; Tamura, Y.; Yoshida, S. The effects of dietary ω−3 fatty acids on the DU-145 transplantable human prostatic tumor. *Anticancer Res.* **1987**, *17*, 1173–1180.

156. Rose, D.P.; Cohen, L.A. Effects of dietary menhaden oil and retinyl acetate on the growth of DU145 human prostatic adenocarcinoma cells transplanted into athymic nude mice. *Carcinogenesis* **1988**, *9*, 603–605. [CrossRef] [PubMed]

157. Rose, D.P.; Connolly, J.M. Dietary fat and breast cancer metastasis by human tumor xenografts. *Breast Cancer Res. Treat.* **1997**, *46*, 225–237. [CrossRef] [PubMed]

158. Kobayashi, N.; Barnard, R.J.; Henning, S.M.; Elashoff, D.; Reddy, S.T.; Cohen, P.; Leung, P.; Hong-Gonzalez, J.; Freedland, S.J.; Said, J.; et al. Effect of altering dietary ω-6/ω-3 fatty acid ratios on prostate cancer membrane composition, cyclooxygenase-2, and prostaglandin E_2. *Clin. Cancer Res.* **2006**, *12*, 4662–4670. [CrossRef] [PubMed]

159. Funahashi, H.; Satake, M.; Hasan, S.; Sawai, H.; Newman, R.A.; Reber, H.A.; Hines, O.J.; Eibl, G. Opposing effects of *n*-6 and *n*-3 polyunsaturated fatty acids on pancreatic cancer growth. *Pancreas* **2008**, *36*, 353–362. [CrossRef] [PubMed]

160. Narayanan, B.A.; Narayanan, N.K.; Desai, D.; Pittman, B.; Reddy, B.S. Effects of a combination of docosahexaenoic acid and 1,4-phenylene bis(methylene) selenocyanate on cyclooxygenase 2, inducible nitric oxide synthase and β-catenin pathways in colon cancer cells. *Carcinogenesis* **2004**, *25*, 2443–2449. [CrossRef] [PubMed]

161. Calviello, G.; Serini, S.; Piccioni, E. *n*-3 polyunsaturated fatty acids and the prevention of colorectal cancer: Molecular mechanisms involved. *Curr. Med. Chem.* **2007**, *14*, 3059–3069. [CrossRef] [PubMed]

162. Sun, H.; Berquin, I.M.; Owens, R.T.; O'Flaherty, J.T.; Edwards, I.J. Peroxisome proliferator-activated receptor γ-mediated up-regulation of syndecan-1 by *n*-3 fatty acids promotes apoptosis of human breast cancer cells. *Cancer Res.* **2008**, *68*, 2912–2919. [CrossRef] [PubMed]

163. Edwards, I.J.; Sun, H.; Hu, Y.; Berquin, I.M.; O'Flaherty, J.T.; Cline, J.M.; Rudel, L.L.; Chen, Y.Q. *In vivo* and *in vitro* regulation of syndecan 1 in prostate cells by *n*-3 polyunsaturated fatty acids. *J. Biol. Chem.* **2008**, *283*, 18441–18449. [CrossRef] [PubMed]

164. O'Flaherty, J.T.; Hu, Y.; Wooten, R.E.; Horita, D.A.; Samuel, M.P.; Thomas, M.J.; Sun, H.; Edwards, I.J. 15-lipoxygenase metabolites of docosahexaenoic acid inhibit prostate cancer cell proliferation and survival. *PLoS ONE* **2012**, *7*, e45480. [CrossRef] [PubMed]

165. Hu, Y.; Sun, H.; O'Flaherty, J.T.; Edwards, I.J. 15-Lipoxygenase-1-mediated metabolism of docosahexaenoic acid is required for syndecan-1 signaling and apoptosis in prostate cancer cells. *Carcinogenesis* **2013**, *34*, 176–182. [CrossRef] [PubMed]

166. Zou, S.; Meng, X.; Meng, Y.; Liu, J.; Liu, B.; Zhang, S.; Ding, W.; Wu, J.; Zhou, J. Microarray analysis of anti-cancer effects of docosahexaenoic acid on human colon cancer model in nude mice. *Int. J. Clin. Exp. Med.* **2015**, *8*, 5075–5084. [PubMed]

167. Sheng, H.; Li, P.; Chen, X.; Liu, B.; Zhu, Z.; Cao, W. ω-3 PUFAs induce apoptosis of gastric cancer cells via ADORA1. *Front. Biosci.* **2014**, *19*, 854–861. [CrossRef]

8

Pork as a Source of Omega-3 (*n*-3) Fatty Acids

Michael E.R. Dugan [1,*], **Payam Vahmani** [1], **Tyler D. Turner** [2], **Cletos Mapiye** [3], **Manuel Juárez** [1], **Nuria Prieto** [1], **Angela D. Beaulieu** [4], **Ruurd T. Zijlstra** [5], **John F. Patience** [6] and **Jennifer L. Aalhus** [1]

Academic Editors: Lindsay Brown, Bernhard Rauch and Hemant Poudyal

[1] Agriculture and Agri-Food Canada, Lacombe Research Centre, Lacombe T4L 1W1, AB, Canada; payam.vahmani@agr.gc.ca (P.V.); manuel.juarez@agr.gc.ca (M.J.); nuria.prieto@agr.gc.ca (N.P.); jennifer.aalhus@agr.gc.ca (J.L.A.)
[2] Josera GmbH & Co. KG, Kleinheubach 63924, Germany; t.turner@josera.de
[3] Department of Animal Sciences, Stellenbosch University, Stellenbosch 7602, South Africa; cmapiye@sun.ac.za
[4] Prairie Swine Centre, Inc., Saskatoon S7H 3J8, SK, Canada; denise.beaulieu@usask.ca
[5] Department of Agricultural, Food and Nutritional Sciences, University of Alberta, Edmonton T6G 2R3, AB, Canada; ruurd.zijlstra@ualberta.ca
[6] Department of Animal Science, Iowa State University, Ames, IA 50011-3150, USA; jfp@iastate.edu
* Correspondence: mike.dugan@agr.gc.ca

Abstract: Pork is the most widely eaten meat in the world, but typical feeding practices give it a high omega-6 (*n*-6) to omega-3 (*n*-3) fatty acid ratio and make it a poor source of *n*-3 fatty acids. Feeding pigs *n*-3 fatty acids can increase their contents in pork, and in countries where label claims are permitted, claims can be met with limited feeding of *n*-3 fatty acid enrich feedstuffs, provided contributions of both fat and muscle are included in pork servings. Pork enriched with *n*-3 fatty acids is, however, not widely available. Producing and marketing *n*-3 fatty acid enriched pork requires regulatory approval, development costs, quality control costs, may increase production costs, and enriched pork has to be tracked to retail and sold for a premium. Mandatory labelling of the *n*-6/*n*-3 ratio and the *n*-3 fatty acid content of pork may help drive production of *n*-3 fatty acid enriched pork, and open the door to population-based disease prevention polices (*i.e.*, food tax to provide incentives to improve production practices). A shift from the status-quo, however, will require stronger signals along the value chain indicating production of *n*-3 fatty acid enriched pork is an industry priority.

Keywords: pig; pork; *n*-3; omega-3; LNA; ETA; EPA; DHA

1. Introduction

Over the last century, changes in agricultural production and patterns of food consumption have led to an increase in the omega-6 (*n*-6) to omega-3 (*n*-3) fatty acid ratio in human diets. The imbalance in the *n*-6 to *n*-3 ratio has been associated with numerous diseases, from cardiovascular and inflammatory diseases to diabetes and autoimmune disorders, and led to calls for rebalancing the ratio in the food supply [1]. Pork is the most widely eaten meat world-wide, accounting for 38% of meat production and over 36% of meat intake in the world [2]. Enriching pork among other meats represents a viable means to increase *n*-3 fatty acid consumption in humans, while leading to concomitant reductions in fatty acids associated with adverse health outcomes (e.g., saturated fatty acids (SFA)). This may be of particular importance in populations that do not consume fish or marine products, where red meat may contribute up to 30% of dietary long chain *n*-3 fatty acids [3]. The objectives of the present review are to examine where pork fits in the human diet, the fatty acid composition of pork, efforts to enrich pork with *n*-3 fatty acids when feeding flaxseed, and examination of practical barriers and possible strategies to help drive *n-3* pork development and entry into the food supply.

2. Pork in Human Diets

The apparent link between plasma cholesterol and cardiovascular disease, and its association with SFA intake, led to recommendations to reduce the intake of SFA rich foods including red meat [4]. In response, swine industries in several countries adopted feeding and breeding strategies to reduce the fat content of pork. Results of these efforts were dramatic, leading to as little as 0.8%–1% intramuscular (marbling) fat, and increasing to a minimum of 1.5% marbling fat has since been recommended to ensure palatability [5]. Even at 2% marbling fat, lean pork contains 120–130 calories per 100 g serving, and only 15% of the calories are from fat. It would take pork marbling levels of 3%–6% to fall into the maximum recommended range of fat intakes for humans (20%–35% of dietary energy, Figure 1) [6]. In addition, if retail pork contains 2% intramuscular fat, the fat typically contains ~35%–40% SFA, equaling 5%–6% of total energy, which is again less than the maximum recommendation of 10% [6]. In light of these facts, and results of a meta-analyses of observational and epidemiological studies indicating SFA intake is not associated with cardiovascular disease risk [7,8], recommendations to substitute other protein sources for lean red meat in the human diet have been questioned [9,10]. On the other hand, even though the low fat and high protein contents of lean pork make it an excellent whole food for inclusion in human diets, complete pork carcasses contain ~47% fat [11], and this fat enters the food supply in the form of sausages, bacon, processed meats, and as lard in baked goods.

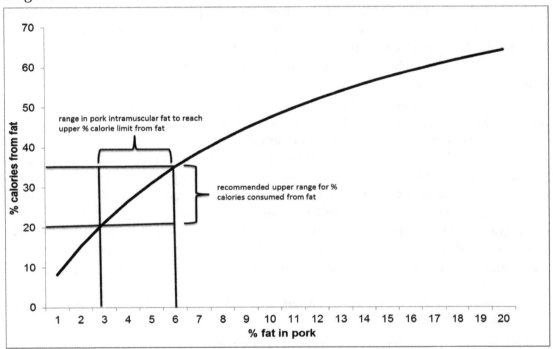

Figure 1. Calories in pork fat relative to recommendations for fat consumption.

Common indicators of the healthfulness of fatty acid profiles (polyunsaturated fatty acid (PUFA)/SFA, and *n-6/n-3* ratios) indicate there may be existing opportunities for their rebalancing in pork. In a survey of retail pork in England, the PUFA/SFA ratio of lean pork was 0.58 [12], which is greater than the 0.4 minimum recommended by the UK Department of Health [13], but an *n-6/n-3* ratio of 7.2:1 was found, exceeding the recommended ratio of 4:1 [13]. Swine diets used in commercial intensive production are typically grain based, with the type of grain fed dependent on local availability and economics. Swine in the US and Canada are typically fed diets based on corn or small grains (barley/wheat). Juárez *et al.* [14] fed pigs on a barley/wheat/soybean based diet for

11 weeks prior to market and found a *longissimus* muscle (*i.e.*, the largest steak/chop muscle running the length of the spine) PUFA/SFA ratio of 0.32 and a *n*-6/*n*-3 ratio of 4.5:1. Romans *et al.* [15] finished pigs using a typical corn/soybean based diet and found a *longissimus* muscle PUFA/SFA ratio of 0.24 and an *n*-6/*n*-3 ratio of 14.3:1. Thus, although lean pork has a desirable nutrient profile with high protein and low fat, there may still be some health benefit to adjusting the fatty acid composition (*i.e.*, reducing the *n*-6/*n*-3 ratio and increasing the PUFA/SFA ratio).

3. Pork Fatty Acid Composition

Lean pork contains a fairly constant proportion of cell membrane phospholipids, which are relatively rich in PUFA [16]. Lean pork also contains variable amounts of neutral lipid, composed mainly of SFA-rich triacyglycerol. The fatty acid composition of pork can thus be improved by reducing its total fat content, but if the fat content is too low, it can lead to palatability issues [17]. The composition of pork can also be influenced by diet, and diet adjustments can be used to improve pork fatty acid profiles without reducing total fat content [18,19]. Opportunities to use diet to change the fatty acid composition of meat are species specific, with major differences found between monogastric and ruminant livestock [20]. Pigs are monogastrics and categorized as homolipoid organisms [21], meaning their fatty acid composition closely reflects the fatty acid composition of their diet. In contrast to ruminant animals, in pigs, fatty acids are not metabolized to any great extent by microbes in the digestive tract prior to lipid digestion and absorption [20]. This makes pork a good candidate for enrichment with *n*-3 fatty acids.

Contrary to popular assumption, fat in red meats, including pork, is not solely composed of SFA (Table 1). When Juárez *et al.* [14] and Turner *et al.* [22] fed pigs a barley/wheat/soybean meal based diet, the *longissimus* muscle (denuded of epimysium and closely associated adipose tissue) was found to contain 2.9% total fat, and the fat contained 39% SFA, 47% monounsaturated fatty acids (MUFA), 11.5% PUFA, and the PUFA were comprised of 9.4% *n*-6 and 2.0% *n*-3 fatty acids. Within the *n*-3 fatty acids, α-linolenic acid (LNA, C18:3*n*-3) was the most concentrated at 22.7 mg/100 g of fresh tissue, and the most abundant long chain (LC) *n*-3 fatty acid was docosapentaenoic acid (DPA, C22:5*n*-3) at 11 mg/100g of fresh tissue. The LC *n*-3 fatty acids most widely studied for their health promoting properties include eicosapentaenoic acid (EPA, C20:5n-3) and docosahexaenoic acid (DHA, C22:6*n*-3) [23,24], and are concentrated in oily fish and marine products (e.g., microalgae). On the other hand, DPA is an intermediate in the pathway during DHA synthesis from EPA (Figure 2), and it is the most abundant LC *n*-3 fatty acid in meat and adipose tissue of terrestrial animals [25]. Docosapentaenoic acid which is freely converted between EPA and DHA, may have beneficial health effects on its own [26]. Consequently, when considering *n*-3 fatty acid nutrition, particularly in populations where oily fish or other LC *n*-3 fatty acid enriched marine products are not consumed, contributions of DPA made by terrestrial animals should be taken into consideration [27].

Table 1. Typical fatty acid composition of *longissimus* muscle and associated tissues in pork from pigs fed a barley/wheat/soybean meal diet.

Fatty Acid	mg/100 g Tissue					% of Fatty Acids				
	LM	AM + E	AM + E + SF	AM +E + SF + SCF	SEM	LM	AM + E	AM + E + SF	AM + E + SF + SCF	SEM
C16:0	718 [d]	1523 [c]	3033 [b]	5782 [a]	227	24.3	24.8	25.6	25.6	0.5
C18:0	378 [d]	822 [c]	1740 [b]	3438 [a]	128	12.8 [c]	13.3 [bc]	14.6 [ab]	15.2 [a]	0.5
ΣSFA	1147 [d]	2458 [c]	5001 [b]	9659 [a]	371	38.8 [b]	39.9 [ab]	42.2 [a]	42.6 [a]	0.9
C16:1-9c	101 [d]	191 [c]	313 [b]	519 [a]	25.8	3.39 [a]	3.09 [a]	2.66 [b]	2.29 [b]	0.12
C18:1-9c	1148 [d]	2430 [c]	4627 [b]	9006 [a]	357	38.6	39.4	39.2	39.9	0.8
C18:1-11c	116 [d]	295 [c]	420 [b]	667 [a]	24.0	3.96 [b]	4.82 [a]	3.59 [c]	2.97 [d]	0.06
ΣMUFA	1409 [d]	3017 [c]	5610 [b]	10652 [a]	415	47.4	49.0	47.5	47.2	0.9
C18:2n-6	189 [d]	422 [c]	822 [b]	1656 [a]	51.4	7.07	7.00	7.09	7.39	0.47
C18:3n-6	8.08 [c]	13.8 [c]	29.8 [b]	66.5 [a]	2.55	0.284 [ab]	0.220 [c]	0.258 [bc]	0.295 [a]	0.012
C20:2n-6	5.54 [d]	15.5 [c]	37.2 [b]	85.9 [a]	2.28	0.205 [d]	0.262 [c]	0.322 [b]	0.385 [a]	0.019
C20:3n-6	6.92 [d]	10.1 [c]	13.4 [b]	21.5 [a]	0.761	0.263 [a]	0.166 [b]	0.115 [bc]	0.095 [c]	0.020
C20:4n-6	46.0 [d]	59.7 [c]	65.8 [b]	75.4 [a]	2.03	1.77 [a]	1.00 [b]	0.580 [c]	0.342 [c]	0.120

Table 1. *Cont.*

Fatty Acid	mg/100 g Tissue					% of Fatty Acids				
	LM	AM + E	AM + E + SF	AM +E + SF + SCF	SEM	LM	AM + E	AM + E + SF	AM + E + SF + SCF	SEM
C22:4n-6	1.35 d	8.66 c	11.8 b	17.1 a	0.59	0.048 d	0.145 a	0.102 b	0.076 c	0.005
Σn-6	249 d	516 c	950 b	1856 a	55.0	9.36	8.57	8.21	8.29	0.61
C18:3n-3	22.7 c	41.3 c	89.5 b	186 a	8.22	0.818	0.669	0.758	0.824	0.067
C20:3n-3	3.01 c	5.75 c	15.6 b	36.7 a	1.22	0.104 c	0.092 c	0.131 b	0.162 a	0.008
C20:5n-3	6.35	5.26	5.72	7.87	0.68	0.235 a	0.0854 b	0.0484 bc	0.0349 c	0.016
C22:3n-3	5.40 a	0.918 c	1.79 bc	2.52 b	0.50	0.204 a	0.0134 b	0.0141 b	0.0108 b	0.011
C22:5n-3	11.0 d	15.4 c	20.8 b	30.4 a	1.1	0.422 a	0.257 b	0.181 bc	0.137 c	0.029
C22:6n-3	5.45 c	6.42 bc	8.71 b	12.7 a	0.88	0.209 a	0.109 b	0.0773 b	0.0581 b	0.024
Σn-3	54.0 c	75.1 c	142 b	276 a	10.8	1.99 a	1.22 b	1.21 b	1.22 b	0.13
ΣPUFA	306 d	596 c	1104 b	2158 a	66	11.5	9.88	9.52	9.63	0.7
TOTAL	2922 d	6140 c	11,795 b	22,577 a	821	100	100	100	100	0
n-6/n-3	4.77 b	7.00 a	6.81 a	6.76 a	0.26					
PUFA/SFA	0.301	0.250	0.228	0.228	0.025					

LM, *longissimus* muscle; AM + E, all muscles in loin + epimysium; AM + E + SF, AM + E + seam fat; AM + E + SF + SCF, AM + E + S + subcutaneous fat; SEM, standard error of the mean. SFA, saturated fatty acids; MUFA, monounsaturated fatty acids; PUFA, polyunsaturated fatty acids. [a,b,c] For mg/100 g and % data, means within a row with different superscripts are significantly different at $p < 0.05$.

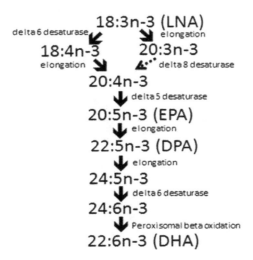

Figure 2. Pathways for *n*-3 fatty acid synthesis. LNA, alpha-linolenic acid; EPA, eicosapentaenoic acid; DPA, docosapentaenoic acid; DHA, docosahexaenoic acid.

The fatty acid composition of pig *longissimus* is the muscle most reported in the literature. Scientifically it is expedient to report fatty acid compositions on pure muscle, but when examining servings of pork, it is important to consider contributions made by various tissues. When Juárez *et al.* [14] and Turner *et al.* [22] combined *longissimus* and other muscles in the primal loin cut, including epimysium and closely associated adipose tissues, the fat content was 6.1% (*i.e.*, increased from 2.9% fat in pure *longissimus* muscle). When intermuscular (seam) fat was further included, the fat content of pork increased to 11.8%, and when 5 mm of overlying backfat was added to complete a commercially trimmed pork chop, the total fat content increased to 22.6%. The addition of fatty tissues to pure muscle also increased the percentage of SFA in total fat, and increased the *n*-6/*n*-3 ratio. In addition, when fatty tissues were included with pure muscle, LNA remained as the most abundant *n*-3 fatty acid, but the second most abundant *n*-3 fatty acid changed from DPA to eicosatrienoic acid (ETA, C20:3*n*-3). Despite the reduction in the %PUFA in the fat because the total fat increased, the actual amount of PUFA on a mg/100 g of fresh tissue basis increased from 306 mg to 2158 mg, and the *n*-3 fatty acids increase from 54 to 276 mg per 100g. Knowing the content of *n*-3 fatty acids in various cuts of pork is therefore of considerable importance as these help define the pig feeding practices required to meet label (enrichment) claims for *n*-3 fatty acids. For example, in Canada to make a retail label claim for *n*-3 fatty acid enrichment, a serving of food must contain at least 300 mg *n*-3 fatty acids [28]. If the serving only contains *longissimus* muscle, the *n*-3 fatty acid content would need to be increased 5–6 fold to reach enrichment status. On the other hand, a commercial loin chop (all muscles, seam and 5 mm of back fat) would likely need limited *n*-3 fatty acid supplementation in pig diets to reach 300 mg *n*-3 fatty acids per serving. Similarly, other higher fat cuts such as back or side ribs and bacon could also meet this label claim with limited supplementation.

As previously mentioned, reducing the marbling fat content of lean pork improves the fatty acid composition by increasing the proportion of PUFA and the PUFA/SFA ratio. If extra-muscular fatty tissues are then added to pork cuts, the proportion of SFA goes up (Table 1). As illustrated in Figure 3, however, when extra-muscular sources of fatty tissue are included in pork cuts, changes in fatty acid composition are not striking. This is because, even when as little as 2.9% intramuscular fat is present, the content of SFA rich triacylglycerols are still enough to overwhelm the contribution made by PUFA rich phospholipids. In practical terms, the fatty acid profile of pork with enough intramuscular fat to ensure palatability is not very different from higher fat products such as pork sausage. The difference in healthfulness is more related to the total fat content rather than the fatty acid profile. It is also worth re-emphasizing that the most abundant class of fatty acids in pork are MUFA, and these are the main fatty acids in the heart healthy Mediterranean diet [29]. Moreover, approximately ~25% of the SFA in pork is stearic acid (C18:0), which is noted to have neutral effects on plasma cholesterol [30].

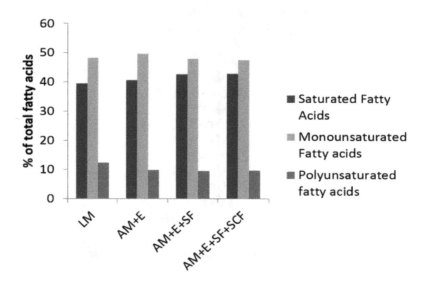

Figure 3. The percentage of saturated fatty acid (SFA), monounsaturated fatty acid (MUFA), and polyunsaturated fatty acid (PUFA) in total fatty acids in cuts of pork loin (LM, *longissimus* muscle; AM+E all loin muscles + epimysium; AM + E + seam fat; AM + E + SF + subcutaneous fat).

4. Enriching Pork with *n*-3 Fatty Acids

4.1. Initial Efforts to Improve Pork Fatty Acid Composition

The idea of modifying the fatty acid composition of pork to make it more healthful is not new. To improve the healthfulness of pork fatty acid profiles, Koch *et al.* [31] fed pigs safflower oil and achieved large increases in pork PUFA in the form of linoleic acid (LA, C18:2*n*-6). Stewart *et al.* [32] also fed a diet rich in LA, and achieved increased PUFA levels in pork and lard. When the LA enriched pork and foods made with LA enriched lard were fed to young women (aged 19–24) they significantly lowered total plasma and low-density lipoprotein (LDL) cholesterol, and increased PUFA and reduced SFA and MUFA in plasma lipids and erythrocytes. The pig diet, however, had *n*-6/*n*-3 fatty acid ratios of ~10:1, and with today's understanding that lower ratios may impart even further benefits, there have been a number of studies conducted attempting to increase pork PUFA by increasing the *n*-3 fatty acid content.

4.2. Efforts to Increase n-3 Fatty Acids in Pork

The ability to substantially alter the *n*-3 fatty acid content of pork was demonstrated in 1972 by Anderson *et al.* [33] when studying LNA turnover. Feeding 20% flaxseed oil for two months to six month old pigs increased fat depot concentrations of LNA from 1% to 15%. Given the understanding that increasing the *n*-3 fatty acid content of pork may benefit consumers, and that feeding flaxseed instead of extracted flaxseed oil may reduce input costs, Cunnane *et al.* [34] fed 5% ground flaxseed to weaned pigs for 8 weeks and found several fold increases in LNA and its elongation and desaturation products in a number of tissues. Since this time, a number of studies have been conducted feeding flaxseed, flaxseed oil or sources of LC *n*-3 fatty acids (*i.e.*, fish meal, fish oil, and marine algae) and results have been extensively reviewed [16,18,19,35,36]. Cherian *et al.* [37], Romans *et al.* [15], Riley *et al.* [38] and Ahn *et al.* [39] conducted intensive studies on the effects of feeding 0 to ~15% flaxseed on pork quality and fatty acid composition, Romans *et al.* [40] and Juárez *et al.* [41] investigated feeding flaxseed for different durations, and Fontanillas *et al.* [42] and Huang *et al.* [43] investigated the evolution of *n*-3 fatty acids in pig tissues over the feeding period. Maximum levels of *n*-3 fatty acid deposition were comparable with enrichments achieved by Anderson *et al.* [33] when feeding flaxseed oil. To date, most studies feeding higher levels of flaxseed or flaxseed oil have found increased tissue contents of LNA, EPA and DPA, but not DHA. For example, Martínez-Ramírez *et al.* [44] found no increase in DHA when feeding pigs diets containing 7%–10% flaxseed, but interestingly, the amounts of other LC *n*-3 fatty acids deposited in pork were independent of whether the flaxseed was fed early or late in the feeding period. When feeding a limited amount of flaxseed (~2%), however, Enser *et al.* [45] found a reduction in the *n*-6/*n*-3 ratio from 9:1 to 5:1 and an increase in DHA. The pathway for *n*-3 fatty acid synthesis from LNA to DHA requires delta-6 desaturation in two places (Figure 2), and the increase in DHA was attributed to the low level of flaxseed supplementation. This means enough LNA was supplied to provide substrate for delta-6 desaturation to C18:4*n*-3, but not enough to out complete for delta-6 desaturase activity later in the pathway (*i.e.*, conversion of C24:5*n*-3 to C24:6*n*-3). Overall, feeding sources of *n*-3 fatty acids to pigs increased their content in pork, but results have been variable, and the differences attributed to the source, amount and type of *n*-3 fatty acids fed, the duration of feeding, the type of feed processing, the weight or age of pigs fed and their gender. Nevertheless, Nguyen *et al.* [46] found the mathematical relationship between the amount of LNA fed and deposited in pork was strong within a study (R^2 = 0.98), but lower when data from several studies are incorporated into a regression (R^2 = 0.68). Consequently, producers seeking to develop a strategy to produce *n*-3 enriched pork will likely be able to achieve consistency, but a standardized feeding program will be required based on in-house development rather than solely on strategies reported in the literature.

4.3. An Example of n-3 Enriched Pork and Post-Production Considerations

Results from Juárez *et al.* [14] and Turner *et al.* [22] provide an example of *n*-3 fatty acid enrichments in pork that might be attained when feeding optimally processed flaxseed to pigs, and factors that need to be considered when developing feeding strategies to meet *n*-3 fatty acid enrichment goals (Table 2). Pigs were fed a diet containing 10% flaxseed co-extruded 50:50 with field peas to optimize LNA digestibility [47]. The diet was fed from 48 to 121 kg body weight over an 11 week period resulting in increased LNA and total *n*-3 fatty acids from 0.82 and 1.99% of total *longissimus* muscle fatty acids to 5.76 and 8.94% respectively. This translated into an increase of LNA and total *n*-3 fatty acids from 22.7 and 54.0 mg per 100 g serving of pork to 145 and 217 mg respectively. These amounts of *n*-3 fatty acids would, however, not qualify for a source claim in a number of countries including Canada and the European Union, but may have potential in the United States. As mentioned previously, to be labelled as a source of *n*-3 fatty acids in Canada, a serving of food serving has to have 300 mg of total *n*-3 fatty acids [28]. In the USA, food servings with ⩾160 mg or ⩾320 mg LNA can be referred to as a "source" or "rich" in LNA respectively, and claims cannot be made for EPA and DHA [48]. In the European Union, foods with 300 mg LNA or 40 mg combined EPA and DHA per serving can be labeled as a source of n-3 fatty acids, and foods with 600 mg LNA or 80 mg combined EPA and DHA can be labeled as rich in n-3 fatty acids [49]. Source claims in all countries would, however, be possible when all muscles and fatty tissues were included in a retail pork chop. In fact, the amount of n-3 fatty acids in commercially trimmed pork chops was 10 times more than required for a source claim in Canada (3360 mg per 100 g serving) [22]. A source claim for combined EPA and DHA could also be made in the European Union (71.5 mg), but could only be considered a rich source if DPA was included in LC n-3 fatty acids (174 mg). The ability to make a source claim is, therefore, dependent on the country, what tissues are included in a serving of pork, the type of cut and the n-3 fatty acids considered to be LC. Consideration should, however, also be given to what consumers actually eat, as often some external fat may be trimmed before consumption. Therefore, ensuring consistent n-3 fatty acid enrichment and consumption might be most easily attained through development of further processed n-3 enriched pork products (e.g., sausages) and secondary products prepared with enriched lard (e.g., baked goods). Notably, when fatty tissues are added to pure muscle, the second most abundant n-3 fatty acid in pork changes from DPA to ETA (up to 381 mg per 100 g serving), and ETA has been shown to have a photo-protective effect in human skin [50]. There is also some limited evidence for delta-8 desaturase activity [51], converting ETA to C20:4n-3 in liver, which may gain importance in LC n-3 fatty acid synthesis as ETA concentrations increase (Figure 2).

Table 2. The fatty acid composition of *longissimus* muscle and associated tissues in pork from pigs fed a diet supplemented with 10% flaxseed.

Fatty Acid	mg/100 g Tissue					% of Fatty Acids				
	LM	AM + E	AM + E + SF	AM + E + SF + SCF	SEM	LM	AM + E	AM + E + SF	AM + E + SF + SCF	SEM
C16:0	571 [d]	1180 [c]	2227 [b]	4169 [a]	152	22.1 [a]	20.1 [b]	20.5 [b]	19.8 [b]	0.3
C18:0	318 [d]	678 [c]	1326 [b]	2545 [a]	102	12.4	11.7	12.2	12.1	0.3
ΣSFA	931 [d]	1953 [c]	3731 [b]	7040 [a]	265	36.0 [a]	33.4 [b]	34.3 [b]	33.5 [b]	0.6
C16:1-9c	66.6 [d]	113 [c]	177 [b]	295 [a]	12.0	2.59 [a]	1.94 [b]	1.68 [bc]	1.41 [c]	0.10
C18:1-9c	873 [d]	1871 [c]	3380 [b]	6727 [a]	218	33.8 [a]	32.2 [b]	31.7 [b]	32.2 [b]	0.5
C18:1-11c	76.7 [d]	196 [c]	265 [b]	419 [a]	14.3	3.06 [b]	3.39 [a]	2.53 [c]	2.01 [d]	0.08
ΣMUFA	1045 [d]	2259 [c]	3991 [b]	7724 [a]	256	40.7 [a]	38.9 [ab]	37.4 [bc]	36.9 [c]	0.6
C18:2n-6	225 [d]	652 [c]	1207 [b]	2470 [a]	55.0	9.68 [b]	11.4 [a]	11.5 [a]	11.9 [a]	0.34
C18:3n-6	6.38 [d]	12.8 [c]	25.1 [b]	53.0 [a]	1.54	0.26	0.223	0.236	0.253	0.011
C20:2n-6	6.40 [d]	24.7 [c]	47.1 [b]	106 [a]	2.75	0.27 [b]	0.437 [a]	0.454 [a]	0.509 [a]	0.025
C20:3n-6	5.86 [c]	7.83 [bc]	10.0 [b]	15.9 [a]	0.79	0.26 [a]	0.141 [b]	0.099 [c]	0.076 [c]	0.012
C20:4n-6	28.2 [c]	34.3 [b]	36.6 [b]	42.3 [a]	1.9	1.35 [a]	0.626 [b]	0.372 [c]	0.205 [c]	0.06
C22:4n-6	1.23 [c]	3.87 [b]	5.27 [b]	7.95 [a]	0.56	0.05 [ab]	0.067 [a]	0.049 [ab]	0.037 [b]	0.007
Σn-6	266 [d]	723 [c]	1306 [b]	2643 [a]	59	11.6	12.7	12.5	12.7	0.4
C18:3n-3	145 [d]	614 [c]	1290 [b]	2800 [a]	71	5.76 [d]	10.6 [c]	12.1 [b]	13.4 [a]	0.30
C20:3n-3	21.5 [d]	82.2 [c]	166 [b]	381 [a]	11.6	0.85 [c]	1.42 [b]	1.55 [b]	1.82 [a]	0.053
C20:5n-3	23.3 [d]	31.9 [c]	38.8 [b]	55.3 [a]	1.7	1.08 [a]	0.573 [b]	0.385 [c]	0.268 [c]	0.05
C22:3n-3	2.48 [b]	2.27 [b]	3.06 [b]	4.75 [a]	0.40	0.10 [a]	0.038 [b]	0.029 [b]	0.023 [b]	0.005
C22:5n-3	21.1 [d]	39.5 [c]	59.7 [b]	102 [a]	3.0	0.95 [a]	0.705 [b]	0.575 [c]	0.491 [c]	0.038
C22:6n-3	3.85 [d]	8.13 [c]	10.6 [b]	16.2 [a]	0.77	0.18 [a]	0.146 [b]	0.105 [c]	0.079 [c]	0.011
Σn-3	217 [d]	778 [c]	1569 [b]	3360 [a]	85	8.94 [d]	13.5 [c]	14.7 [b]	16.1 [a]	0.39
ΣPUFA	486 [d]	1506 [c]	2883 [b]	6018 [a]	143	20.6 [c]	26.3 [b]	27.4 [ab]	28.9 [a]	0.7
TOTAL	2519 [d]	5788 [c]	10,683 [b]	20,881 [a]	627	100	100	100	100	0
n-6/n-3	1.28 [a]	0.935 [b]	0.850 [c]	0.788 [c]						
PUFA/SFA	0.581 [b]	0.796 [a]	0.807 [a]	0.869 [a]						

LM, *longissimus* muscle; AM+E, all muscles in loin + epimysium; AM + E + SF, AM + E + seam fat; AM + E + SF + SCF, AM + E + S + subcutaneous fat; SEM, standard error of the mean. SFA, saturated fatty acids; MUFA, monounsaturated fatty acids; PUFA, polyunsaturated fatty acids. [a,b,c] For mg/100 g and % data, means within a row with different superscripts are significantly different at $p < 0.05$.

Currently, production of pork enriched with n-3 fatty acids is possible, but it is not clear which n-3 fatty acid should be enriched, to what extent they should be enriched and in what tissues. Feeding pigs a limited amount of flaxseed can rebalance the n-6/n-3 ratio in pork [45], but a healthier n-6/n-3 ratio is not something that can be advertised or put on a label in most countries. Feeding increased amounts of flaxseed can yield pork that can be labelled as a source, or rich source of n-3 fatty acids, but if consumers trim visible fat or the fat is lost during cooking, purchased pork may differ from pork consumed. Even when pork is enriched with enough n-3 fatty acids to allow for a source claim, beneficial effects of consuming such pork have not been extensively investigated. Coats et al. [52] found regular consumption of pork enriched with LC n-3 fatty acids by feeding fish meal increased erythrocyte DHA by 15%, and compared to a control group, serum triacylglycerol decreased to a greater extent and thromboxane production increased to a lesser extent. Using a rabbit model, Vossen et al. [53] fed pork enriched with LNA or LNA plus LC n-3, and found only pork enriched with LNA plus LC n-3 fatty acids reduced the total plasma cholesterol to high-density lipoprotein cholesterol (HDL-C) ratio. Clearly, it would be of benefit to conduct additional clinical trials to establish the health effects of consuming commercial pork compared to pork enriched with n-3 fatty acids, and factors considered should include the n-6/n-3 ratio, the amount and composition of n-3 fatty acids and the overall fat content of the pork in different meat cuts.

5. Practical Barriers Limiting n-3 Pork Development and Entry into the Food Supply

5.1. The Call for n-3 Enriched Meat Unfulfilled to Date

Simopoulos [54] indicated that it is essential in the process of returning the n-3 fatty acids into the food supply, that the balance of n-6/n-3 fatty acids in the diet that existed during human evolution is maintained. To date fish-meal, flaxseed, and marine algae in poultry feeds have increased the n-3 fatty acid content of egg yolks and led to the supply of n-3 fatty acid-enriched eggs in the marketplace [55]. Simopoulos [54] noted research on the production of n-3 fatty acid-enriched products from poultry, beef, lamb, pork, milk and bakery products was ongoing. Taking advancements in the ability to enrich animal products with n-3 fatty acids into account, Givens and Gibbs [56] estimated potential dietary intakes of EPA+DHA from foods derived from animals fed enriched diets would be ~231 mg/day, which would double current intakes in the UK, and help meet the recommend intake of 450 mg/day. Currently, however, in most countries, despite the technological capability to do so, the availability of n-3 enriched meats, including pork, is not widespread.

5.2. Why Production of n-3 Enriched Pork Has Not Been Adopted

5.2.1. Visibility

When the SFA content of red meat was associated with increased plasma cholesterol and cardiovascular disease in the 1960s, consumers could visually identify and select meats with lower fat contents, and animal producers selected and fed animals to meet consumer demands for leaner meat. In developed countries, sweeping changes in pork production took place within a value chain geared to produce commodity pork for mass markets. The cost of pork production and the retail price of pork were not increased due to changes in production strategies. Currently, even though the production of n-3 fatty acid enriched meats, including pork, has been encouraged, changing fat composition in retail pork has not been as successful as previous efforts to reduce the total fat content of pork. As opposed to the total fat content, the fatty acid composition of retail pork is not visible to consumers.

5.2.2. Challenges along the Value Chain

There are several challenges to producing n-3 enriched pork along the value chain. Increasing the n-3 fatty acid content of pork can lead to increased input costs depending on feedstuffs available and requirements for processing. Entry into the n-3 pork market may also have lagged because feeding high levels of n-3 fatty acids can lead to fat softness and palatability problems [14]. Effects on freshly cooked pork chops have, however, been limited [14,39,57] and most negative effects have been found in cooked/reheated pork chops and freshly cooked ground pork with excessive

n-3 fatty acid enrichments. Once n-3 fatty acid enriched pork is produced, it also requires vertical integration from production to retail, along with differentiated marketing and higher prices to cover input costs, distribution costs and profits for producers. Producing n-3 fatty acid enriched pork to meet source claims also requires regulatory approval for package labelling, defining what will be included in portions, what production strategies are needed to meet enrichment requirements, and also added costs for fatty acid analysis of feeds and pork during product development and for quality control. Strategies to drive an industry-wide shift towards n-3 fatty acid enriched pork must, therefore, be developed if a clear goal for producers is widespread production and marketing of n-3 enriched pork.

6. Strategies to Encourage Production and Market Availability of n-3 Fatty Acid Enriched Pork

Strategies to encourage production and market availability of n-3 fatty acid enriched pork will likely require concerted efforts along the value chain. Producer entry into the n-3 fatty acid enriched pork market may be enhanced with the understanding that only limited supplementation of n-3 fatty acids in diets is required to meet label claims when contributions of all tissues in a serving are included [22]. This also opens possibilities for feeding oils or oilseeds that may not be as highly enriched with LNA as flaxseed (e.g., whole canola or canola oil). An industry-wide shift in pork production practices might also be driven by mandatory labelling of n-3 fatty acids and the n-6/n-3 ratio in meat, making these visible to consumers. When consumers know the n-3 fatty acid and n-6/n-3 ratio in foods, it provides the opportunity to select more healthful foods, and impetus to the industry to find lower cost production strategies. In this way, pork may not have to reach specified amounts of n-3 fatty acids to meet regulatory approval as a source of n-3 fatty acids, but could contribute a greater quantity of n-3 fatty acids to the human diet, and at the very least, not further imbalance in the n-6/n-3 ratio. Analyzing the fatty acid composition of pork in the packing house or at retail by traditional means (i.e., gas chromatography) would not be cost effective or practical, but newer non-invasive technologies including near infra-red reflectance spectrophotometry (NIRS), NIRS hyperspectral imaging, or Raman spectroscopy [58–61] may hold promise to deliver analyses in seconds *versus* days, and coupled to new tracking systems, such as radio frequency identifier tags, may be able to deliver this information to the consumer at retail. Mandatory labelling of n-3 fatty acids and the n-6/n-3 ratio might also open the door to population-based prevention policies (i.e., food tax to drive nutritional improvements through changes in production practices), which could generate health gains while paying for themselves through future reductions of health-care expenditures [62], or by providing incentives to producers with specified amounts and types of n-3 fatty acids in their pig feed. Market pull could also be generated through inclusion of healthier sources of fatty acids (i.e., n-3 enriched lard) in baked goods, and further processed products that already qualify for nutritional labels, and this might in turn result in healthier pork meat as a byproduct. For all the strategies, however, it is clear that there needs to be more defined incentives provided to producers, and a stronger signal that changes are required along the value chain.

7. Conclusions

Currently retail pork is not considered a source of n-3 fatty acids, and in fact suffers from an imbalanced n-6/n-3 fatty acid ratio related to modern feeding practices. Pork is the most consumed meat in the world, and its fatty acid content and composition is directly influenced by diet. There have been calls to correct the imbalanced n-6/n-3 ratio in foods, including pork, and although this correction would seem to be a simple fix by modifying pig diets, adoption of such practices is not widespread. Producing n-3 enriched pork may increase production costs, enriched pork has to be tracked to retail, and the pork must be sold at a premium to recover added costs and provide profit for the effort. Labelling pork as a source of n-3 fatty acids also requires regulatory approval, development costs and costs for quality control to maintain enrichment status. As a result, n-3 enriched pork will likely continue to command a limited market share, and only be available to those willing to pay a premium. Several strategies to drive an industry wide shift towards *n*-3 fatty acid enriched pork production are possible including mandatory labelling of the *n*-3 fatty acid content and *n*-6/*n*-3 ratio, and development of population based prevention polices. This would allow consumers to make choices based on valued attributes, and provide for natural market segmentation without having to reach specific amounts of *n*-3 fatty acids per serving. When coupled with improvements in the speed of non-invasive fatty acid analyses and tracking technologies, we could be on the verge of meeting health conscious consumers growing demand for nutritional information, while providing impetus to pork value chain to make producing pork with a higher *n*-3 fatty acid content and lower *n*-6/*n*-3 ratio an industry wide priority.

Author Contributions: The authors are all part of a collaborative group which has been involved in several research trials developing flaxseed feeding strategies to enrich *n*-3 fatty acids in pork. M.E.R.D. is the lead author on the review, and all co-authors contributed by providing comments and suggested revisions to the manuscript.

References

1. Simopoulos, A.P. Importance of the omega-6/omega-3 balance in health and disease: Evolutionary aspects of diet. *World Rev. Nutr. Diet.* **2011**, *102*, 10–21. [PubMed]
2. FAO Sources of Meat. Available online: http://www.fao.org/ag/againfo/themes/en/meat/backgr_sources.html (accessed on 2 September 2015).
3. Ollis, T.E.; Meyer, B.J.; Howe, P.R. Australian food sources and intakes of omega–6 and omega–3 polyunsaturated fatty acids. *Ann. Nutr. Metab.* **1999**, *43*, 346–355. [CrossRef] [PubMed]
4. Teicholz, N. *The Big Fat Surprise: Why Butter, Meat and Cheese belong in a Healthy Diet*; Simon and Schuster: New York, NY, USA, 2014.
5. Fortin, A.; Robertson, W.; Tong, A. The eating quality of canadian pork and its relationship with intramuscular fat. *Meat Sci.* **2005**, *69*, 297–305. [CrossRef] [PubMed]
6. U.S. Department of Health and Human Services; U.S. Department of Agriculture. *Dietary Guidelines for Americans*; US Government Printing Office: Washington, DC, USA, 2010.
7. Siri-Tarino, P.W.; Sun, Q.; Hu, F.B.; Krauss, R.M. Meta-analysis of prospective cohort studies evaluating the association of saturated fat with cardiovascular disease. *Am. J. Clin. Nutr.* **2010**, *98*, 535–546. [CrossRef] [PubMed]
8. Chowdhury, R.; Warnakula, S.; Kunutsor, S.; Crowe, F.; Ward, H.A.; Johnson, L.; Franco, O.H.; Butterworth, A.S.; Forouhi, N.G.; Thompson, S.G.; *et al.* Association of dietary, circulating, and supplement fatty acids with coronary risk: A systematic review and meta-analysis. *Ann. Intern. Med.* **2014**, *160*, 398–406. [CrossRef] [PubMed]
9. Barendse, W. Should animal fats be back on the table? A critical review of the human health effects of animal fat. *Anim. Prod. Sci.* **2014**, *54*, 831–855.
10. Binnie, M.A.; Barlow, K.; Johnson, V.; Harrison, C. Red meats: Time for a paradigm shift in dietary advice. *Meat Sci.* **2014**, *98*, 445–451. [CrossRef] [PubMed]
11. Heinz, G.; Hautzinger, P. Meat Processing Technology for Small to Medium Scale Producers. Available online: http://www.fao.org/docrep/010/ai407e/ai407e00.htm (accessed on 2 September 2015).
12. Enser, M.; Hallett, K.; Hewitt, B.; Fursey, G.A.J.; Wood, J.D. Fatty acid content and composition of english beef, lamb and pork at retail. *Meat Sci.* **1996**, *42*, 443–456. [CrossRef]
13. Cardiovascular Review Group, Great Britain—Department of Health. *Nutritional Aspects of Cardiovascular Disease*; HMSO: Richmond, UK, 1994.
14. Juárez, M.; Dugan, M.E.R.; Aldai, N.; Aalhus, J.L.; Patience, J.F.; Zijlstra, R.T.; Beaulieu, A.D. Increasing omega-3 levels through dietary co-extruded flaxseed supplementation negatively affects pork palatability. *Food Chem.* **2011**, *126*, 1716–1723. [CrossRef] [PubMed]
15. Romans, J.R.; Johnson, R.C.; Wulf, D.M.; Libal, G.W.; Costello, W.J. Effects of ground flaxseed in swine diets on pig performance and on physical and sensory characteristics and omega-3 fatty acid content of pork: I. Dietary level of flaxseed. *J. Anim. Sci.* **1995**, *73*, 1982–1986.
16. Wood, J.D.; Enser, M.; Fisher, A.V.; Nute, G.R.; Sheard, P.R.; Richardson, R.I.; Hughes, S.I.; Whittington, F.M. Fat deposition, fatty acid composition and meat quality: A review. *Meat Sci.* **2008**, *78*, 343–358. [CrossRef] [PubMed]

17. Savell, J.; Cross, H. The role of fat in the palatability of beef, pork, and lamb. In *Designing Foods: Animal Product Options in the Marketplace*; National Academy Press: Washington, DC, USA, 1988; pp. 345–355.

18. Raes, K.; de Smet, S.; Demeyer, D. Effect of dietary fatty acids on incorporation of long chain polyunsaturated fatty acids and conjugated linoleic acid in lamb, beef and pork meat: A review. *Anim. Feed Sci. Technol.* **2004**, *113*, 199–221. [CrossRef]

19. Woods, V.B.; Fearon, A.M. Dietary sources of unsaturated fatty acids for animals and their transfer into meat, milk and eggs: A review. *Livest. Sci.* **2009**, *126*. [CrossRef]

20. Doreau, M.; Chilliard, Y. Digestion and metabolism of dietary fat in farm animals. *Br. J. Nutr.* **1997**, *78*, S15–S35. [CrossRef] [PubMed]

21. Shorland, F.B. Effect of the dietary fat on the composition of depot fats of animals. *Nature* **1950**, *165*. [CrossRef]

22. Turner, T.D.; Mapiye, C.; Aalhus, J.L.; Beaulieu, A.D.; Patience, J.F.; Zijlstra, R.T.; Dugan, M.E.R. Flaxseed fed pork: *N*-3 fatty acid enrichment and contribution to dietary recommendations. *Meat Sci.* **2014**, *96*, 541–547. [CrossRef] [PubMed]

23. Narayan, B.; Miyashita, K.; Hosakawa, M. Physiological effects of eicosapentaenoic acid (EPA) and docosahexaenoic acid (DHA)—A review. *Food Rev. Int.* **2006**, *22*, 291–307. [CrossRef]

24. Swanson, D.; Block, R.; Mousa, S.A. Omega-3 fatty acids EPA and DHA: Health benefits throughout life. *Adv. Nutr.* **2012**, *3*. [CrossRef] [PubMed]

25. Howe, P.; Meyer, B.; Record, S.; Baghurst, K. Dietary intake of long-chain omega-3 polyunsaturated fatty acids: Contribution of meat sources. *Nutrition* **2006**, *22*, 47–53. [CrossRef] [PubMed]

26. Miller, E.; Kaur, G.; Larsen, A.; Loh, S.P.; Linderborg, K.; Weisinger, H.S.; Turchini, G.M.; Cameron-Smith, D.; Sinclair, A.J. A short-term *n*-3 DPA supplementation study in humans. *Eur. J. Nutr.* **2013**, *52*, 895–904. [CrossRef] [PubMed]

27. Vahmani, P.; Mapiye, C.; Prieto, N.; Rolland, D.C.; McAllister, T.A.; Aalhus, J.L.; Dugan, M.E. The scope for manipulating the polyunsaturated fatty acid content of beef: A review. *J. Anim. Sci. Biotechnol.* **2015**, *6*. [CrossRef] [PubMed]

28. Canadian Food Inspection Agency (CFIA): Omega-3 and Omega-6 Polyunsaturated Fatty Acid Claims. Available online: http://www.inspection.gc.ca/food/labelling/food-labelling-for-industry/nutrient-content/specific-claim-requirements/eng/1389907770176/1389907817577?chap=7 (accessed on 9 September 2015).

29. Kris-Etherton, P.M. Monounsaturated fatty acids and risk of cardiovascular disease. *Circulation* **1999**, *100*, 1253–1258. [CrossRef] [PubMed]

30. Yu, S.; Derr, J.; Etherton, T.D.; Kris-Etherton, P. Plasma cholesterol-predictive equations demonstrate that stearic acid is neutral and monounsaturated fatty acids are hypocholesterolemic. *Am. J. Clin. Nutr.* **1995**, *61*, 1129–1139. [PubMed]

31. Koch, D.E.; Pearson, A.M.; Magee, W.T.; Hoefer, J.A.; Schweigert, B.S. Effect of diet on the fatty acid composition of pork fat. *J. Anim. Sci.* **1968**, *27*, 360–365.

32. Stewart, J.W.; Kaplan, M.L.; Beitz, D.C. Pork with a high content of polyunsaturated fatty acids lowers LDL cholesterol in women. *Am. J. Clin. Nutr.* **2001**, *74*, 179–187. [PubMed]

33. Anderson, D.B.; Kauffman, R.G.; Benevenga, N.J. Estimate of fatty acid turnover in porcine adipose tissue. *Lipids* **1972**, *7*, 488–489. [CrossRef] [PubMed]

34. Cunnane, S.C.; Stitt, P.A.; Sujata, G.; Armstrong, J.K. Raised omega-3 fatty acid levels in pigs fed flax. *Can. J. Anim. Sci.* **1990**, *70*, 251–254. [CrossRef]

35. Kouba, M.; Enser, M.; Whittington, F.M.; Nute, G.R.; Wood, J.D. Effect of a high-linolenic acid diet on lipogenic enzyme activities, fatty acid composition, and meat quality in the growing pig. *J. Anim. Sci.* **2003**, *81*, 1967–1979. [PubMed]

36. Corino, C.; Rossi, R.; Cannata, S.; Ratti, S. Effect of dietary linseed on the nutritional value and quality of pork and pork products: Systematic review and meta-analysis. *Meat Sci.* **2014**, *98*, 679–688. [CrossRef] [PubMed]

37. Cherian, G.; Sim, J.S. Dietary alpha-linolenic acid alters the fatty acid composition of lipid classes in swine tissues. *J. Agric. Food Chem.* **1995**, *43*, 2911–2916. [CrossRef]

38. Riley, P.A.; Enser, M.; Nute, G.R.; Wood, J.D. Effects of dietary linseed on nutritional value and other quality aspects of pig muscle and adipose tissue. *Anim. Sci.* **2000**, *71*, 483–500.

39. Ahn, D.U.; Lutz, S.; Sim, J.S. Effects of dietary alpha-linolenic acid on the fatty acid composition, storage stability and sensory characteristics of pork loin. *Meat Sci.* **1996**, *43*, 291–299. [CrossRef]

40. Romans, J.R.; Wulf, D.M.; Johnson, R.C.; Libal, G.W.; Costello, W.J. Effects of ground flaxseed in swine diets on pig performance and on physical and sensory characteristics and omega-3 fatty acid content of pork: II. Duration of 15% dietary flaxseed. *J. Anim. Sci.* **1995**, *73*, 1987–1999. [PubMed]

41. Juárez, M.; Dugan, M.; Aldai, N.; Aalhus, J.; Patience, J.; Zijlstra, R.; Beaulieu, A. Feeding co-extruded flaxseed to pigs: Effects of duration and feeding level on growth performance and backfat fatty acid composition of grower–finisher pigs. *Meat Sci.* **2010**, *84*, 578–584. [CrossRef] [PubMed]

42. Fontanillas, R.; Barroeta, A.; Baucells, M.D.; Guardiola, F. Backfat fatty acid evolution in swine fed diets high in either cis-monounsaturated, trans, or (*n*-3) fats. *J. Anim. Sci.* **1998**, *76*, 1045–1055. [PubMed]

43. Huang, F.R.; Zhan, Z.P.; Luo, J.; Liu, Z.X.; Peng, J. Duration of dietary linseed feeding affects the intramuscular fat, muscle mass and fatty acid composition in pig muscle. *Livest. Sci.* **2008**, *118*, 132–139. [CrossRef]

44. Martínez-Ramírez, H.R.; Kramer, J.K.G.; de Lange, C.F.M. Retention of *n*-3 polyunsaturated fatty acids in trimmed loin and belly is independent of timing of feeding ground flaxseed to growing-finishing female pigs. *J. Anim. Sci.* **2014**, *92*, 238–249. [CrossRef] [PubMed]

45. Enser, M.; Richardson, R.I.; Wood, J.D.; Gill, B.P.; Sheard, P.R. Feeding linseed to increase the *n*-3 pufa of pork: Fatty acid composition of muscle, adipose tissue, liver and sausages. *Meat Sci.* **2000**, *55*, 201–212. [CrossRef]

46. Nguyen, L.Q.; Nuijens, M.C.G.A.; Everts, H.; Salden, N.; Beynen, A.C. Mathematical relationships between the intake of *n*-6 and *n*-3 polyunsaturated fatty acids and their contents in adipose tissue of growing pigs. *Meat Sci.* **2003**, *65*, 1399–1406. [CrossRef]

47. Htoo, J.K.; Meng, X.; Patience, J.F.; Dugan, M.E.R.; Zijlstra, R.T. Effects of coextrusion of flaxseed and field pea on the digestibility of energy, ether extract, fatty acids, protein, and amino acids in grower-finisher pigs. *J. Anim. Sci.* **2008**, *86*, 2942–2951. [CrossRef] [PubMed]

48. U.S. Department of Health and Human Services (HHS). Food labeling: Nutrient content claims; alpha-linolenic acid, eicosapentaenoic acid, and docosahexaenoic acid omega-3 fatty acids. *Fed. Regist.* **2014**, *79*, 23262–23273.

49. European Food Safety Authority (EFSA). Scientific opinion: Labelling reference intake values for *n*-3 and *n*-6 polyunsaturated fatty acids. *EPSA J.* **2009**, *1176*, 1–11.

50. Kim, E.J.; Kim, M.-K.; Jin, X.-J.; Oh, J.-H.; Kim, J.E.; Chung, J.H. Skin aging and photoaging alter fatty acids composition, including 11,14,17-eicosatrienoic acid, in the epidermis of human skin. *J. Korean Med. Sci.* **2010**, *25*, 980–983. [CrossRef] [PubMed]

51. Schenck, P.A.; Rakoff, H.; Emken, E.A. δ8 desaturation *in vivo* of deuterated eicosatrienoic acid by mouse liver. *Lipids* **1996**, *31*, 593–600. [CrossRef] [PubMed]

52. Coates, A.M.; Sioutis, S.; Buckley, J.D.; Howe, P.R. Regular consumption of *n*-3 fatty acid-enriched pork modifies cardiovascular risk factors. *Br. J. Nutr.* **2009**, *101*, 592–597. [CrossRef] [PubMed]

53. Vossen, E.; Raes, K.; Maertens, L.; Vandenberge, V.; Haak, L.; Chiers, K.; Ducatelle, R.; de Smet, S. Diets containing *n*-3 fatty acids-enriched pork: Effect on blood lipids, oxidative status and atherosclerosis in rabbits. *J. Food Biochem.* **2012**, *36*, 359–368. [CrossRef]

54. Simopoulos, A.P. New products from the agri-food industry: The return of *n*-3 fatty acids into the food supply. *Lipids* **1999**, *34*, S297–S301. [CrossRef] [PubMed]

55. Lewis, N.M.; Seburg, S.; Flanagan, N.L. Enriched eggs as a source of *n*-3 polyunsaturated fatty acids for humans. *Poult. Sci.* **2000**, *79*, 971–974. [CrossRef] [PubMed]

56. Givens, D.; Gibbs, R. Very long chain *n*-3 polyunsaturated fatty acids in the food chain in the uk and the potential of animal-derived foods to increase intake. *Nutr. Bull.* **2006**, *31*, 104–110. [CrossRef]

57. Bryhni, E.A.; Kjos, N.P.; Ofstad, R.; Hunt, M. Polyunsaturated fat and fish oil in diets for growing-finishing pigs: Effects on fatty acid composition and meat, fat, and sausage quality. *Meat Sci.* **2002**, *62*. [CrossRef]

58. Damcz, J.-L.; Clerjon, S. Quantifying and predicting meat and meat products quality attributes using electromagnetic waves: An overview. *Meat Sci.* **2013**, *95*, 879–896. [CrossRef] [PubMed]

59.   Prieto, N.; Dugan, M.E.R.; López-Campos, O.; McAllister, T.A.; Aalhus, J.L.; Uttaro, B. Near infrared reflectance spectroscopy predicts the content of polyunsaturated fatty acids and biohydrogenation products in the subcutaneous fat of beef cows fed flaxseed. *Meat Sci.* **2012**, *90*, 43–51. [CrossRef] [PubMed]

60.   Prieto, N.; Uttaro, B.; Mapiye, C.; Turner, T.; Dugan, M.; Zamora, V.; Young, M.; Beltranena, E. Predicting fat quality from pigs fed reduced-oil corn dried distillers grains with solubles by near infrared reflectance spectroscopy: Fatty acid composition and iodine value. *Meat Sci.* **2014**, *98*, 585–590. [CrossRef] [PubMed]

61.   Berhe, D.T.; Eskildsen, C.E.; Lametsch, R.; Hviid, M.S.; van den Berg, F.; Engelsen, S.B. Prediction of total fatty acid parameters and individual fatty acids in pork backfat using raman spectroscopy and chemometrics: Understanding the cage of covariance between highly correlated fat parameters. *Meat Sci.* **2016**, *111*, 18–26. [CrossRef] [PubMed]

62.   Cecchini, M.; Sassi, F.; Lauer, J.A.; Lee, Y.Y.; Guajardo-Barron, V.; Chisholm, D. Tackling of unhealthy diets, physical inactivity, and obesity: Health effects and cost-effectiveness. *Lancet* **2010**, *376*, 1775–1784. [CrossRef]

9

Is there a Role for Alpha-Linolenic Acid in the Fetal Programming of Health?

Alicia I. Leikin-Frenkel [1,2]

1   The Sackler Faculty of Medicine, Tel Aviv University, Tel Aviv 69978, Israel; alicial@post.tau.ac.il;

2   Bert Strassburger Lipid Center, Sheba, Tel Hashomer, Ramat Gan 52621, Israel

Academic Editors: Lindsay Brown, Bernhard Rauch and Hemant Poudyal

Abstract: The role of ω3 alpha linolenic acid (ALA) in the maternal diet during pregnancy and lactation, and its effect on the prevention of disease and programming of health in offspring, is largely unknown. Compared to ALA, ω3 docosahexaenoic (DHA) and eicosapentaenoic (EPA) acids have been more widely researched due to their direct implication in fetal neural development. In this literature search we found that ALA, the essential ω3 fatty acid and metabolic precursor of DHA and EPA has been, paradoxically, almost unexplored. In light of new and evolving findings, this review proposes that ALA may have an intrinsic role, beyond the role as metabolic parent of DHA and EPA, during fetal development as a regulator of gene programming for the prevention of metabolic disease and promotion of health in offspring.

Keywords: alpha linolenic acid; maternal diet; fetal programming; metabolic syndrome; gene expression; ω3 fatty acids

1. Introduction

More than 80 years ago, Burr *et al.* [1] described the essential fatty acids (EFA) linoleic acid (ω6 LA) and alpha linolenic acid (ω3 ALA) in animals. Their research contributed to the knowledge and concept that normal growth, development and health in mammals depends on EFA nutritional supply. Both EFA share enzymes like the Δ6 desaturase and elongases, and, thus, compete as substrates in this metabolic pathway (Figure 1). The genetic variants of desaturases determine the nutritional requirements for the supply of fatty acids and consequently, health and/or disease, as previously reviewed [2,3].

During the course of mammalian development, fatty acids (FA) are transferred to the fetus through the placenta [4] and their composition depends, to a great extent, on the maternal diet [5]. Maternal nutrition during pregnancy-lactation can induce significant changes in body composition, physiology and metabolism in offspring. Thus, the Fetal Origins Hypothesis was inspired by evidence showing that adult cardiovascular disease begins through developmental activation of a set of genes and metabolic pathways in the offspring in response to *in utero* under- or over-nutrition [6]. FAs play a primary role in growth and development and it is now accepted that imbalances in their intake during pregnancy and lactation may result in permanent changes that affect appetite control, neuroendocrine function and energy metabolism in the fetus; thus, influencing the metabolic programming [7]. However, the roles of EFAs and the mechanisms by which they impact the long-term health of the offspring remains to be determined [8]. The importance of the FA composition in the diet and the significant differences between ALA and its metabolic products DHA and EPA has been spotted both in adults [9] and in maternal diets during pregnancy [10]. Some recent reviews even reinforce the importance of maternal dietary FA quality for the health outcomes in offspring [7,8,11,12].

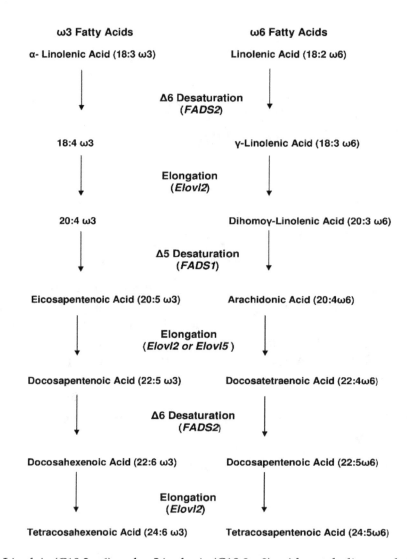

Figure 1. Linoleic (C18:2*n*-6) and α-Linolenic (C18:3*n*-3) acid metabolism and elongation.

Beyond the existing differences between human and animals, the basic tissue, physiological and morphological placental developments are conserved between species. Therefore, animal models can be considered suitable when researching the impact of nutritional FAs on development and their long-term influence on the offspring's susceptibility to metabolic diseases, including obesity, insulin resistance (IR), and cardiovascular risk [13]. Importantly, when looking for a comprehensive understanding of the role of nutritional FAs on development for the prevention of adult disease, a nutrigenetics approach is recommended [14,15].

2. Dietary ω3 Fatty Acids and Health

DHA and EPA: As defined by Burr [1], ALA is the only ω3 essential FA for mammals, while DHA and EPA are its downstream metabolic products. The benefits of consumption or supplementation of ω3 polyunsaturated fatty acids (PUFAs) by adults on the prevention and treatment of obesity, metabolic syndrome (MS), and cardiovascular disease (CVD) have been reported [16,17]. Most of the reviewed studies were randomized-controlled intervention trials suggesting that supplementation with ω3 PUFA might improve some obesity-associated metabolic syndrome features such as insulin resistance, hypertension and dyslipidemia by decreasing plasma triglycerides [18]. Similarly, they also confer cardio protection by lowering blood pressure and through their benefits on vascular and anti-inflammatory properties [19]. The efficacy of ω3 PUFA on reducing myocardial infarction, arrhythmia, cardiac and sudden death, or stroke is, however, controversial [20]. Although it is now widely accepted that DHA and EPA have beneficial effects on CVD, it is not yet clear if these benefits are directly or exclusively related to DHA and EPA [21,22]. Other benefits of DHA and EPA, such as reversion of neuropathies, have also been described [23,24] for both plant and marine ω-3 FAs.

ALA: The relationship between ALA and chronic disease is unclear. As supported by human studies [22–24], high intake of ALA is protective against fatal ischemic heart disease. In later years, the use of ALA-rich oils deserved attention in the search for nutritional ways of preventing or ameliorating cardiovascular disease and metabolic syndrome. Rodriguez-Leyva *et al.* reported that epidemiological randomized studies using flaxseed oil as a preventive intervention in a healthy population or in subjects identified as "at risk" for CVD are missing [25]. Baxheinrich *et al.* reported the beneficial effects of ALA rich rapeseed oil on body weight, systemic inflammation and endothelial function in patients with MS traits [26,27]. These past works showed that providing ALA significantly contributed to reductions in systolic blood pressure, total cholesterol, LDL-cholesterol and insulin levels after six months. Moreover, ALA was shown to significantly decrease body fat mass, as well as improve both vascular function and inflammation.

The effects of ALA, as well as those of EPA and DHA, on the metabolic syndrome have been further reviewed by Poudyal *et al.* [28]. They addressed ALA, DHA and EPA as individual entities, and provided evidence of potentially independent effects for each of the ω3 FAs on cardiovascular health. These same authors also reported that the three ω3 FA could each reduce inflammation in cardiac fibrosis and hepatic steatosis in a high-fat diet induced model of metabolic syndrome in rats. Those effects were associated to a complete suppression of Stearoyl CoA desaturase (SCD1) function. In those studies, ALA induced comparatively different FA redistribution of retroperitoneal fat, skeletal muscle and liver. Furthermore, it was suggested that the accumulation of the ω3 FA in adipose tissue, as well as in skeletal muscle, may account for their crucial role in the reduction of abdominal fat, inflammation, dyslipidemia and IR [28]. Conversely, recommendations for ALA intake in pregnant women for the prevention of metabolic diseases in offspring are limited [29–33].

3. How Efficient Is ALA Conversion to EPA and DHA in Humans?

Dietary ALA is metabolically converted into acetate or CO_2 through β-oxidation, or desaturated and elongated into EPA, ω3 DPA and DHA [34]. ALA conversion to longer products in tracer studies has been observed in nearly all humans studied from birth through late middle-aged men and women [34,35].

It is clear that the metabolism of ω3 FA depends on other nutrients, in particular ω6 FAs, due to their competition for the same enzymes and transport systems [2]. They also compete for incorporation into more complex lipids that comprise mammalian tissues, where high levels of ω6 PUFA replace and reduce ω3 PUFA levels. Early studies of rat liver microsomes showed that the Δ-6 desaturase activity measured *in vitro* was subject to competitive inhibition by other substrates. In particular, desaturation of ALA to ω3 eicosatrienoic acid was shown to be inhibited by LA and, conversely, LA conversion to ω6 gamma linolenic acid was inhibited by ALA [36,37].

When studying the impact of ALA on the improvement of the metabolic syndrome, the following question arises: is the conversion of ALA into EPA and DHA responsible for the observed effects? This question was addressed by Truong *et al.* [32] in relation to genetic variants in the Δ6 desaturase gene (*Fads2*). Adipose tissue was used as a biomarker of ALA intake in adult humans, and the authors showed that high concentrations of ALA in adipose tissue were associated with lower prevalence ratios of the metabolic syndrome compared to low ALA. Although an interaction between ALA and *Fads2* genotype (T-del) was borderline significant, it nevertheless suggested that genetic variation may play an important role along with diet in the development of metabolic syndrome, at least in the studied population. A variety of models have confirmed that ALA accumulates significantly and is converted into longer ω3 FA in humans [34]. According to the ISSFAL official statement #5, studies in healthy adults showed that supplementing ALA to Western diets containing LA raises DHA and EPA levels in blood and breast milk [38]. In addition, these and other studies have provided evidence indicating that FA accumulation is tissue-dependent [38] suggesting that metabolism may be based upon a tissue-selective need for longer ω3 FA, such as DHA.

As claimed by Anderson *et al.* [39], clarification of ALA's involvement in health and disease is essential. Indeed, it is insufficient to assume that ALA exerts its beneficial effects through conversion to EPA and DHA. More thorough research is required to identify the differential effects of ALA on metabolic disease like IR and CVD and to differentiate the possible heterogeneous effects of ALA *versus* DHA and EPA. The use of developed animal models such as the Δ6 knockout mouse [40] that inhibits the conversion of ALA into EPA, and EPA into DHA, could be highly useful in this regard. No such work has been performed to date.

4. Adults

It has been observed that humans of all ages, from preterm and even fetuses to adults, convert ALA to DHA. However, the efficiency of conversion seems to decrease as infants mature [35]. ALA is partitioned to β-oxidation as energy source, for metabolic conversion to longer PUFA and for incorporation into tissues [39,41,42]. Importantly, studies were also reported in which a significant increase in plasma DHA levels was achieved by altering the oils in the diet and changing both ALA and LA content [43].

There seems to be an agreement that the partitioning of ALA towards β-oxidation in humans is lower in women than in men [44,45], an effect attributed to estrogen [34], which may explain the higher conversion of ALA to longer-chain PUFA in women [32,41]. The explanation for the preferred use of ALA for β-oxidation seems to be the greater affinity of carnitine palmitoyl transferase-1, the rate limiting enzyme in mitochondrial β-oxidation, for this EFA compared to other PUFA [41]. Most studies examining ALA have been performed in young men. The few studies focused specifically on women of reproductive age showed that conversion of ALA to EPA and DHA is 2.5× greater in women compared to age-matched men [43–45]. This is ascribed not only to the differential partitioning towards β-oxidation, but also to an up-regulation of the translocation of very long metabolic products towards the peroxisome in women [34]. It has been suggested that ALA conversion increases in pregnancy, which is supported by data in pregnant rats [44–46].

Clearly, gender differences exist and are of importance when recommending ω3 FA to men or women and, in this case of the latter, whether they are pregnant or not [41]. Work performed by Childs and others [46,47] have provided further support for this concept. The examination of whether there are sex differences in the long-chain ω3 FA response to increased ALA intake in humans showed that women have a higher increase than men in the EPA content of plasma phospholipids after six months. The gender differences in ALA use, metabolism and destination, warrant further investigation.

5. Fatty Acids Quality and Early Life

Pregnancy is supposed to be a period of high requirement for DHA in humans due to the fetus' need for rapid growth and neural development [34]. FA levels in the embryo and newborn babies are directly associated with maternal FA levels and composition; therefore, any variation in the maternal intake of FAs susceptible to genetic variability is pivotal for fetal growth, development and health [47]. There is some evidence suggesting that the influence of genetic variation in *FADS* genes on both circulating and tissue FA profiles, which can influence disease risk, may have a trans-generational effect [48,49]. Moreover, it has been shown that breastfeeding also exposes babies to the maternal genetic Fads variations through their effects on milk quality and quantity of fatty acids that, in turn, affect the baby health and intelligence quotient [50]. Consequently, these studies show that the influence of *FADS2* polymorphisms in the mother is of uttermost importance for the array of FAs transferred from mother to child during uterine development and breastfeeding. This knowledge reinforces the importance of a nutritional adjustment during the critical perinatal period.

DHA and EPA: The effects of different qualities of dietary FAs during pregnancy and/or lactation on fetal development and offspring metabolism have been recently reviewed [7]. Maternal consumption of diets rich in ω3 PUFA in particular showed benefits for the development of offspring and it was even suggested that they exert epigenetic regulation for the prevention of obesity, insulin resistance and cardiovascular diseases [51,52]. The consumption of DHA and EPA during crucial periods of fetal development has beneficial physiologic and metabolic effects on the health of offspring by protecting them from the onset of metabolic diseases [7,11]. Nevertheless, results in the field are controversial, and the independent effects of ALA have not been studied enough.

ALA: During pregnancy there is a reduction of DHA in maternal serum while, at the same time, an increased requirement of DHA and EPA for fetal brain development [38,49]. The solution to compensate for this supposed imbalance can be to either provide ALA, the precursor for DHA and EPA, or these end products directly. Not enough scientific information exists comparing for the benefits of either supplementation. From the clinical aspect, criticism is raised regarding the claim of support for fetal cognitive health and brain function improvement associated with DHA and EPA supplementation [53].

Larque *et al.* [12] reported a somewhat positive relationship between maternal or cord serum DHA percentages and cognitive skills in young children. Unfortunately, valuable information was missing from this study: ALA is not mentioned amongst ω3 FAs and the blood FA composition of mothers and/or children was not described.

During the literature search described here, only one study was found indicating a negative effect of maternal over-consumption of ω3 FAs on life span and auditory brainstem response in older adult offspring. As in several papers, the term ω3 FA was broadly used, without specifying the dietary FA composition and without mentioning the specific effects of ALA [54].

6. Perinatal Manipulation of ALA

In relation to perinatal metabolism, significant FA desaturase activities have been detected in fetuses and preterm infants, indicating the existence of the molecular pathways at early stages of life [55,56].

Published research regarding the positive effects of DHA and EPA has been reviewed showing that they are essential for proper fetal development [57]. Supplementation of ω3 PUFA during pregnancy has been linked to decreased incidence of allergies [58]. An interesting study using flaxseed oil in mice questions whether ALA provision during gestation and lactation could induce epigenetic changes in maternal and offspring livers [58]. In this study, the authors described an interaction between ALA dietary content and the FA metabolism, through down-regulation of the expression of enzymes involved in the elongation (*Elovl2*) and desaturation (*Fads1*) of FAs in maternal livers. A positive correlation between *Fads2* promoter methylation in maternal livers and offspring livers with changes in the expression of DNA methyltransferases at day 19 of pregnancy was described. Even though the work was inconclusive, the authors suggested that the maternal availability of ALA during gestation-lactation could differentially alter the metabolism of ω3 and ω6 FAs, as well as the epigenetic status of *Fads2* in maternal and offspring' livers.

Research focusing on ALA content in the maternal diet and the long-term side effects on metabolic syndrome in the offspring is scarce. Our laboratory has begun focusing on those effects and showed that maternal dietary enrichment of ALA, compared to SFA, led to lower body weight gain, liver fat accumulation, and homeostasis model assessment (HOMA) index, as well as reduced SCD1 in the adult offspring exposed to a high fat diet [59]. Those results suggested that the relative increase in dietary ALA during pregnancy and lactation may have the potential to prevent obesity and insulin resistance in the offspring. Furthermore, Shomonov-Wagner *et al.* [60] compared the effects of dietary enrichment in ω3 ALA, DHA or EPA, compared to saturated fatty acids (SFA). That work showed that SFA, independent of total fat amount or calories, induced liver lipid accumulation and IR in offspring at weaning, while ALA was the most efficient ω3 FA to prevent the induced metabolic alterations. That work proposed that not only ALA and SFA have divergent effects on IR and liver lipid levels, but also that each of ALA, DHA and EPA behaved differently. Furthermore, ALA preventive effects were, apparently, unrelated to its conversion into DHA and EPA. Consequently, we conclude that ω3 ALA, DHA and EPA should be studied and referred to individually and not as a group.

Recently published results seem to indicate that ALA, as opposed to SFA, up-regulates the expression of genes involved in lipid oxidation and in the circadian rhythm [61].

7. Regulatory Mechanisms

The ω3 FA family seems to have distinct abilities to modulate metabolic functions and gene expression [62]. Deckelman et al. [63] mentioned that the longer chain length and higher number of double bonds give these FAs unique properties and suggested that they relate to modulation of enzymes associated with signaling pathways/incorporation of EPA and DHA into membrane phospholipids and direct effects on gene expression, amongst others. However, ALA has not been studied enough, and the molecular interactions between ALA and genes, are only now beginning to be described [61].

Maternal dietary enrichment with ALA and the long terms effects on offspring susceptibility to obesity and metabolic syndrome are an important and urgent subject waiting to be investigated. Also important to consider are FA-gene interactions. Based on the literature found, we may assume that ALA has beneficial effects during gestation, presumably on the prevention of obesity-associated disease in offspring [61]. Ahmed [64] described a proteomics approach to examine the regulatory roles of ω3 FAs. By using mice fed high or low ω3 FA containing diets, some affected proteins were identified related to lipid, glucose and protein metabolism. Unfortunately their work excluded ALA, but their information hints at the interaction between FAs and protein targets for the regulation of metabolic pathways. These results, together with preliminary evolving information, warrant more studies that would benefit from testing ALA, DHA and EPA separately.

8. Epigenetics

Environmental factors such as diet during fetal development can induce long-term modifications in the genes of the fetus. Human epidemiological data and controlled animal studies corroborate the impact of diet in the perinatal period and its lasting effect on gene expression and metabolism [65]. The question, "how do FAs influence the establishment of an epigenotype" [66], is intriguing and stimulating. It is proposed that the peroxisome proliferator-activated receptor alpha (PPARa), an abundant nuclear receptor transcription factor, may be a candidate to be regulated by maternal dietary FAs in embryonic life. Wang et al. [67] described the way maternal and, possibly, paternal imbalanced over- and under-nutrition may induce epigenetic modifications. Thus, DNA methylation, histone modification and miRNAs, may regulate genome activity and gene expression leading to proteins that affect fetal programming and organ physiology with lifelong consequences, sex-dependent in some cases. The developmental adaptations that permanently change structure, physiology and metabolism in offspring would thereby predispose for metabolic and cardiovascular risk later in adult life. Vickers's [68] analyzed not only the in utero, but also the trans-generational, possibilities for epigenetic modifications and its consequences. Niculescu et al. [58] showed epigenetic modifications induced specifically by ALA in an in vitro study. ALA was shown to alter the distribution of cells by influencing cell cycle phases, apoptosis and gene and protein expression of DNA methyl transferases 1 and 3. However, no modifications in global DNA methylation were found.

Burdge et al. [69] reviewed the interaction between FAs and the epigenome to conclude that it is not known, at present, how FAs modify the epigenome. Some of the existing limitations include the lack of definition of the experimental diets and the susceptibility of histone deacetylases to inhibition by short chain FAs present in most experimental diets. Nevertheless, the mechanisms underpinning transmission of developmental programming urgently require further research.

9. Final Thoughts and Recommendations

The importance of ω3 FAs for the development and long-term health of offspring is widely recognized. The importance of ALA, specifically, is only now beginning to be recognized; however, more thorough research is necessary in order to better understand its independent role in developmental programming.

Based on ongoing research [28,61] we propose here the concept that ALA may have a role in the programming of health. Specifically, it may have intrinsic regulatory properties on gene expression during fetal development that extend beyond its simple metabolic conversion to DHA and EPA.

Although the human conversion of ALA to DHA and EPA is gender-related and relatively low (up to 4%) [41], a higher consumption of ALA related to LA may increase it. Besides, individual DHA and EPA are not easily available and expensive. Moreover, DHA- and EPA-rich fish oil has some health disadvantages [22] due to contaminating factors such as heavy metals, teratogens, and others.

Due to the widespread use of the general term "ω3 FA", that is sometimes misleading, we propose that scientific publications apply a more precise nomenclature to identify the specific FAs tested (*i.e.*, ALA, DHA, and EPA).

In order to enlarge the understanding of ALA's role in fetal development and programming, we recommend to analyze the effects of a maternal diet enriched in each of the individual ω3 FAs, in simple nutritional animal models that examine the tissue distribution, as well as gene expression and metabolic outcomes, in offspring.

Acknowledgments: Alicia I. Leikin-Frenkel is grateful to Dror Harats, Director of the Bert Strassburger Lipid Center, for providing the infrastructure and conditions for working on this manuscript. She is also grateful to David M. Mutch for carefully reading the manuscript.

Abbreviations

ALA	ω3 alpha linolenic acid
FA	fatty acid
CVD	cardiovascular risk disease
DHA	docosahexenoic acid
DPA	docosapentenoic acid
EFA	essential fatty acid
EPA	eicosapentenoic acid
Fads2	gene of Δ6 desaturase enzyme
IR	insulin resistance
LA	linoleic acid
LDL	low density lipoproteins
Ppargc1a/*Ppargc1a*	peroxisome proliferative activated receptor gamma coactivator1a enzyle and gene, respectively
PUFA	polyunsaturated fatty acid
SCD1/*Scd1*	stearoyl-CoA desaturase 1 enzyme and gene, respectively
SFA	saturated fatty acid

References

1. Burr, G.O.; Burr, M.M. The nature and role of the fatty acids essential in nutrition. *J. Biol. Chem.* **1930**, *86*, 587–621. [CrossRef]

2. Sinopolus, A. Genetic variants in the metabolism of omega-6 and omega-3 fatty acids: Their role in the determination of nutritional requirements and chronic disease risk. *Exp. Biol. Med.* **2010**, *235*, 785–795.

3. Merino, D.M.; Ma, D.W.L.; Mutch, D.M. Genetic variation in lipid desaturases and its impact on the development of human disease. *Lipids Health Dis.* **2010**, *9*, 63. [CrossRef] [PubMed]

4. Innis, S.M. Essential fatty acid transfer and fetal development. *Placenta* **2005**, *26*, 570–575. [CrossRef] [PubMed]

5. Hornstra, G. Essential fatty acids in mothers and their neonates. *Am. J. Clin. Nutr.* **2000**, *71*, 1262S–1269S. [PubMed]

6. Barker, D.J.P. Fetal origins of coronary heart disease. *BJM* **1995**, *311*, 171–174. [CrossRef]

7.   Mennitti, L.V.; Oliveira, J.L.; Morais, C.A.; Estadella, D.; Oyama, L.M.; Nascimento, C.M.D.; Pisani, L.P. Type of fatty acids in maternal diets during pregnancy and/or lactation and metabolic consequences of the offspring. *J. Nutr. Biochem.* **2015**, *26*, 99–111. [CrossRef] [PubMed]

8.   Kabaran, S.; TanjuBesler, H.T. Do fatty acids affect fetal programming? *J. Health Popul. Nutr.* **2015**, *33*, 14. [CrossRef] [PubMed]

9.   Alfaradhi, M.; Ozanne, S.E. Developmental programming in response to maternal overnutrition. *Front. Genet.* **2011**, *27*, 1–13. [CrossRef] [PubMed]

10.   Valenzuela, R.; Bascuñán, K.A.; Chamorro, R.; Barrera, C.; Sandoval, J.; Puigrredon, C.; Parraguez, G.; Orellana, P.; Gonzalez, V.; Valenzuela, A. Modification of Docosahexaenoic Acid Composition of Milk from Nursing Women Who Received Alpha Linolenic Acid from Chia Oil during Gestation and Nursing. *Nutrients* **2015**, *7*, 6405–6424. [CrossRef] [PubMed]

11.   Swanson, D.; Block, R.; Mousa, S.A. Omega-3 fatty acids EPA and DHA: Health benefits throughout life. *Adv. Nutr.* **2012**, *3*, 1–7. [CrossRef] [PubMed]

12.   Larque, E.; Gil-Sanchez, A.; Prieto-Sanchez, M.T.; Koletzko, B. Omega 3 fatty acids, gestation and pregnancy outcomes. *Br. J. Nutr.* **2012**, *107*, S77–S84. [CrossRef] [PubMed]

13.   Fonseca, B.M.; Correia-da-Silva, G.; Teixeira, N.A. The rat as an animal model for fetoplacental development: A reappraisal of the post-implantation period. *Reprod. Biol.* **2012**, *12*, 97–118. [CrossRef]

14.   Brennan, R.O.; Mulligan, W.C. *Nutrigenetics: New Concepts for Relieving Hypoglycemia*; M Evans & Co.: New York, NY, USA, 1975; p. 258.

15.   Mutch, D.M.; Wahli, W.; Williamson, G. Nutrigenomics and nutrigenetics: The emerging faces of Nutrition. *FASEB.* **2005**, *19*, 1602–1616. [CrossRef] [PubMed]

16.   Dayton, S.; Pearce, M.L.; Goldman, H. Controlled trial of a diet high in unsaturated fat for prevention of atherosclerotic complications. *Lancet* **1968**, *16*, 1060–1062. [CrossRef]

17.   Lorente-Cebrián, S.; Costa, A.G.; Navas-Carretero, S.; Zabala, M.; Martínez, J.A.; Moreno-Aliaga, M.J. Role of omega-3 fatty acids in obesity, metabolic syndrome, and cardiovascular diseases: A review of the evidence. *Physiol. Biochem.* **2013**, *69*, 633–651. [CrossRef] [PubMed]

18.   Gebauer, S.K.; Psota, T.L.; Harris, W.S.; Kris-Etherton, P.M. n-3 Fatty acid dietary recommendations and food sources to achieve essentiality and cardiovascular benefits. *Am. J. Clin. Nutr.* **2006**, *83*, S1526–S1535.

19.   Poudyal, H.; Panchal, S.K.; Diwan, V.; Brown, L. Omega-3 fatty acids and metabolic syndrome: Effects and emerging mechanisms of action. *Prog. Lipid Res.* **2011**, *50*, 372–387. [CrossRef] [PubMed]

20.   Abeywardena, M.W.; Patten, G.S. Role of ω3 Long chain Polyunsaturated Fatty Acids in Reducing Cardio-Metabolic Risk Factors. *Endocr. Metab. Immune Disord. Drug Targets* **2011**, *11*, 232–246. [CrossRef] [PubMed]

21.   Larsson, S.C.; Orsini, N.; Wolk, A. Long-chain omega-3 polyunsaturated fatty acids and risk of stroke: A meta-analysis. *Eur. J. Epidemiol.* **2012**, *27*, 895–901. [CrossRef] [PubMed]

22.   Kris-Etherton, P.M.; Harris, W.S.; Appel, L.J. Fish Consumption, Fish Oil, Omega-3 Fatty Acids, and Cardiovascular Disease. *Circulation* **2002**, *106*, 2747–2757. [CrossRef] [PubMed]

23.   Coste, T.C.; Gerbi, A.; Vague, P.; Pieroni, G.; Raccah, D. Neuroprotective Effect of Docosahexaenoic Acid-Enriched Phospholipids in Experimental Diabetic Neuropathy. *Diabetes* **2003**, *52*, 2578–2585. [CrossRef] [PubMed]

24.   Barceló-Coblijn, G.; Murphy, E.J. Alpha-linolenic acid and its conversion to longer chain n-3 fatty acids: Benefits for human health and a role in maintaining tissue n-3 fatty acid levels. *Prog. Lipid Res.* **2009**, *48*, 355–374. [CrossRef] [PubMed]

25.   Rodriguez-Leyva, D.; Bassett, C.M.C.; McCullough, R.; Pierce, P. The cardiovascular effects of flaxseed and its omega-3 fatty acid, alpha-linolenic acid. *Can. J. Cardiol.* **2010**, *26*, 489–496. [CrossRef]

26.   Baxheinrich, A.; Stratmann, B.; Lee-Barkey, Y.H.; Tschoepe, D.; Wahrburg, U. Effects of an energy-restricted diet rich in plant-derived a-linolenic acid on systemic inflammation and endothelial function in overweight-to-obese patients with metabolic syndrome traits. *Br. J. Nutr.* **2014**, *112*, 1315–1322.

27.   Egert, S.; Baxheinrich, A.; Lee-Barkey, Y.H.; Tschoepe, D.; Wahrburg, U.; Stratmann, B. Effects of a rapeseed oil-enriched hypoenergetic diet with a high content of α-linolenic acid on body weight and cardiovascular risk profile in patients with the metabolic syndrome. *Br. J. Nutr.* **2012**, *108*, 682–691.

28.   Poudyal, H.; Panchal, S.K.; Ward, L.C.; Brown, L. Effects of ALA, EPA and DHA in high-carbohydrate, high-fat diet-induced metabolic syndrome in rats. *J. Nutr. Biochem.* **2013**, *24*, 1041–1052. [CrossRef] [PubMed]

29. Commor, W.E.; Bendich, A. Highly unsaturated fatty acids in nutrition and disease prevention. *Am. J. Clin. Nutr.* **2000**, *71* (Suppl. 1), 169S–398S.

30. Hu, F.B.; Stampfer, M.J.; Manson, J.A.E.; Rimm, E.B.; Wolk, A.; Colditz, G.A.; Hennekens, C.H.; Willett, W.C. Dietary intake of a-linolenic acid and risk of fatal ischemic heart disease among women. *Am. J. Clin. Nutr.* **1999**, *69*, 890–897. [PubMed]

31. Truong, H.; di Bello, J.R.; Ruiz-Narvaez, E.; Kraft, P.; Campos, H.; Baylin, A. Does genetic variation in the $\Delta6$-desaturase promoter modify the association between α-linolenic acid and the prevalence of metabolic syndrome? *Am. J. Clin. Nutr.* **2009**, *89*, 920–925. [CrossRef] [PubMed]

32. Fleming, J.A.; Kris-Etherton, P.M. The evidence for α-linolenic acid and cardiovascular disease benefits: Comparisons with eicosapentaenoic acid and docosahexaenoic acid. *Adv. Nutr.* **2014**, *5*, 863S–876S. [CrossRef] [PubMed]

33. Decsi, T.; Koletzko, B. *n*-3 Fatty acids and pregnancy outcomes. *Curr. Opin. Clin. Nutr. Metab. Care* **2005**, *8*, 161–166. [CrossRef] [PubMed]

34. Brenna, J.T. Efficiency of conversion of α-linolenic acid to long chain *n*-3 fatty acids in man. *Curr. Opin. Clin. Nutr. Metab. Care* **2002**, *5*, 127–132. [CrossRef]

35. Burdge, G.C. Metabolism of α-linolenic acid in humans. *Prostaglandins Leukot. Essent. Fat. Acids* **2006**, *75*, 161–168. [CrossRef] [PubMed]

36. Mohrhauer, H.; Holman, R.T. Effect of linolenic acid upon the metabolism of linoleic acid. *J. Nutr.* **1963**, *81*, 67–74. [PubMed]

37. Brenner, R.R.; Peluffo, R.O. Effect of saturated and unsaturated fatty acids on the desatu-ration *in vitro* of palmitic, stearic, oleic, linoleic, and linolenic acids. *J. Biol. Chem.* **1966**, *241*, 5213–5219. [PubMed]

38. Brenna, J.T.; Salem, N., Jr.; Sinclair, A.J.; Cunnane, S.C. Alpha-Linolenic acid supplementation and conversion to n-3 long-chain polyunsaturated fatty acids in humans. *Prostaglandins Leukot Essent Fatty Acids.* **2009**, *80*, 85–91. [CrossRef] [PubMed]

39. Anderson, B.M.; Ma, D.W. Are all *n*-3 polyunsaturated fatty acids created equal? *Lipids Health Dis.* **2009**, *10*, 33. [CrossRef] [PubMed]

40. Stoffel, W.; Holz, B.; Jenke, B.; Binczek, E.; Gunter, R.H.; Kiss, C.; Karakesisoglou, I.; Thevis, M.; Weber, A.A.; Arnhold, S.; *et al.* Delta6-desaturase (FADS2) deficiency unveils the role of omega3- and omega6-polyunsaturated fatty acids. *EMBO J.* **2008**, *27*, 2281–2292. [CrossRef] [PubMed]

41. Burdge, G. Alpha-linolenic acid metabolism in men and women: Nutritional and biological implications. *Curr. Opin. Clin. Nutr. Metab. Care* **2004**, *7*, 137–144. [CrossRef] [PubMed]

42. DeLany, J.P.; Windhauser, M.M.; Champagne, C.M.; Bray, G.A. Differential oxidation of individual dietary fatty acids in humans. *Am. J. Clin. Nutr.* **2000**, *72*, 905–911. [PubMed]

43. Burdge, G.C.; Jones, A.E.; Wootton, S.A. Eicosapentaenoic and docosapentaenoic acids are the principal products of α-linolenic acid metabolism in young men. *Br. J. Nutr.* **2002**, *88*, 355–363. [CrossRef] [PubMed]

44. Burdge, G.C.; Wootton, S.A. Conversion of α-linolenic acid to eicosapentaenoic, docosapentaenoic and docosahexaenoic acids in young women. *Br. J. Nutr.* **2002**, *88*, 411–420. [CrossRef] [PubMed]

45. Burdge, G.C.; Calder, P.C. Conversion of alpha-linolenic acid to longer-chain polyunsaturated fatty acids in human adults. *Reprod. Nutr. Dev.* **2005**, *45*, 581–597. [CrossRef] [PubMed]

46. Childs, C.; Kew, E.S.; Finnegan, Y.E.; Minihane, A.M.; Leigh-Firban, E.C.; Williams, C.M.; Calder, P.C. Increased dietary α-linolenic acid has sex-specific effects upon eicosapentaenoic acid status in humans: Re-examination of data from a randomized, placebo-controlled, parallel study. *Nutr. J.* **2014**, *13*, 113–117. [CrossRef] [PubMed]

47. Molto-Puigmarti, C.; Plat, J.; Mensink, R.P.; Muller, A.; Jansen, E.; Zeegers, M.P.; Thijs, C. FADS1 FADS2 gene variants modify the association between fishintake and the docosahexaenoic acid proportions in human milk. *Am. J. Clin. Nutr.* **2010**, *91*, 1368–1376. [CrossRef] [PubMed]

48. Xie, L.; Innis, S. Genetic variants of the FADS1 FADS2 gene cluster are associated with altered (*n*-6) and (*n*-3) essential fatty acids in plasma and erythrocyte phospholipids in women during pregnancy and in breast milk during lactation. *J. Nutr.* **2008**, *138*, 2222–2228. [CrossRef] [PubMed]

49. Caspi, A.; Williams, B.; Kim-Cohen, J.; Craig, I.W.; Milne, B.J.; Poulton, R.; Schalkwyk, L.C.; Taylor, A.; Werts, H.; Moffitt, T.E. Moderation of breastfeeding effects on the IQ by genetic variation in fatty acid metabolism. *Proc. Natl. Acad. Sci. USA* **2007**, *104*, 18860–18865. [CrossRef] [PubMed]

50.   Burdge, G.; Calder, P.C. Dietary α-linolenic acid and health-related outcomes: A metabolic perspective. *Nutr. Res. Rev.* **2006**, *19*, 26–52. [CrossRef] [PubMed]

51.   Arterburn, L.M.; Hall, E.B.; Oken, H. Distribution, interconversion, and dose response of *n*-3 fatty acids in humans. *Am. J. Clin. Nutr.* **2006**, *83*, S1467–1476S.

52.   Niculescu, M.D.; Lupu, D.S.; Craciunescu, C.N. Perinatal manipulation of α-linolenic acid intake induces epigenetic changes in maternal and offspring livers. *FASEB J.* **2013**, *27*, 350–358. [CrossRef] [PubMed]

53.   Koren, G. Polyunsaturated fatty acids and fetal brain development Unfulfilled promises. *Can. Fam. Phys.* **2015**, *61*, 41–42.

54.   Church, M.W.; Jen, K.-L.C.; Anumba, J.I.; Jackson, D.A.; Adams, B.R.; Hotra, J.W. Excess Omega-3 Fatty Acid Consumption by Mothers during Pregnancy and Lactation Caused Shorter Life Span and Abnormal ABRs in Old Adult Offspring. *Neurotoxicol. Teratol.* **2010**, *32*, 171–181. [CrossRef] [PubMed]

55.   Uauy, R.; Mena, P.; Wegher, B.; Nieto, S.; Salem, N. Long chain polyunsaturated fatty acid formation in neonates: Effect of gestational age and intrauterine growth. *Pediatr. Res.* **2000**, *47*, 127. [CrossRef] [PubMed]

56.   Rodriguez, A.; Sarda, P.; Nessmann, C.; Boulot, P.; Poisson, J.P.; Leger, C.L.; Descomps, B. Fatty acid desaturase activities and polyunsaturated fatty acid composition in human liver between the seventeenth and thirty-sixth gestational weeks. *Am. J. Obstet. Gynecol.* **1998**, *179*, 1063–1070. [CrossRef]

57.   Miles, E.A.; Calder, P.C. Omega-6 and omega-3 polyunsaturated fatty acids and allergic diseases in infancy and childhood. *Curr. Pharm. Des.* **2014**, *20*, 946–953. [CrossRef] [PubMed]

58.   Niculescu, M.D. Alpha-Linolenic Acid Alters Cell Cycle, Apoptosis, and DNA Methyltransferase Expression in Mouse Neural Stem Cells, but Not Global DNA Methylation. *J. Hum. Nutr. Food Sci.* **2014**, *2*, 1026.

59.   Hollander, K.S.; TempelBrami, C.; Konikoff, F.M.; Fainaru, M.; Leikin-Frenkel, A. Dietary enrichment with alpha-linolenic acid during pregnancy attenuates insulin resistance in adult offspring in mice. *Arch. Physiol. Biochem.* **2014**, *120*, 99–111. [CrossRef] [PubMed]

60.   Shomonov-Wagner, L.; Raz, A.; Leikin-Frenkel, A. Alpha linolenic acid in maternal diet halts the lipid disarray due to saturated fatty acids in the liver of mice offspring at weaning. *Lipids Health Dis.* **2015**, *14*, 14. [CrossRef] [PubMed]

61.   Leikin-Frenkel, A.; Shomonov-Wagner, L.; Juknat, A.; Pasmanik-Chor, M. Maternal Diet Enriched with alpha-Linolenic or Saturated Fatty Acids Differentially Regulates Gene Expression in the Liver of Mouse Offspring. *J. Nutrigenet. Nutrigenom.* **2015**, *8*, 185–194.

62.   Clarke, S.D. Polyunsaturated Fatty Acid Regulation of Gene Transcription: A Molecular Mechanism to Improve the Metabolic Syndrome. *J. Nutr.* **2001**, *131*, 1129–1132. [CrossRef]

63.   Deckelbaum, R.J.; Worgall, T.S.; Seo, T. *n*-3 Fatty acids and gene expression. *J. Clin. Nutr.* **2006**, *83* (Suppl. 6), 1520S–1525S.

64.   Ahmed, A.A.; Balogun, K.A.; Bykova, N.V.; Cheema, S.K. Novel regulatory roles of omega-3 fatty acids in metabolic pathways: A proteomics approach. *Nutr. Metab.* **2014**, *11*, 6. [CrossRef] [PubMed]

65.   Ong, T.P.; Ozanne, S.E. Developmental programming of type 2 diabetes: Early nutrition and epigenetic mechanisms. *Curr. Opin. Clin. Nutr. Metab. Care* **2015**, *18*, 354–360. [CrossRef] [PubMed]

66.   Waterland, R.A.; Rached, M.-T. Developmental establishment of epigenotype: A role for dietary fatty acids? *Scand. J. Food Nutr.* **2006**, *50* (Suppl. 2), 21–26. [CrossRef]

67.   Wang, J.; Wu, Z.; Li, D.; Li, N.; Dindot, S.V.; Satterfield, M.C.; Bazer, F.W.; Wu, G. Nutrition Epigenetics and Metabolic Syndrome. *Antioxid. Redox Signal.* **2012**, *17*, 282–301. [CrossRef] [PubMed]

68.   Vickers, M.H. Early Life Nutrition, Epigenetics and Programming of Later Life Disease. *Nutrients* **2004**, *6*, 2165–2178. [CrossRef] [PubMed]

69.   Burdge, G.C.; Lillycrop, K.A. Fatty acids and epigenetics. *Curr. Opin. Clin. Nutr. Metab. Care* **2014**, *17*, 156–161. [CrossRef] [PubMed]

10

Using *Caenorhabditis elegans* to Uncover Conserved Functions of Omega-3 and Omega-6 Fatty Acids

Jennifer L. Watts

School of Molecular Biosciences and Center for Reproductive Biology, College of Veterinary Medicine, Washington State University, Pullman, WA 99164, USA; jwatts@vetmed.wsu.edu

Academic Editors: Lindsay Brown, Bernhard Rauch and Hemant Poudyal

Abstract: The nematode *Caenorhabditis elegans* is a powerful model organism to study functions of polyunsaturated fatty acids. The ability to alter fatty acid composition with genetic manipulation and dietary supplementation permits the dissection of the roles of omega-3 and omega-6 fatty acids in many biological process including reproduction, aging and neurobiology. Studies in *C. elegans* to date have mostly identified overlapping functions of 20-carbon omega-6 and omega-3 fatty acids in reproduction and in neurons, however, specific roles for either omega-3 or omega-6 fatty acids are beginning to emerge. Recent findings with importance to human health include the identification of a conserved Cox-independent prostaglandin synthesis pathway, critical functions for cytochrome P450 derivatives of polyunsaturated fatty acids, the requirements for omega-6 and omega-3 fatty acids in sensory neurons, and the importance of fatty acid desaturation for long lifespan. Furthermore, the ability of *C. elegans* to interconvert omega-6 to omega-3 fatty acids using the FAT-1 omega-3 desaturase has been exploited in mammalian studies and biotechnology approaches to generate mammals capable of exogenous generation of omega-3 fatty acids.

Keywords: *C. elegans*; polyunsaturated fatty acids; fat-1; omega-3 desaturase

1. Introduction

The adage "you are what you eat" is especially true regarding fat. Specific types of fat in the human diet have important biological consequences on health and wellness. Long chain polyunsaturated fatty acids (PUFAs) are dietary requirements for humans and other mammals. Essential fatty acids can be classified as omega-6, or omega-3, depending on the position of the terminal double bond relative to the methyl end of the fatty acids. For example, the omega-6 fatty acid linoleic acid (LA, 18:2) is an 18-carbon fatty acid with double bonds at carbons 9 and 12, while the omega-3 fatty acid alpha-linolenic acid (ALA, 18:3) is an 18-carbon fatty acid with double bonds at carbons 9, 12, and 15. The essential fatty acids can be elongated and further desaturated to generate a range of 20- and 22-carbon omega-6 and omega-3 fatty acids [1]. Omega-6 fatty acids are prevalent in vegetable oils, especially corn, safflower, and soybean oil, while omega-3 fatty acids are found in fishes such as salmon and tuna. Because humans cannot interconvert omega-6 and omega-3 fatty acids, the ratio of omega-6 to omega-3 fatty acids is determined by dietary intake [2]. This is important because, in spite of their structural similarity, the biological functions of omega-6 and omega-3 fatty acids can be quite divergent [3].

Long chain fatty acids from the omega-3 and omega-6 families play crucial roles in membrane structure and function [4]. For example, the *cis* double bonds influence lipid packing, membrane fluidity [5], and membrane protein activity [6]. Omega-3 and omega-6 fatty acids are precursors for potent signaling molecules, and signals produced from omega-3 *versus* omega-6 PUFAs can sometimes have opposing effects [3]. Upon stimulation, long chain omega-6 and omega-3 fatty acids are cleaved from membrane lipids by phospholipases and oxygenated by cyclooxygenase, lipoxygenase, or cytochrome P450 enzymes to form a wide range of prostaglandins, leukotrienes, lipoxins, as well as hydroxy-, epoxy-, and hydroperoxy-derivatives [7,8]. These molecules, collectively termed "eicosanoids" act as powerful short range hormones affecting inflammation, immune responses, and reproductive processes [9].

PUFAs are important components of endocannabinoids, which are ethanolamide derivatives of phospholipids that bind to endocannabinoid receptors to regulate memory, appetite, mood, and pain sensation [10,11]. Finally, both omega-3 and omega-6 PUFAs and their eicosanoid derivatives are ligands for transcription factors, and therefore they influence gene expression. In addition to known receptors for eicosanoid and ethanolamide derivatives, an omega-3 fatty acid receptor, GPR120, has recently been identified [12,13]. Substantial evidence exists for opposing functions of omega-3 and omega-6 fatty acids in the regulation of inflammation, primarily that eicosanoids derived from most omega-6 fatty acids have pro-inflammatory effects, while those derived from omega-3 fatty acids do not (reviewed in [3]). However, opposing functions for omega-3 and omega-6 fatty acids in non-inflammatory processes are not well defined.

2. Why Study Fatty Acid Functions Using *C. elegans*?

An attractive animal model for studies of fatty acid function is the roundworm *C. elegans*. This popular model organism is easy and inexpensive to maintain in the lab, and its well-understood developmental programs, simple anatomy, short lifespan, well-annotated genome, and ease of genetic analysis allow for studies of diverse biological processes, including those related to human nutrition and disease [14]. In the lab, the nematodes grow on petri plates on lawns of *Escherichia coli* bacteria, which provide dietary nutrients, including proteins, carbohydrates, and saturated and mono-unsaturated fatty acids derived from digestion of bacterial membranes [15].

However, *C. elegans* are capable of synthesizing all necessary fatty acids *de novo*, and the core enzymes of fatty acid biosynthesis are conserved, including acetyl CoA carboxylase, fatty acid synthase, and a range of fatty acid desaturase and elongase activities, enabling *C. elegans* to synthesize long chain PUFAs including arachidonic acid (AA, 20:4) and eicosapentaenoic acid (EPA, 20:5) [16] (Figure 1A). Unlike most other animal species, the *C. elegans* genome encodes an omega-3 desaturase enzyme that can convert 18-carbon and 20-carbon omega-6 fatty acids into omega-3 fatty acids [17], along with a Δ12 desaturase, which catalyzes the formation of LA from oleic acid (OA, 18:1) [18]. Thus, *C. elegans* does not have any dietary fatty acid requirements. Like most other animals, *C. elegans* also possesses Δ6 and Δ5 desaturase enzymes, which act, in conjunction with fatty acid elongases, on similar substrates used by mammals and other animals to form 20-carbon PUFAs [19]. However, *C. elegans* lacks the specific elongase activity to produce 22-carbon PUFAs. Strains containing mutations in genes of the fatty acid desaturation pathway facilitate functional studies of PUFAs, because fatty acid composition can be manipulated both genetically and through the diet [20–22].

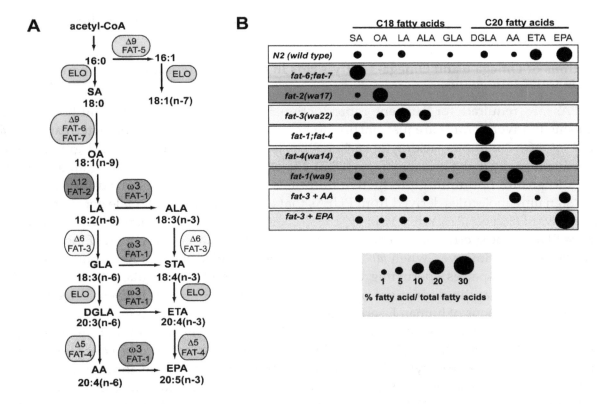

Figure 1. (A) Biosynthesis of omega-6 and omega-3 fatty acids in *C. elegans*. Unlike most other animals, *C. elegans* possesses Δ12 desaturase and ω3 desaturase enzymes, and therefore does not require essential dietary fatty acids to synthesize a range of omega-6 and omega-3 fatty acids; **(B)** Mutant strains lacking functional desaturase enzymes are depleted in specific polyunsaturated fatty acids. The area of each circle represents the ratio of specific fatty acids relative to total fatty acid content. Data shown are representative examples of multiple GC/MS measurements. Abbreviations: ELO, elongase; SA, stearic acid; OA, oleic acid; LA, linoleic acid; ALA, alpha-linolenic acid; GLA, gamma-linolenic acid; STA, stearidonic acid; DGLA, dihommo gamma-linolenic acid; ETA, eicosatrienoic acid; AA, arachidonic acid; EPA, eicosapentaenoic acid. Figure is modified from [23].

3. *C. elegans* Mutants Lacking Fatty Acid Desaturase Activity Are Useful for Studies of Conserved Functions of Omega-6 and Omega-3 Fatty Acids

The *C. elegans* genome contains single genes encoding the Δ12, Δ5, Δ6, and omega-3 desaturase enzymes necessary for the biosynthesis of a range of omega-6 and omega-3 PUFAs. There are three genes encoding the Δ9 desaturases, which convert saturated fatty acids into monounsaturated fatty acids (MUFAs). One Δ9 desaturase, FAT-5, uses palmitic acid (16:0) as a substrate to produce palmitoleic acid (16:1), while the other two Δ9 desaturases, FAT-6 and FAT-7 use both 16:0 and stearic acid (18:0) as substrates to produce (16:1) and oleic acid (18:1) [24]. Mutant strains lacking functional desaturase enzymes have been isolated and used for many studies of functions of specific fatty acids in reproduction, longevity and neurobiology. Because roundworms do not have blood vessels, nor do they express inflammatory markers such as TNFα and NFκβ, the roles of omega-6 and omega-3 PUFAs can be studied independently of their inflammatory functions. As might be expected, strains carrying mutations in the desaturase genes acting early in the pathway, such as Δ9 desaturases (*fat-6;fat-7* double mutants), Δ12 desaturase (*fat-2* mutants), and Δ6 desaturase (*fat-3* mutants) have more severe lipid composition changes, as well as more severe phenotypic consequences, such as growth, movement, and reproductive defects, than strains carrying mutations in desaturases acting later in the pathway, such as the Δ5 desaturase [20,21,25] (Figure 1B). *C. elegans* has been a powerful model for unraveling mechanisms of development, neurobiology, and longevity, and the studies reviewed below demonstrate how fatty acid function is involved in these fundamental biological processes.

4. Functions of Omega-6 and Omega-3 Fatty Acids in *C. elegans* Reproduction: Sperm Guidance and Germ Cell Maintenance

PUFAs are required for efficient reproduction in many animal species, although specific mechanisms in invertebrates are just starting to be elucidated [26]. Initial characterization of *fat-2*, *fat-3* and *fat-6;fat-7* mutants lacking 20-carbon PUFAs revealed slow growth and greatly reduced reproductive capacity in the mutant strains [20,21,25]. It is likely that PUFAs are required for multiple processes to ensure optimum reproductive output. One process characterized by the Miller lab involves signaling molecules derived from PUFAs that are required in the female germ line for sperm guidance toward oocytes [27]. When wild-type males were mated to *fat-2* mutants, which are unable to synthesize PUFAs, the sperm failed to migrate toward the spermatheca, the region of the uterus where fertilization occurs. However, when *fat-2* mutants were provided dietary 20-carbon PUFAs, either omega-3 or omega-6 species, sperm migration greatly improved [27]. It is likely that the signaling is mediated by prostaglandin derivatives of omega-3 and omega-6 PUFAs, because directly injecting nanomolar concentrations of human F-series prostaglandins promoted sperm movement [28]. A range of F-series prostaglandins are synthesized in the *C. elegans* germ line, including those derived from both omega-3 and omega-6 PUFAs [29]. Interestingly, *C. elegans* does not encode a clear homolog of the mammalian cyclooxygenase enzyme that is the rate-limiting step of prostaglandin synthesis. Instead, metabolite analysis revealed an alternative prostaglandin synthesis pathway that does not involve prostaglandin-D or -E intermediates [29,30]. The Miller lab took full advantage of whole-organism genetic approaches to discover that the synthesis of F-series prostaglandins is regulated by both insulin signaling in the intestine and TGF-β signaling in sensory neurons in order to finely control reproductive output [28,31]. Both of these signaling pathways respond to food availability, thus, during food scarcity, prostaglandin biosynthesis is reduced, leading to reduced efficiency of sperm locating the fertilization site, ultimately resulting in a lower fertilization rate. Interestingly, the alternative Cox-independent prostaglandin pathway may be conserved in mammals, because F-class prostaglandins have been detected in Cox double knockout mice [31].

While 20-carbon omega-6 and omega-3 PUFAs are redundant in their ability to promote proper sperm migration to oocytes, a role for divergent activities of omega-6 and omega-3 PUFAs in reproduction is suggested by dietary studies. Watts and Browse discovered that dietary supplementation of the omega-6 PUFA dihomogamma linolenic acid (DGLA, 20:3*n*-6) resulted in sterility due to the destruction of germ cells [32]. Supplementation of arachidonic acid (AA, 20:4*n*-6) also led to germ cell death, although at a much higher concentration than DGLA. On the contrary, supplementation with omega-3 fatty acids, such as eicosapentaenoic acid (EPA, 20:5*n*-3) had no adverse effects on the nematodes [32]. Genetic analyses revealed a large number of gene mutations that altered the sensitivity to DGLA. For example, the *fat-1* mutant strain, which cannot convert omega-6 fatty acids to omega-3 fatty acids, was more sensitive to dietary DGLA than wild type [32]. On the other hand, stress resistant strains, such as the insulin-like growth factor receptor *daf-2* mutants, did not become sterile when exposed to DGLA [33]. The *daf-2* mutants showed increased transcription of genes involved in detoxification and stress resistance, suggesting that the negative effects of DGLA may be due to a toxic product derived from DGLA [33,34]. A recent study from the Watts lab showed that the negative effects of DGLA in the *C. elegans* germ line are likely due to the production of specific epoxide derivatives of DGLA, the synthesis of which depend on the cytochrome P450 (CYP) enzyme CYP-33E2 [35]. Direct injection of specific epoxides derived from DGLA, but not those derived from EPA, triggered germ cell abnormalities resembling cell fusion or failed cytokinesis, which ultimately lead to apoptosis and germ cell death. Interestingly, even though knockdown of CYP-33E2 in *C. elegans* led to reduced germ cell death and higher reproductive outputs during DGLA feeding, the CYP-33E2 knock-down worms had a lower brood size when fed a normal diet [35]. This suggests that CYP-33E2 may be producing beneficial epoxides from other PUFAs, such as EPA, that could be required for optimal reproduction.

5. Functions of Omega-6 and Omega-3 Fatty Acids in Longevity: Critical Roles for Δ9 Desaturases

Because of its small size, short lifespan, and ease of genetic manipulation, *C. elegans* has been a premier organism for discoveries of genetic and physiological mechanisms regulating aging and longevity [36,37]. Recent lipidomics and genetic studies suggest roles for specific fatty acids in promoting longevity in *C. elegans* [38]. PUFAs contain more double bonds than saturated or MUFAs, therefore they are more likely to undergo peroxidation, which in turn leads to propagation of reactive oxygen species (ROS), which cause further damage to proteins and nucleic acids. In many organisms the degree of membrane unsaturation negatively correlates with lifespan [39]. This concept is supported by a *C. elegans* study showing a correlation between long-lived mutants in the insulin signaling pathway and changes in unsaturated fatty acid composition [40]. The mutants examined had increased (MUFAs) with decreased PUFAs. Additionally, high concentrations of dietary fish oil was shown to lead to higher levels of lipid peroxidation products and shorter lifespan [40,41]. In contrast, another study showed that supplementation of omega-6 PUFAs activates autophagy and promotes long lifespan [42]. Furthermore, several long-lived mutant strains express higher levels of Δ9 desaturases than wild type [34]. The Δ9 desaturases synthesize MUFAs in mammals, but are the first step in the synthesis of PUFAs in *C. elegans*. Thus, the roles of PUFAs in aging are still not clear.

Importantly, the oxidative damage theory of aging, which states that the accumulation of molecular damage due to ROS is a key contributor to aging, is currently undergoing a paradigm shift based on experiments in *C. elegans* [43]. Studies in which worms were grown under oxygen levels ranging from 2%–40% did not show significant changes in lifespan [44]. In addition, growth of m in the presence of antioxidants did not always increase lifespan [43], and specific mutations in antioxidant genes did not always lead to reduced lifespan [43,45,46]. Furthermore, treatment with low levels of chemicals that induce ROS actually produced increased resistance to oxidative stress and increased lifespan through the process of stress-induced hormesis [47,48]. Thus, while it is clear that high levels of ROS cause cellular damage, regulated ROS release and fluctuations in ROS are important for inducing both signaling and protection pathways [49–52]. This might explain why lower concentrations of dietary fish oil led to slightly longer lifespans [41]. It is also crucial to consider that membranes undergo constant remodeling and turnover. A recent study demonstrated that PUFAs in *C. elegans* membranes turn over very rapidly, such that the majority of PUFAs and other membrane lipids are replaced each day, suggesting that oxidized fatty acids are rapidly removed [53]. Knock-down of Δ9 desaturase activity reduces membrane turn-over, which might lead to increased lipid peroxidation in spite of lower PUFA production [53]. It appears that the beneficial functions of omega-6 and omage-3 PUFAs might outweigh the potential for oxidative damage conferred by the high degree of unsaturation.

In animals, dietary resources must be allocated between reproduction and somatic maintenance, thus reproduction and life span are metabolically linked. In *C. elegans*, removal of the germ line results in worms with increased fat stores and longer lifespan (reviewed in [54,55]). Several recent studies implicate fatty acid metabolism in long lifespan in germ-line ablated animals. Two nuclear hormone receptor homologs, NHR-80 and NHR-49, regulate the expression of Δ9 desaturases [56,57], and these two nuclear receptor proteins, as well as the FAT-6 and FAT-7 Δ9 desaturases are required for long lifespan in animals lacking a germ line [58,59]. Additionally, the lysosomal lipase LIPL-4 and intact autophagy pathways are required for extended longevity in germ-line less nematodes [60,61]. A recent metabolomic analysis revealed that a specific lipid species, oleoylethanolamide, accumulates in worms over-expressing the lipase LIPL-4. This ethanolamide derivative of oleic acid then directly binds to the lysosomal lipid chaperone LPB-8, which is then translocated to the nucleus. Oleoylethanolamide also binds to and activates the nuclear receptor NHR-80, activating transcription of Δ9 desaturases and promoting longevity [62]. Thus, lipid signaling from the lysosome to the nucleus has long lasting physiological effects, including lifespan extension.

In humans, diets high in sugars lead to excess lipid storage and ultimately cause adverse health effects, including obesity, diabetes, and cardiovascular coronary heart disease [63,64]. In *C. elegans*, dietary glucose causes shortened lifespan [65,66]. Two transcriptional regulators of Δ9 desaturases, MDT-15 and SBP-1 were recently shown to protect *C. elegans* from glucose-induced accelerated aging by preventing the accumulation of saturated fat [67]. Glucose feeding increases the saturated fatty acid composition of *C. elegans*, and MDT-15 and SBP-1 activate Δ9 and other fatty acid desaturases to prevent saturated fatty acid-induced lipotoxicity by converting saturated fatty acids into MUFAs and PUFAs [67–70].

A key transcription factor required for increased longevity in germ-line ablated worms is SKN-1/Nrf. This transcription factor is most studied for its roles in stress responses, especially to oxidative stress [71]. Interestingly, SKN-1 also regulates the transcription of lipid metabolism genes that are up-regulated in germ-line deficient animals, including fatty acid desaturases [71]. When SKN-1 is over-expressed, lipids are depleted from somatic, but not germ-line tissues [72]. This phenotype is similar to that seen in wild type worms upon nutrient depletion or exposure to pro-oxidants, and is also seen in *fat-6;fat-7* double mutants lacking 20-carbon PUFAs, as well as in *fat-1;fat-4* double mutants, which accumulate DGLA, but cannot synthesize EPA or AA. Supplementation with OA, AA, and EPA, but not other fatty acids, suppressed the somatic depletion of lipids, suggesting that specific fatty acid species may be involved in the allocation of germline *versus* somatic lipids, thereby influencing both reproduction and longevity [72].

6. Functions of Omega-6 and Omega-3 Fatty Acids in *C. elegans* Neurons: Synaptic Vesicle Formation, Signal Transduction in Sensory Neurons, and Complex Behavioral Responses to Alcohol and Oxygen

Other than adipose tissue, human brain tissue contains the highest proportion of lipids, with brain phospholipids containing high levels of both omega-6 and omega-3 PUFAs. Diets deficient in omega-3 and other PUFAs lead to defective neural function (reviewed in [73,74]). *C. elegans* has a simplified nervous system consisting of 302 neurons, and the network of neurons and their connections has been thoroughly mapped [75]. The *fat-3* mutant strain, which lacks 20-carbon omega-6 and omega-3 PUFAs, shows uncoordinated movement and defective egg laying behavior, phenotypes which are controlled by motor neurons and hermaphrodite-specific serotonergic vulva neurons [21,76]. Lesa *et al.* showed that *fat-3* mutants display defects in neurotransmitter release, and that synaptic vesicles were depleted in neuronal termini at the neuromuscular junction, indicating that 20-carbon PUFAs are required for synaptic vesicle formation and accumulation [76].

Sensory neurons are also affected in *fat-3* and *fat-1;fat-4* double mutants, which exhibit defects in olfactory chemotaxis behavior to volatile odorants sensed by AWC neurons, but less or no defective chemotaxis behavior to odorants sensed by AWA neurons [23]. This genetic evidence implicates PUFAs in specific neuronal signal transduction pathways. The AWA neurons possess TRPV type channels to respond to stimulatory signals, whereas the AWC neurons, which are not affected by PUFA deficiency, use cyclic nucleotide gated channels. Similarly, the ASH sensory neurons use TRPV channels to respond to noxious stimuli, and stimulate rapid escape behavior to heavy metals, high osmolarity, and nose touch. The *fat-3* and *fat-1;fat-4* double mutants showed behavioral defects upon exposure to these stimuli, and were rescued by dietary supplementation of both omega-6 and omega-3 fatty acids, indicating that PUFAs are also necessary for function in ASH neurons [23]. Direct calcium imaging of ASH neuronal response in *fat-3* mutants showed diminished calcium responses, while exogenous EPA elicited calcium responses and avoidance responses in *fat-3* mutants, bypassing the PUFA biosynthesis defects, and providing evidence for 20-carbon omega-6 and omega-3 PUFAs as regulators of *in vivo* TRPV channel activity [23].

Olfactory adaptation is the process where sensory neurons reduce their response to prolonged stimulation. Even though sensory response to volatile odorants sensed by AWC neurons was nearly normal in PUFA-deficient mutants, adaptation to volatile odorants mediated by AWC neurons was abnormal in *fat-3* and *fat-1;fat-4* mutant strains, and this defect was rescued by dietary PUFAs [77]. Similar to the findings described above for AWA neurons, this study linked the roles of PUFAs in olfactory adaptation in AWC neurons to TRPV channels, which in AWC neurons function downstream of the nuclear accumulation of the cGMP-dependent protein kinase EGL-4 [77].

In the research described above, omega-6 and omega-3 fatty acids play redundant roles in their ability to rescue the neuronal defects, indicating that both omega-6 and omega-3 fatty acids perform the required cellular functions. Several recent studies suggest specific roles for omega-6 and omega-3 fatty acids in neuronal processes. A *C. elegans* mutant in fatty acid amide hydrolase activity (*faah-1*) is defective in the regeneration of axons after laser surgery [78]. Fatty acid amide hydrolase breaks down endocannabinoids, such as arachidonyl ethanolamide (AEA). In *C. elegans*, AEA appears to inhibit axon regeneration via the Goα subunit GOA-1 [78]. Surprisingly, eicosapentaenoyl ethanolamide (EPEA), derived from EPA, shows less inhibitory activity, even though EPEA is much more abundant in *C. elegans* tissues than AEA [79]. On the other hand, omega-3 fatty acids are specifically required for the process of alcohol tolerance [80], a neuroadaptive process that compensates for the effects of alcohol in humans and in *C. elegans* [81]. This study showed that unlike wild type nematodes, *fat-3*, *fat-4*, and *fat-1* mutants did not recover movement after exposure to ethanol. EPA, but not AA supplementation was necessary and sufficient for the neuroplasticity required to compensate for the effects of alcohol intoxication in *C. elegans* [80]. Finally, AA in phospholipids, but not EPA, is required for neurons responding to light touch [82]. The Goodman lab found that *fat-3* and *fat-4* mutants, neither of which can synthesize AA, showed reduced response to touch. AA, but not EPA, rescued touch sensitivity in *fat-3* and *fat-4* mutants. Interestingly, eicosatetraynoic acid (EYTA), a non-metabolizable structural analog of AA, also rescued the touch response phenotype. The ability of EYTA to rescue touch response indicates that AA is not required to be oxidized into an eicosanoid for its activity. In addition to mutant and dietary supplementation analysis, the researchers used dynamic force spectroscopy to reveal that AA in phospholipids modulates biophysical properties of touch receptor neuron membranes to allow for optimal function [82]. Taken together, these recent studies reveal that omega-6 and omega-3 PUFAs can have distinct roles in neurological processes.

In addition to the alternative prostaglandin synthesis pathway described above, recent studies demonstrate that in *C. elegans*, omega-3 and omega-6 fatty acids are modified into eicosanoid-like molecules by the actions of CYP enzymes, and that these CYP-derived eicosanoids have important biological functions. Studies from Menzel's group revealed that CYP-33E2, which is most closely related to human CYP2J2, prefers EPA over AA as a substrate, and produces epoxyeicosatetraenoic acid (17,18-EEQ) as its main product [83]. CYP-29A3 is most closely related to human CYP4, and it uses AA to produce the hydroxyl derivative 20-HETE [84]. These eicosanoids have opposing effects on pharyngeal pumping and food uptake, with 17,18-EEQ mimicking the effects of the neurohormone serotonin on fasted worms, where both the eicosanoid and serotonin stimulate pharyngeal pumping. In contrast, 20-HETE and octopamine reduced pharyngeal pumping and food intact in well-fed worms [85]. Furthermore, 17,18-EEQ synthesis is increased upon serotonin supplementation, while 20-HETE synthesis increases upon application of octopamine [85], implicating eicosanoids as mediators of neurohormones affecting food intake. Another CYP enzyme, CYP-13A12, acts on PUFAs to respond oxygen levels [86]. In humans, reoxygenzation after oxygen deprivation causes tissue damage due to inflammation [87]. The *C. elegans* study showed that CYP-13A12 responds to the oxygen-dependent enzyme EGL-9 and hypoxia-inducible factor (HIF-1) to facilitate a movement response to reoxygenation after oxygen deprivation [86]. CYP-13A12 generates epoxy and hydroxyl eicosanoids from AA and EPA, including 14,15-epoxyeicosatrienoic acid (14,15-EET) from AA and 17,18-EEQ from EPA [88]. This research implicates conserved roles for omega-6 and omega-3 PUFAs and eicosanoid formation in ischemia and reperfusion.

7. Using the *C. elegans Fat-1* Gene for Studies in Mammals: Endogenous Omega-3 Functions and Biotechnology Applications

The discovery of the first animal omega-3 desaturase, the *C. elegans* FAT-1 desaturase [17], enabled Kang to construct the *fat-1* transgenic mouse, which expresses the *C. elegans* omega-3 desaturase and permits the conversion endogenous omega-6 to omega-3 fatty acids in mammalian tissues [89]. Lipidomic analysis revealed hundreds of specific lipid species that are altered between wild type and the *fat-1* mouse, including EPA and DHA-containing phospholipids and cholesterol esters, as well as many species of EPA-derived epoxides and diols formed via CYP enzymes [90]. Studies using the *fat-1* mouse model now appear in numerous publications in which researchers examined the effects of endogenously synthesized, as opposed to dietary, omega-3 fatty acids on a range of processes in a mammalian model. This research provides evidence that increased production of omega-3 PUFAs, coupled with a reduction in omega-6 PUFAs, protects mammals from a range of diseases, including cancer, diabetes and inflammatory diseases (reviewed in [91–95]). Recent studies reveal new insights into molecular mechanisms in which omega-3 PUFAs protect against various disease outcomes as diverse as diabetic neuropathy [96], fatty liver disease [97], pancreatic beta cell death [98], and vascular inflammation [99]. Thus, the *fat-1* mouse model promises to be central to unraveling the mechanisms of omega-3 and omega-6 fatty acids in health and disease.

The success of expressing the *C. elegans fat-1* omega-3 desaturase gene in mice led the way for expression of *fat-1* in other mammals. Because modern diets are thought to be deficient in omega-3 fatty acids, increasing omega-3 fatty acids in human food is desirable [100]. Concerns regarding heavy metal contamination of marine fish [101], as well as depletion of ocean fish stocks due to overfishing, lead to a desire for alternative sources of omega-3 fatty acids in human diets. The creation of transgenic farm animals, such as pigs [102–104] and cattle [105,106], set the stage for using nematode *fat-1* genes to someday provide milk and meat with higher omega-3 content to human consumers. However, more studies are needed to ensure the safety of food produced from transgenic animals. In addition, altering the omega-3/omega-6 ratio in farm animals might have adverse effects on their reproduction, as lower brood size was observed in mice expressing *fat-1* in their mammary glands [107].

8. Conclusions and Future Studies

Discoveries made using model organisms have had significant impact on human medicine. For example, *C. elegans* research has been crucial for the elucidation of genetic pathways underlying programmed cell death, longevity, and signal transduction pathways that occur during development as well as during carcinogenesis (reviewed in [14]). This research has led to the discovery of drug targets and novel therapeutics in humans. Studies in *C. elegans* regarding non-inflammatory functions of PUFAs clearly demonstrate that 20-carbon PUFAs play key roles in reproduction and in the nervous system. While it appears that many functions of 20-carbon omega-6 and omega-3 fatty acids are redundant, examples of specific functions for DGLA, AA and EPA are beginning to emerge [35,42,80,82,85]. Genetic analysis and simple physiology render the *C. elegans* model especially useful for studies of PUFA functions in reproduction, development, and longevity, because vertebrate models are much more difficult, time consuming, and expensive to manipulate. Roles of PUFAs in longevity are just starting to be examined, and several studies suggest that Δ9 desaturase is a pro-longevity factor. Future studies are needed to determine if PUFA activity depends on being metabolized into eicosanoids or other signaling molecules, or whether their functions are derived from membrane biophysical properties or direct interactions with membrane proteins. Similarly, the identification of *C. elegans* receptors for PUFAs and eicosanoids, as well as the identification of specific signal transduction pathways that are affected by PUFA composition, will allow for more mechanistic studies. It is likely that mammalian studies using the *fat-1* transgenic mouse will continue to be fruitful because the transgene can be crossed into numerous genetic models of disease, thereby examining the effects of endogenous omega-3 fatty acid production on many different disease outcomes. In summary,

C. elegans is a powerful model for the integration of dietary and genetic studies for PUFA function in reproduction, development, neuroscience and aging.

Acknowledgments: The author thanks Marshall Deline and Jason Watts for helpful comments on the manuscript. Research in the Watts lab is supported by the National Institute of Diabetes and Digestive and Kidney Diseases of the National Institutes of Health under award number R01DK074114.

References

1.   Wallis, J.G.; Watts, J.L.; Browse, J. Polyunsaturated fatty acid synthesis: What will they think of next? *Trends Biochem. Sci.* **2002**, *27*, 467. [CrossRef]

2.   Simopoulos, A.P. Genetic variants in the metabolism of omega-6 and omega-3 fatty acids: Their role in the determination of nutritional requirements and chronic disease risk. *Exp. Biol. Med.* **2010**, *235*, 785–795. [CrossRef] [PubMed]

3.   Schmitz, G.; Ecker, J. The opposing effects of *n*-3 and *n*-6 fatty acids. *Prog. Lipid Res.* **2008**, *47*, 147–155. [CrossRef] [PubMed]

4.   Antonny, B.; Vanni, S.; Shindou, H.; Ferreira, T. From zero to six double bonds: Phospholipid unsaturation and organelle function. *Trends Cell Biol.* **2015**, *25*, 427–436. [CrossRef] [PubMed]

5.   Bigay, J.; Antonny, B. Curvature, lipid packing, and electrostatics of membrane organelles: Defining cellular territories in determining specificity. *Dev. Cell* **2012**, *23*, 886–895. [CrossRef] [PubMed]

6.   Niu, S.L.; Mitchell, D.C.; Lim, S.Y.; Wen, Z.M.; Kim, H.Y.; Salem, N., Jr.; Litman, B.J. Reduced G protein-coupled signaling efficiency in retinal rod outer segments in response to *n*-3 fatty acid deficiency. *J. Biol. Chem.* **2004**, *279*, 31098–31104. [CrossRef] [PubMed]

7.   Funk, C.D. Prostaglandins and leukotrienes: Advances in eicosanoid biology. *Science* **2001**, *294*, 1871–1875. [CrossRef] [PubMed]

8.   Spector, A.A.; Kim, H.Y. Cytochrome p450 epoxygenase pathway of polyunsaturated fatty acid metabolism. *Biochim. Biophys. Acta* **2015**, *1851*, 356–365. [CrossRef] [PubMed]

9.   Nebert, D.W.; Wikvall, K.; Miller, W.L. Human cytochromes P450 in health and disease. *Philos. Trans. R. Soc. Lond. Ser. B Biol. Sci.* **2013**, *368*, 20120431. [CrossRef] [PubMed]

10. Xu, J.Y.; Chen, C. Endocannabinoids in synaptic plasticity and neuroprotection. *Neuroscientist* **2015**, *21*, 152–168. [CrossRef] [PubMed]

11. Maccarrone, M.; Bab, R.; Biro, T.; Cabral, G.A.; Dey, S.K.; di Marzo, V.; Konje, J.C.; Kunos, G.; Mechoulam, R.; Pacher, P.; *et al.* Endocannabinoid signaling at the periphery: 50 years after THC. *Trends Pharmacol. Sci.* **2015**, *36*, 277–296. [CrossRef] [PubMed]

12. Oh, D.Y.; Olefsky, J.M. Omega 3 fatty acids and GPR120. *Cell Metab.* **2012**, *15*, 564–565. [CrossRef] [PubMed]

13. Im, D.S. Functions of omega-3 fatty acids and FFA4 (GPR120) in macrophages. *Eur. J. Pharmacol.* **2015**. [CrossRef] [PubMed]

14. Corsi, A.K.; Wightman, B.; Chalfie, M. A transparent window into biology: A primer on *Caenorhabditis elegans*. *Genetics* **2015**, *200*, 387–407. [CrossRef] [PubMed]

15. Brooks, K.K.; Liang, B.; Watts, J.L. The influence of bacterial diet on fat storage in *C. elegans*. *PLoS ONE* **2009**, *4*, e7545. [CrossRef] [PubMed]

16. Watts, J.L. Fat synthesis and adiposity regulation in *Caenorhabditis elegans*. *Trends Endocrinol. Metab.* **2009**, *20*, 58–65. [CrossRef] [PubMed]

17. Spychalla, J.P.; Kinney, A.J.; Browse, J. Identification of an animal omega-3 fatty acid desaturase by heterologous expression in arabidopsis. *Proc. Natl. Acad. Sci. USA* **1997**, *94*, 1142–1147. [CrossRef] [PubMed]

18. Peyou-Ndi, M.M.; Watts, J.L.; Browse, J. Identification and characterization of an animal delta(12) fatty acid desaturase gene by heterologous expression in *Saccharomyces cerevisiae*. *Arch. Biochem. Biophys.* **2000**, *376*, 399–408. [CrossRef] [PubMed]

19. Watts, J.L.; Browse, J. Isolation and characterization of a delta 5-fatty acid desaturase from *Caenorhabditis elegans*. *Arch. Biochem. Biophys.* **1999**, *362*, 175–182. [CrossRef] [PubMed]

20. Watts, J.L.; Browse, J. Genetic dissection of polyunsaturated fatty acid synthesis in *Caenorhabditis elegans*. *Proc. Natl. Acad. Sci. USA* **2002**, *99*, 5854–5859. [CrossRef] [PubMed]

21. Watts, J.L.; Phillips, E.; Griffing, K.R.; Browse, J. Deficiencies in C20 polyunsaturated fatty acids cause behavioral and developmental defects in *Caenorhabditis elegans* fat-3 mutants. *Genetics* **2003**, *163*, 581–589. [PubMed]

22. Deline, M.L.; Vrablik, T.L.; Watts, J.L. Dietary supplementation of polyunsaturated fatty acids in *Caenorhabditis elegans. J. Vis. Exp.* **2013**. [CrossRef] [PubMed]

23. Kahn-Kirby, A.H.; Dantzker, J.L.; Apicella, A.J.; Schafer, W.R.; Browse, J.; Bargmann, C.I.; Watts, J.L. Specific polyunsaturated fatty acids drive TRPV-dependent sensory signaling *in vivo. Cell* **2004**, *119*, 889–900. [CrossRef] [PubMed]

24. Watts, J.L.; Browse, J. A palmitoyl-CoA-specific delta9 fatty acid desaturase from *Caenorhabditis elegans. Biochem. Biophys. Res. Commun.* **2000**, *272*, 263–269. [CrossRef] [PubMed]

25. Brock, T.J.; Browse, J.; Watts, J.L. Fatty acid desaturation and the regulation of adiposity in *Caenorhabditis elegans. Genetics* **2007**, *176*, 865–875. [CrossRef] [PubMed]

26. Vrablik, T.L.; Watts, J.L. Polyunsaturated fatty acid derived signaling in reproduction and development: Insights from *Caenorhabditis elegans* and *Drosophila melanogaster. Mol. Reprod. Dev.* **2013**, *80*, 244–259. [CrossRef] [PubMed]

27. Kubagawa, H.M.; Watts, J.L.; Corrigan, C.; Edmonds, J.W.; Sztul, E.; Browse, J.; Miller, M.A. Oocyte signals derived from polyunsaturated fatty acids control sperm recruitment *in vivo. Nat. Cell Biol.* **2006**, *8*, 1143–1148. [CrossRef] [PubMed]

28. Edmonds, J.W.; Prasain, J.K.; Dorand, D.; Yang, Y.; Hoang, H.D.; Vibbert, J.; Kubagawa, H.M.; Miller, M.A. Insulin/FOXO signaling regulates ovarian prostaglandins critical for reproduction. *Dev. Cell* **2010**, *19*, 858–871. [CrossRef] [PubMed]

29. Hoang, H.D.; Prasain, J.K.; Dorand, D.; Miller, M.A. A heterogeneous mixture of F-series prostaglandins promotes sperm guidance in the *Caenorhabditis elegans* reproductive tract. *PLoS Genet.* **2013**, *9*, e1003271. [CrossRef] [PubMed]

30. Prasain, J.K.; Wilson, L.; Hoang, H.D.; Moore, R.; Miller, M.A. Comparative lipidomics of *Caenorhabditis elegans* metabolic disease models by swath non-targeted tandem mass spectrometry. *Metabolites* **2015**, *5*, 677–696. [CrossRef] [PubMed]

31. McKnight, K.; Hoang, H.D.; Prasain, J.K.; Brown, N.; Vibbert, J.; Hollister, K.A.; Moore, R.; Ragains, J.R.; Reese, J.; Miller, M.A. Neurosensory perception of environmental cues modulates sperm motility critical for fertilization. *Science* **2014**, *344*, 754–757. [CrossRef] [PubMed]

32. Watts, J.L.; Browse, J. Dietary manipulation implicates lipid signaling in the regulation of germ cell maintenance in *C. elegans. Dev. Biol.* **2006**, *292*, 381–392. [CrossRef] [PubMed]

33. Webster, C.M.; Deline, M.L.; Watts, J.L. Stress response pathways protect germ cells from omega-6 polyunsaturated fatty acid-mediated toxicity in *Caenorhabditis elegans. Dev. Biol.* **2013**, *373*, 14–25. [CrossRef] [PubMed]

34. Murphy, C.T.; McCarroll, S.A.; Bargmann, C.I.; Fraser, A.; Kamath, R.S.; Ahringer, J.; Li, H.; Kenyon, C. Genes that act downstream of DAF-16 to influence the lifespan of *Caenorhabditis elegans. Nature* **2003**, *424*, 277–283. [CrossRef] [PubMed]

35. Deline, M.; Keller, J.; Rothe, M.; Schunck, W.H.; Menzel, R.; Watts, J.L. Epoxides derived from dietary dihomo-gamma-linolenic acid induce germ cell death in *C. elegans. Sci. Rep.* **2015**, *5*, 15417. [CrossRef] [PubMed]

36. Amrit, F.R.; Ratnappan, R.; Keith, S.A.; Ghazi, A. The *C. elegans* lifespan assay toolkit. *Methods* **2014**, *68*, 465–475. [CrossRef] [PubMed]

37. Kenyon, C.J. The genetics of ageing. *Nature* **2010**, *464*, 504–512. [CrossRef] [PubMed]

38. Schroeder, E.A.; Brunet, A. Lipid profiles and signals for long life. *Trends Endocrinol. Metab.* **2015**, *26*, 589–592. [CrossRef] [PubMed]

39. Hulbert, A.J.; Kelly, M.A.; Abbott, S.K. Polyunsaturated fats, membrane lipids and animal longevity. *J. Comp. Physiol. B Biochem.Syst. Environ. Physiol.* **2014**, *184*, 149–166. [CrossRef] [PubMed]

40. Shmookler-Reis, R.J.; Xu, L.; Lee, H.; Chae, M.; Thaden, J.J.; Bharill, P.; Tazearslan, C.; Siegel, E.; Alla, R.; Zimniak, P.; *et al.* Modulation of lipid biosynthesis contributes to stress resistance and longevity of *C. elegans* mutants. *Aging* **2011**, *3*, 125–147. [PubMed]

41. Sugawara, S.; Honma, T.; Ito, J.; Kijima, R.; Tsuduki, T. Fish oil changes the lifespan of *Caenorhabditis elegans* via lipid peroxidation. *J. Clin. Biochem. Nutr.* **2013**, *52*, 139–145. [CrossRef] [PubMed]

42. O'Rourke, E.J.; Kuballa, P.; Xavier, R.; Ruvkun, G. Omega-6 polyunsaturated fatty acids extend life span through the activation of autophagy. *Genes Dev.* **2013**, *27*, 429–440. [CrossRef] [PubMed]

43. Gems, D.; Doonan, R. Antioxidant defense and aging in *C. elegans*: Is the oxidative damage theory of aging wrong? *Cell Cycle* **2009**, *8*, 1681–1687. [CrossRef] [PubMed]

44. Honda, S.; Ishii, N.; Suzuki, K.; Matsuo, M. Oxygen-dependent perturbation of life span and aging rate in the nematode. *J. Gerontol.* **1993**, *48*, B57–B61. [CrossRef] [PubMed]

45. Zhou, K.I.; Pincus, Z.; Slack, F.J. Longevity and stress in *Caenorhabditis elegans*. *Aging* **2011**, *3*, 733–753. [PubMed]

46. Van Raamsdonk, J.M.; Hekimi, S. Deletion of the mitochondrial superoxide dismutase SOD-2 extends lifespan in *Caenorhabditis elegans*. *PLoS Genet.* **2009**, *5*, e1000361. [CrossRef] [PubMed]

47. Cypser, J.R.; Johnson, T.E. Multiple stressors in *Caenorhabditis elegans* induce stress hormesis and extended longevity. *J. Gerontol. A Biol. Sci. Med. Sci.* **2002**, *57*, B109–B114. [CrossRef] [PubMed]

48. Cypser, J.R.; Tedesco, P.; Johnson, T.E. Hormesis and aging in *Caenorhabditis elegans*. *Exp. Gerontol.* **2006**, *41*, 935–939. [CrossRef] [PubMed]

49. Schaar, C.E.; Dues, D.J.; Spielbauer, K.K.; Machiela, E.; Cooper, J.F.; Senchuk, M.; Hekimi, S.; van Raamsdonk, J.M. Mitochondrial and cytoplasmic ROS have opposing effects on lifespan. *PLoS Genet.* **2015**, *11*, e1004972. [CrossRef] [PubMed]

50. Back, P.; Braeckman, B.P.; Matthijssens, F. ROS in aging *Caenorhabditis elegans*: Damage or signaling? *Oxid. Med. Cell. Longev.* **2012**, *2012*, 608478. [CrossRef] [PubMed]

51. Yee, C.; Yang, W.; Hekimi, S. The intrinsic apoptosis pathway mediates the pro-longevity response to mitochondrial ROS in *C. elegans*. *Cell* **2014**, *157*, 897–909. [CrossRef] [PubMed]

52. Shadel, G.S.; Horvath, T.L. Mitochondrial ros signaling in organismal homeostasis. *Cell* **2015**, *163*, 560–569. [CrossRef] [PubMed]

53. Dancy, B.C.; Chen, S.W.; Drechsler, R.; Gafken, P.R.; Olsen, C.P. 13C- and 15N-Labeling strategies combined with mass spectrometry comprehensively quantify phospholipid dynamics in *C. elegans*. *PLoS ONE* **2015**, *10*, e0141850. [CrossRef] [PubMed]

54. Kenyon, C. A pathway that links reproductive status to lifespan in *Caenorhabditis elegans*. *Ann. N. Y. Acad. Sci.* **2010**, *1204*, 156–162. [CrossRef] [PubMed]

55. Hansen, M.; Flatt, T.; Aguilaniu, H. Reproduction, fat metabolism, and life span: What is the connection? *Cell Metab.* **2013**, *17*, 10–19. [CrossRef] [PubMed]

56. Brock, T.J.; Browse, J.; Watts, J.L. Genetic regulation of unsaturated fatty acid composition in *C. elegans*. *PLoS Genet.* **2006**, *2*, e108. [CrossRef] [PubMed]

57. Van Gilst, M.R.; Hadjivassiliou, H.; Jolly, A.; Yamamoto, K.R. Nuclear hormone receptor NHR-49 controls fat consumption and fatty acid composition in *C. elegans*. *PLoS Biol.* **2005**, *3*, e53. [CrossRef] [PubMed]

58. Ratnappan, R.; Amrit, F.R.; Chen, S.W.; Gill, H.; Holden, K.; Ward, J.; Yamamoto, K.R.; Olsen, C.P.; Ghazi, A. Germline signals deploy NHR-49 to modulate fatty-acid beta-oxidation and desaturation in somatic tissues of *C. elegans*. *PLoS Genet.* **2014**, *10*, e1004829. [CrossRef] [PubMed]

59. Goudeau, J.; Bellemin, S.; Toselli-Mollereau, E.; Shamalnasab, M.; Chen, Y.; Aguilaniu, H. Fatty acid desaturation links germ cell loss to longevity through NHR-80/HNF4 in *C. elegans*. *PLoS Biol.* **2011**, *9*, e1000599. [CrossRef] [PubMed]

60. Lapierre, L.R.; Gelino, S.; Melendez, A.; Hansen, M. Autophagy and lipid metabolism coordinately modulate life span in germline-less *C. elegans*. *Curr. Biol.* **2011**, *21*, 1507–1514. [CrossRef] [PubMed]

61. Wang, M.C.; O'Rourke, E.J.; Ruvkun, G. Fat metabolism links germline stem cells and longevity in *C. elegans*. *Science* **2008**, *322*, 957–960. [CrossRef] [PubMed]

62. Folick, A.; Oakley, H.D.; Yu, Y.; Armstrong, E.H.; Kumari, M.; Sanor, L.; Moore, D.D.; Ortlund, E.A.; Zechner, R.; Wang, M.C. Aging. Lysosomal signaling molecules regulate longevity in *Caenorhabditis elegans*. *Science* **2015**, *347*, 83–86. [CrossRef] [PubMed]

63. DiNicolantonio, J.J.; Lucan, S.C.; O'Keefe, J.H. The evidence for saturated fat and for sugar related to coronary heart disease. *Prog. Cardiovasc. Dis.* **2015**. [CrossRef] [PubMed]

64. Kolderup, A.; Svihus, B. Fructose metabolism and relation to atherosclerosis, type 2 diabetes, and obesity. *J. Nutr. Metab.* **2015**, *2015*, 823081. [CrossRef] [PubMed]

65. Lee, S.J.; Murphy, C.T.; Kenyon, C. Glucose shortens the life span of *C. elegans* by downregulating DAF-16/FOXO activity and aquaporin gene expression. *Cell Metab.* **2009**, *10*, 379–391. [CrossRef] [PubMed]

66. Schulz, T.J.; Zarse, K.; Voigt, A.; Urban, N.; Birringer, M.; Ristow, M. Glucose restriction extends *Caenorhabditis elegans* life span by inducing mitochondrial respiration and increasing oxidative stress. *Cell Metab.* **2007**, *6*, 280–293. [CrossRef] [PubMed]

67. Lee, D.; Jeong, D.E.; Son, H.G.; Yamaoka, Y.; Kim, H.; Seo, K.; Khan, A.A.; Roh, T.Y.; Moon, D.W.; Lee, Y.; *et al.* SREBP and MDT-15 protect *C. elegans* from glucose-induced accelerated aging by preventing accumulation of saturated fat. *Genes Dev.* **2015**, *29*, 2490–2503. [CrossRef] [PubMed]

68. Taubert, S.; van Gilst, M.R.; Hansen, M.; Yamamoto, K.R. A mediator subunit, MDT-15, integrates regulation of fatty acid metabolism by NHR-49-dependent and -independent pathways in *C. elegans*. *Genes Dev.* **2006**, *20*, 1137–1149. [CrossRef] [PubMed]

69. Walker, A.K.; Jacobs, R.L.; Watts, J.L.; Rottiers, V.; Jiang, K.; Finnegan, D.M.; Shioda, T.; Hansen, M.; Yang, F.; Niebergall, L.J.; *et al.* A conserved SREBP-1/phosphatidylcholine feedback circuit regulates lipogenesis in metazoans. *Cell* **2011**, *147*, 840–852. [CrossRef] [PubMed]

70. Yang, F.; Vought, B.W.; Satterlee, J.S.; Walker, A.K.; Jim Sun, Z.Y.; Watts, J.L.; DeBeaumont, R.; Saito, R.M.; Hyberts, S.G.; Yang, S.; *et al.* An ARC/mediator subunit required for SREBPP control of cholesterol and lipid homeostasis. *Nature* **2006**, *442*, 700–704. [CrossRef] [PubMed]

71. Steinbaugh, M.J.; Narasimhan, S.D.; Robida-Stubbs, S.; Moronetti Mazzeo, L.E.; Dreyfuss, J.M.; Hourihan, J.M.; Raghavan, P.; Operana, T.N.; Esmaillie, R.; Blackwell, T.K. Lipid-mediated regulation of SKN-1/Nrf in response to germ cell absence. *eLife* **2015**, *4*. [CrossRef] [PubMed]

72. Lynn, D.A.; Dalton, H.M.; Sowa, J.N.; Wang, M.C.; Soukas, A.A.; Curran, S.P. Omega-3 and -6 fatty acids allocate somatic and germline lipids to ensure fitness during nutrient and oxidative stress in *Caenorhabditis elegans*. *Proc. Natl. Acad. Sci. USA* **2015**, *112*, 15378–15383. [CrossRef] [PubMed]

73. Bazinet, R.P.; Laye, S. Polyunsaturated fatty acids and their metabolites in brain function and disease. *Nat. Rev. Neurosci.* **2014**, *15*, 771–785. [CrossRef] [PubMed]

74. Sinclair, A.J.; Begg, D.; Mathai, M.; Weisinger, R.S. Omega 3 fatty acids and the brain: Review of studies in depression. *Asia Pac. J. Clin.Nutr.* **2007**, *16*, 391–397. [PubMed]

75. White, J.G.; Southgate, E.; Thomson, J.N.; Brenner, S. The structure of the nervous system of the nematode *Caenorhabditis elegans*. *Philos. Trans. R. Soc. Lond. Ser. B Biol. Sci.* **1986**, *314*, 1–340. [CrossRef]

76. Lesa, G.M.; Palfreyman, M.; Hall, D.H.; Clandinin, M.T.; Rudolph, C.; Jorgensen, E.M.; Schiavo, G. Long chain polyunsaturated fatty acids are required for efficient neurotransmission in *C. elegans*. *J. Cell Sci.* **2003**, *116*, 4965–4975. [CrossRef] [PubMed]

77. O'Halloran, D.M.; Altshuler-Keylin, S.; Lee, J.I.; L'Etoile, N.D. Regulators of AWC-mediated olfactory plasticity in *Caenorhabditis elegans*. *PLoS Genet.* **2009**, *5*, e1000761. [CrossRef] [PubMed]

78. Pastuhov, S.I.; Fujiki, K.; Nix, P.; Kanao, S.; Bastiani, M.; Matsumoto, K.; Hisamoto, N. Endocannabinoid-goalpha signalling inhibits axon regeneration in *Caenorhabditis elegans* by antagonizing gqalpha-PKC-JNK signalling. *Nat. Commun.* **2012**, *3*, 1136. [CrossRef] [PubMed]

79. Lucanic, M.; Held, J.M.; Vantipalli, M.C.; Klang, I.M.; Graham, J.B.; Gibson, B.W.; Lithgow, G.J.; Gill, M.S. *N*-Acylethanolamine signalling mediates the effect of diet on lifespan in *Caenorhabditis elegans*. *Nature* **2011**, *473*, 226–229. [CrossRef] [PubMed]

80. Raabe, R.C.; Mathies, L.D.; Davies, A.G.; Bettinger, J.C. The omega-3 fatty acid eicosapentaenoic acid is required for normal alcohol response behaviors in *C. elegans*. *PLoS ONE* **2014**, *9*. [CrossRef]

81. Davies, A.G.; Bettinger, J.C.; Thiele, T.R.; Judy, M.E.; McIntire, S.L. Natural variation in the NPR-1 gene modifies ethanol responses of wild strains of *C. elegans*. *Neuron* **2004**, *42*, 731–743. [CrossRef] [PubMed]

82. Vasquez, V.; Krieg, M.; Lockhead, D.; Goodman, M.B. Phospholipids that contain polyunsaturated fatty acids enhance neuronal cell mechanics and touch sensation. *Cell Rep.* **2014**, *6*, 70–80. [CrossRef] [PubMed]

83. Kosel, M.; Wild, W.; Bell, A.; Rothe, M.; Lindschau, C.; Steinberg, C.E.; Schunck, W.H.; Menzel, R. Eicosanoid formation by a cytochrome P450 isoform expressed in the pharynx of *Caenorhabditis elegans*. *Biochem. J.* **2011**, *435*, 689–700. [CrossRef] [PubMed]

84. Kulas, J.; Schmidt, C.; Rothe, M.; Schunck, W.H.; Menzel, R. Cytochrome P450-dependent metabolism of eicosapentaenoic acid in the nematode *Caenorhabditis elegans*. *Arch. Biochem. Biophys.* **2008**, *472*, 65–75. [CrossRef] [PubMed]

85. Zhou, Y.; Falck, J.R.; Rothe, M.; Schunck, W.H.; Menzel, R. Role of CYP eicosanoids in the regulation of pharyngeal pumping and food uptake in *Caenorhabditis elegans*. *J. Lipid Res.* **2015**, *56*, 2110–2123. [CrossRef] [PubMed]

86. Ma, D.K.; Rothe, M.; Zheng, S.; Bhatla, N.; Pender, C.L.; Menzel, R.; Horvitz, H.R. Cytochrome P450 drives a HIF-regulated behavioral response to reoxygenation by *C. elegans*. *Science* **2013**, *341*, 554–558. [CrossRef] [PubMed]

87. Eltzschig, H.K.; Eckle, T. Ischemia and reperfusion-from mechanism to translation. *Nat. Med.* **2011**, *17*, 1391–1401. [CrossRef] [PubMed]

88. Keller, J.; Ellieva, A.; Ma, D.K.; Ju, J.J.; Nehk, E.; Konkel, A.; Falck, J.R.; Schunck, W.H.; Menzel, R. CYP-13A12 of the nematode *Caenorhabditis elegans* is a PUFA-epoxygenase involved in behavioural response to reoxygenation. *Biochem. J.* **2014**, *464*, 61–71. [CrossRef] [PubMed]

89. Kang, J.X.; Wang, J.; Wu, L.; Kang, Z.B. Transgenic mice: Fat-1 mice convert *n*-6 to *n*-3 fatty acids. *Nature* **2004**, *427*, 504. [CrossRef] [PubMed]

90. Astarita, G.; Kendall, A.C.; Dennis, E.A.; Nicolaou, A. Targeted lipidomic strategies for oxygenated metabolites of polyunsaturated fatty acids. *Biochim. Biophys. Acta* **2015**, *1851*, 456–468. [CrossRef] [PubMed]

91. Kang, J.X. From fat to fat-1: A tale of omega-3 fatty acids. *J. Membr. Biol.* **2005**, *206*, 165–172. [CrossRef] [PubMed]

92. Kang, J.X. Fat-1 transgenic mice: A new model for omega-3 research. *Prostaglandins Leukot Essent Fat. Acids* **2007**, *77*, 263–267. [CrossRef] [PubMed]

93. Kang, J.X. The omega-6/omega-3 fatty acid ratio in chronic diseases: Animal models and molecular aspects. *World Rev. Nutr. Diet.* **2011**, *102*, 22–29. [PubMed]

94. Kang, J.X.; Liu, A. The role of the tissue omega-6/omega-3 fatty acid ratio in regulating tumor angiogenesis. *Cancer Metastasis Rev.* **2013**, *32*, 201–210. [CrossRef] [PubMed]

95. Kang, J.X.; Weylandt, K.H. Modulation of inflammatory cytokines by omega-3 fatty acids. *Sub-Cell. Biochem.* **2008**, *49*, 133–143.

96. Bak, D.H.; Zhang, E.; Yi, M.H.; Kim, D.K.; Lim, K.; Kim, J.J.; Kim, D.W. High omega3-polyunsaturated fatty acids in fat-1 mice prevent streptozotocin-induced purkinje cell degeneration through bdnf-mediated autophagy. *Sci. Rep.* **2015**, *5*, 15465. [CrossRef] [PubMed]

97. Huang, W.; Wang, B.; Li, X.; Kang, J.X. Endogenously elevated *n*-3 polyunsaturated fatty acids alleviate acute ethanol-induced liver steatosis. *BioFactors* **2015**, *41*, 453–462. [PubMed]

98. Hwang, W.M.; Bak, D.H.; Kim, D.H.; Hong, J.Y.; Han, S.Y.; Park, K.Y.; Lim, K.; Lim, D.M. Attenuation of streptozotocin-induced pancreatic beta cell death in transgenic fat-1 mice via autophagy activation. *Endocrinol. Metab.* 2015. Available online: http://e-enm.org/DOIx.php?id=10.3803/EnM.2015.30.e24 (accessed on 2 February 2016).

99. Li, X.; Ballantyne, L.L.; Che, X.; Mewburn, J.D.; Kang, J.X.; Barkley, R.M.; Murphy, R.C.; Yu, Y.; Funk, C.D. Endogenously generated omega-3 fatty acids attenuate vascular inflammation and neointimal hyperplasia by interaction with free fatty acid receptor 4 in mice. *J. Am. Heart Assoc.* **2015**, *4*, e001856. [CrossRef] [PubMed]

100. Simopoulos, A.P. Human requirement for *n*-3 polyunsaturated fatty acids. *Poult. Sci.* **2000**, *79*, 961–970. [CrossRef] [PubMed]

101. Rice, K.M.; Walker, E.M., Jr.; Wu, M.; Gillette, C.; Blough, E.R. Environmental mercury and its toxic effects. *J. Prev. Med. Public Health* **2014**, *47*, 74–83. [CrossRef] [PubMed]

102. Lai, L.; Kang, J.X.; Li, R.; Wang, J.; Witt, W.T.; Yong, H.Y.; Hao, Y.; Wax, D.M.; Murphy, C.N.; Rieke, A.; *et al.* Generation of cloned transgenic pigs rich in omega-3 fatty acids. *Nat. Biotechnol.* **2006**, *24*, 435–436. [CrossRef] [PubMed]

103. Zhang, P.; Zhang, Y.; Dou, H.; Yin, J.; Chen, Y.; Pang, X.; Vajta, G.; Bolund, L.; Du, Y.; Ma, R.Z. Handmade cloned transgenic piglets expressing the nematode fat-1 gene. *Cell. Reprogram.* **2012**, *14*, 258–266. [PubMed]

104. Zhou, Y.; Lin, Y.; Wu, X.; Feng, C.; Long, C.; Xiong, F.; Wang, N.; Pan, D.; Chen, H. The high-level accumulation of *n*-3 polyunsaturated fatty acids in transgenic pigs harboring the *n*-3 fatty acid desaturase gene from caenorhabditis briggsae. *Transgenic Res.* **2014**, *23*, 89–97. [CrossRef] [PubMed]

105. Guo, T.; Liu, X.F.; Ding, X.B.; Yang, F.F.; Nie, Y.W.; An, Y.J.; Guo, H. Fat-1 transgenic cattle as a model to study the function of omega-3 fatty acids. *Lipids Health Dis.* **2011**, *10*, 244. [CrossRef] [PubMed]

106. Wu, X.; Ouyang, H.; Duan, B.; Pang, D.; Zhang, L.; Yuan, T.; Xue, L.; Ni, D.; Cheng, L.; Dong, S.; *et al.*
      Production of cloned transgenic cow expressing omega-3 fatty acids. *Transgenic Res.* **2012**, *21*, 537–543.
      [CrossRef] [PubMed]
107. Pohlmeier, W.E.; Hovey, R.C.; Van Eenennaam, A.L. Reproductive abnormalities in mice expressing omega-3
      fatty acid desaturase in their mammary glands. *Transgenic Res.* **2011**, *20*, 283–292. [CrossRef] [PubMed]

11

Supplementation with Omega-3 Fatty Acids in Psychiatric Disorders

Paola Bozzatello, Elena Brignolo, Elisa De Grandi and Silvio Bellino *

Centre for Personality Disorders, Department of Neuroscience, University of Turin, 10126 Turin, Italy; paola.bozzatello@unito.it (P.B.); elena.brignolo@yahoo.com (E.B.); elisa.degrandi@gmail.com (E.D.G.)
* Correspondence: silvio.bellino@unito.it

Academic Editors: Lindsay Brown, Bernhard Rauch and Hemant Poudyal

Abstract: A new application for omega-3 fatty acids has recently emerged, concerning the treatment of several mental disorders. This indication is supported by data of neurobiological research, as highly unsaturated fatty acids (HUFAs) are highly concentrated in neural phospholipids and are important components of the neuronal cell membrane. They modulate the mechanisms of brain cell signaling, including the dopaminergic and serotonergic pathways. The aim of this review is to provide a complete and updated account of the empirical evidence of the efficacy and safety that are currently available for omega-3 fatty acids in the treatment of psychiatric disorders. The main evidence for the effectiveness of eicosapentaenoic acid (EPA) and docosahexaenoic acid (DHA) has been obtained in mood disorders, in particular in the treatment of depressive symptoms in unipolar and bipolar depression. There is some evidence to support the use of omega-3 fatty acids in the treatment of conditions characterized by a high level of impulsivity and aggression and borderline personality disorders. In patients with attention deficit hyperactivity disorder, small-to-modest effects of omega-3 HUFAs have been found. The most promising results have been reported by studies using high doses of EPA or the association of omega-3 and omega-6 fatty acids. In schizophrenia, current data are not conclusive and do not allow us either to refuse or support the indication of omega-3 fatty acids. For the remaining psychiatric disturbances, including autism spectrum disorders, anxiety disorders, obsessive-compulsive disorder, eating disorders and substance use disorder, the data are too scarce to draw any conclusion. Concerning tolerability, several studies concluded that omega-3 can be considered safe and well tolerated at doses up to 5 g/day.

Keywords: polyunsaturated fatty acids; omega-3 fatty acids; mood disorders; schizophrenia; borderline personality disorder; attention deficit hyperactivity disorder; eating disorders; substance use disorder; tolerability

1. Introduction

The role of omega-3 highly unsaturated fatty acids (HUFAs) in human mental health has been widely studied in the last two decades.

Omega-3 fatty acids eicosapentaenoic acid (EPA) and docosahexaenoic acid (DHA) are derived from alpha-linolenic acid (ALA) and are dietary essential fatty acids. They cannot be synthetized de novo by mammals and are provided by supplementation, such as fish oil.

EPA and DHA act as competitive inhibitors of omega-6 fatty acids causing a reduction in the synthesis of pro-inflammatory mediators [1]. In fact, the omega-6 family of fatty acids is converted to arachidonic acid and then into prostaglandins and leukotrienes, which are responsible of the pro-inflammatory effects. Therefore, a diet rich in fish oil has been shown to decrease the incidence of inflammatory diseases.

In addition, HUFAs slow coronary atherosclerosis by optimizing cholesterol concentrations and lowering plasma triglyceride levels. HUFAs also have antithrombotic, antiarrhythmic and vasodilatory properties, providing the protection of the cardiovascular system and significantly diminishing cardiovascular mortality. These effects of omega-3 fatty acids have supported indications in the secondary prevention of hypertension, coronary heart disease, type 2 diabetes and in some cases of rheumatoid arthritis, Crohn's disease, ulcerative colitis, chronic obstructive pulmonary disease and renal disease [2,3].

EPA and DHA are important for fetal development, including neuronal, retinal and immune functions [4].

In recent years, the interest of omega-3 fatty acids has grown in psychiatry, and their role in the treatment of several mental diseases has been investigated. HUFAs are important components of phospholipids and cholesterol esters of the neuronal cell membrane, especially of dendritic and synaptic membranes. The rationale for the use of these new agents in psychiatric disorders stemmed from their primary action in producing modification of the synaptic membrane [5]. Indeed, they modulate and are involved in brain cell signaling, including monoamine regulation [6–10], modification of receptor properties or the activation of signal transduction by receptors.

Among psychiatric diseases, long-chain omega-3 fatty acids have been tested in the treatment of schizophrenia, unipolar and bipolar mood disorders, anxiety disorders, obsessive-compulsive disorder, attention deficit hyperactivity disorder (ADHD), autism, aggression, hostility and impulsivity, borderline personality disorder, substance abuse and anorexia nervosa. The aim of this review is to provide an updated account of the empirical evidence of the efficacy and safety that are currently available for omega-3 fatty acids in the treatment of mental disorders. In particular, we focused on the data of efficacy and the adverse effects of different doses of HUFAs in the treatment of mental disorders, to determine which dose levels of single or combined fatty acids are related to a good clinical response of specific mental disorders with a low risk of significant adverse effects.

2. Methods

This review presents and critically evaluates data from clinical trials, systematic reviews and meta-analyses published from 1980 to September 2015, after a systematic research on the Medline database provided by the U.S. National Library of Medicine (http://www.ncbi.nlm.nih.gov/pubmed?otool=iitutolib). The search terms were: omega-3 fatty acids; HUFAs; eicosapentaenoic acid; docosahexaenoic acid; ethyl-eicosapentaenoic acid; α-lipoic acid; α-linoleic acid; psychiatric disorders; psychotic disorders; schizophrenia; mood disorders; anxiety disorders; obsessive-compulsive disorder; attention deficit hyperactivity disorder; autism spectrum disorders; aggression, hostility, impulsivity; personality disorders; borderline personality disorder; substance dependence; anorexia nervosa; adverse effects; dose.

2.1. Schizophrenia

Studies of post mortem samples have shown that patients with schizophrenia have often low levels of EPA and DHA in their brain cells. The level of fatty acids is considered important to maintain the correct nerve cell-membrane metabolism [11]. The evidence is strong enough to have led to a 'membrane phospholipid hypothesis' of schizophrenia [12,13]. Based on findings that in individuals with schizophrenia or related psychotic disorders, certain omega-3 and omega-6 HUFA levels are reduced compared to healthy control samples, the idea that restoration of HUFA resources could be used as a treatment option in psychotic disorders has been widely discussed [14].

To date, there are 13 RCTs available concerning the role of omega-3 fatty acids supplementation in schizophrenia or related disorders. For ethical and clinical reasons, most trials used the add-on strategy, including patients who already received neuroleptics or atypical antipsychotics. Two exceptions are the studies published by Amminger [15] and Markulev [16], which considered patients at high risk for developing psychosis. Peet et al. [17] and Emsley et al. [18] designed trials with omega-3 HUFAs as a monotherapy, but in both cases, almost all patients needed to be treated also with an antipsychotic drug during the course of the trial. Only six RCTs [15,17,19–22] reported that HUFAs had a benefit on positive or negative symptoms. The sample size of all of the reviewed studies was small, and the population investigated suffered from a considerable degree of heterogeneity. In fact, not only patients with a diagnosis of schizophrenia were included, but also subjects with schizoaffective disorder [23], first episode of psychosis [21,24] and resistant schizophrenia [19]. The omega-3 supplementation has been administered in a dosage ranging from 1–4 g/day. The duration of the trials has been limited to 8–16 weeks in the majority of the studies. The main issue is that no conclusions could be drawn regarding the medium- to long-term effects of HUFAs in schizophrenia, according to the findings of the four meta-analysis available on this topic [25–28] (Table 1).

Table 1. Double-blind controlled trials of highly unsaturated fatty acids (HUFAs) as an add-on strategy in the treatment of schizophrenia. PANSS, Positive and Negative Syndrome Scale; E-EPA, ethyl-EPA.

Study	Drug and Dose	Sample	Treatment Duration	Results
Peet et al., 2001 [17]	EPA or DHA 2 g/day	45 patients	12 weeks	↓ psychotic symptoms measured with PANSS in the group treated with EPA
Peet et al., 2001 [17]	EPA 2 g/day	30 patients	12 weeks	↓ positive symptoms measured with PANSS
Peet and Horrobin, 2002 [19]	E-EPA 1–4 g/day	115 patients	12 weeks	↓ positive symptoms measured with PANSS, ↓ depressive symptoms
Jamilian et al., 2014 [20]	1 g/day	60 patients	8 weeks	↓ psychotic symptoms measured with PANSS
Fenton et al., 2001 [23]	ethyl-EPA 3 g/day	87 patients	16 weeks	no significant differences in positive, negative symptoms, mood or cognition
Berger et al., 2007 [24]	ethyl-EPA 2 g/day	69 patients	12 weeks	no efficacy on specific psychotic symptoms
Amminger et al., 2010 [15]	EPA 700 mg/day + DHA 480 mg/day	76 individuals "UHR"	12 weeks	↓ progression in psychosis in young UHR patients
Pawelzcyk et al., 2016 [21]	EPA + DHA 2.2 g/day	71 patients with FEP	26 weeks	↓ psychotic symptoms measured with PANSS ↓ depressive symptoms ↑ level of functioning
Bentsen et al., 2013 [22]	ethyl-EPA 2 g/day	99 patients	16 weeks	↓ impairment of the course of psychosis
Emsley et al., 2014 [18]	EPA 2 g/day + DHA 1 g/day + α-LA 300 mg/day	33 patients	2 years	relapse prevention of psychotic symptoms
Emsley et al., 2002 [29]	ethyl-EPA 3 g/day	40 patients	12 weeks	↓ positive symptoms and negative symptoms measured with PANSS

Abbreviations: EPA = eicosapentaenoic acid; DHA = docosahexaenoic acid; ethyl-EPA = ethyl-eicosapentaenoic acid; α-LA = α-lipoic acid; UHR = ultra-high-risk; FEP = first episode of psychosis; ↓ = decrease of; ↑ = increase of.

Peet and colleagues [17] performed a 12-week placebo-controlled trial in 30 males and 15 females on stable antipsychotic medication who were still symptomatic. Only 35 patients completed the trial. The authors found that EPA was more effective at the reduction of symptoms as assessed with the Positive and Negative Syndrome Scale (PANSS) in comparison to DHA and placebo. In the same year, Peet and colleagues [17] conducted a second RCT to test EPA (dose: 2 g/day) as a monotherapy for schizophrenia. Thirty patients who never assumed an antipsychotic agent with a recent diagnosis of schizophrenia were recruited. For ethical reasons, antipsychotic medications were permitted, so at the end of the study, only two patients remained without an antipsychotic treatment. The results indicated that patients treated with EPA, but also antipsychotics, improved more than placebo-treated subjects in psychopathology measured with the PANSS. In 2002, Peet and Horrobin [19] administered ethyl-EPA to patients with resistant schizophrenia for 12 weeks. One hundred and fifteen subjects, who were already in treatment with clozapine, olanzapine, risperidone, quetiapine or a neuroleptic, were randomly assigned to placebo or 1, 2 or 4 g/day of ethyl-EPA arm in addition to antipsychotic drugs. Authors reported a significant improvement of the PANSS total score and subscales scores in the 2 g/day EPA-treated group, but there was also a large effect of placebo in patients receiving only typical or new generation antipsychotics. In contrast, in patients on clozapine, there was little placebo response, but a significant effect of augmentation with ethyl-EPA on all rating scales, PANSS, PANSS subscales and the Montgomery-Asberg Depression Rating Scale (MADRS).

More recently, Jamilian and colleagues [20] compared 1 g/day of non-specified omega-3 with placebo in 60 patients with schizophrenia who already assumed a standard antipsychotic medication. Omega-3 outperformed placebo significantly, based on the PANSS score.

Less encouraging findings were presented by Fenton and colleagues [23] who designed a 16-week study to evaluate the efficacy of ethyl-EPA (3 g/day) vs. placebo in 87 patients with schizophrenia or schizoaffective disorder with residual symptoms in treatment with conventional antipsychotics. The results indicated no significant differences in positive or negative symptoms, mood and cognition. Similar results were reported by Berger and colleagues [24], who performed an RCT including 69 patients with first-episode psychosis who were treated for 12 weeks with a flexible dose of antipsychotic medication (risperidone, olanzapine or quetiapine) plus ethyl-EPA (E-EPA) (2 g/day) or placebo. The authors suggested that E-EPA may accelerate treatment response and ameliorate the tolerability of antipsychotics, but they remained skeptical about the specific efficacy of EPA in early psychosis.

Early treatment of the prodromal period of psychotic disorders has been linked to more favorable outcomes. The term 'ultra-high-risk' (UHR) identifies individuals who are at increased risk of developing full blown psychotic symptoms. Treatment with omega-3 HUFAs may be an interesting treatment option for UHR subjects due to the low incidence of adverse effects.

Amminger and colleagues [15] performed an RCT on 76 individuals with high risk for developing psychosis comparing omega-3 HUFAs (1.2 g/day) to placebo during a period of 12 weeks. This phase was followed by a further 40-week monitoring period. This study showed that fatty acids may prevent the progression in psychosis in young UHR patients. Recently, in a multicenter double-blind randomized study, 304 participants meeting the 'at-risk' criteria were allocated to treatment with either omega-3 plus cognitive-behavioral case management (CBCM) or placebo plus CBCM. The total length of treatment was six months. The data collected are still under evaluation [16].

Another recent RCT was designed by Pawelczyk et al. [21] to compare the efficacy of 2.2 g/day of HUFAs or olive oil placebo added on to an antipsychotic medication with regard to symptom severity in patients suffering from first-episode schizophrenia. An improvement in psychopathology and the level of functioning was observed.

In the last few years, the first placebo-controlled trial on the association of omega-3 fatty acid and redox regulators for treating schizophrenia was conducted for 16 weeks by Bentsen and colleagues [22]. The participants were 99 patients with a diagnosis of schizophrenia or related psychoses who were divided in four groups (double placebo, active vitamins, active EPA or double active). The psychotic symptoms were assessed with PANSS. The results showed that adding E-EPA 2 g/day or vitamin E 364 mg· day/1 plus vitamin C 1000 mg/day to antipsychotic drugs prevented the course of psychosis, but only among patients with low levels of erythrocyte HUFAs. On the contrary, combining EPA and the vitamins neutralized this detrimental effect. Emsley and colleagues [18] tested a combination of omega-3 polyunsaturated fatty acids (EPA 2 g/day and DHA 1 g/day) and a metabolic antioxidant, alpha-lipoic acid (α-LA 300 mg/day), as prevention treatment of relapse after antipsychotic discontinuation in subjects who were successfully treated for 2–3 years after a first-episode of schizophrenia or schizoaffective disorder. Unfortunately, this study was affected by a small sample size and by premature termination of recruitment due to the high relapse rates and the severity of the relapse episodes. Finally, the results failed to support evidence that HUFAs + α-LA could be a worthwhile tool to maintenance antipsychotic treatment in relapse prevention.

Emsley et al. [29,30] also investigated the efficacy of long-chain fatty acids in reducing side effects due to conventional antipsychotic treatment in two randomized controlled trials. In particular, they verified the effects of omega-3 fatty acids supplementation on extrapyramidal symptoms. The first study [29] found some beneficial effects of E-EPA (3 g/day) as add-on treatment in 40 patients with chronic schizophrenia, who had received a stable antipsychotic medication for at least six months on extrapyramidal symptoms assessed with the Extrapyramidal Symptoms Rating Scale. Moreover, the authors in this study also found a significant improvement of positive and negative symptoms measured with the PANSS. Unfortunately, the second study [30], disconfirmed these results in a larger sample of 77 patients with schizophrenia or schizoaffective disorders and tardive dyskinesia. In this trial, patients received E-EPA (2 g/day) or placebo for 12 weeks. The E-EPA arm had an initial improvement in dyskinesia, but this result was not stable beyond six weeks.

Four meta-analyses [25–28] of RCTs were conducted in order to establish if the available data support the use of omega-3 fatty acids in patients affected by schizophrenia or other psychotic disorders. The authors concluded that the evidence in favor of omega-3s as psychotropic agents in schizophrenia is preliminary, and the findings remain yet inconclusive.

2.2. Major Depressive Disorder

In 1998, Hibbeln [31] discovered a direct and powerful inverse association between fish consumption and the prevalence of major depression in a study aimed to test the hypothesis that a high consumption of fish could be correlated with a lower annual prevalence of major depression. One year later, it was established that depression often co-occurs with cardiovascular disease, which is associated with elevated cholesterol and lower fatty acids plasma levels [32]. After this discovery, abnormal fatty acid compositions in the peripheral tissues (e.g., plasma, serum and red blood cells) of patients with depression have been reported extensively [33,34].

Twenty randomized controlled trials were conducted in order to evaluate the effectiveness of omega-3, EPA and DHA, in the treatment of mild or moderate depressive disorder. Fatty acids were administered both as a monotherapy and as supplementation to ongoing pharmacotherapy or psychotherapy. Doses ranged from 0.4–4.4 g/day of EPA and from 0.2–2.4 g/day of DHA. Ten RCTs investigated the efficacy of omega-3 fatty acids as an individual treatment strategy, but only seven of them reported that EPA and/or DHA had a positive effect on core depressive symptoms. Seven RCTs aimed to determine whether administering omega-3 fatty acids provides any additional benefit to conventional patient treatment (e.g., fluoxetine, citalopram or sertraline) for major depression. Five of these studies obtained a significant improvement of depressive symptoms [35–39]. However, the validity of these findings is limited by the heterogeneity of methods among different studies, including the use of unstandardized assessment instruments of depressive symptoms, as well as considerable differences in doses and ratios of omega-3 fatty acids, the duration of the trials and the demographic and clinical characteristics of the samples. Further studies are needed to better understand the mechanisms of the antidepressant effects of HUFAs and to explain the reason for the discordant results published until now.

Peet and Horrobin [35] conducted a 12-week study that showed improvement in patients treated with 1 g/day of ethyl-EPA (E-EPA) and who were refractory to selective serotonin uptake inhibitor monotherapy for major depression. Findings showed that only 1 g/day of omega-3, but not 2 or 4 g/day, was effective in reducing depressive symptoms measured with the Hamilton Depression Rating Scale (HDRS), the MADRS and the Back Depression Inventory (BDI) (effect size: 0.92) in adults with ongoing depression. Nemets et al. [40] designed a four-week placebo-controlled study on 20 subjects already undergoing antidepressant therapy and found better outcome results in the treatment group with E-EPA at the dosage of 2 g/day. The effect of omega-3 was significant from the second week of treatment, similarly to the time of response to antidepressants and resulting in an improvement of core depressive symptoms on the HDRS. The same authors [41] suggested that omega-3 may have a therapeutic benefit in 6–12-year-old children with major depression.

Of the 20 patients who entered data analysis, 10 received placebo and 10 received omega-3 (0.4 g/day of EPA plus 0.2 g/day of DHA) for 16 weeks. Depression symptoms were assessed with the Childhood Depression Rating Scale, the Childhood Depression Inventory and the Clinical Global Impression (CGI). Su and colleagues [36] conducted an eight-week RCT comparing EPA (at the dose of 4.4 g/day) plus DHA (at the dose of 2.2 g/day) with placebo in augmentation to antidepressant in 22 patients with major depression. They found encouraging results: participants who were treated with omega-3 fatty acids had a significantly lower score of the HDRS. An interesting study on 36 pregnant women with major depressive disorder [42] compared omega-3 HUFAs monotherapy (2.2 g/day of EPA plus 1.2 g/day of DHA) with placebo. Twenty-four patients who finished the trial showed significantly lower depressive symptoms' ratings on the HDRS, the Edinburgh Postnatal Depression Scale (EPDS), and the BDI. The findings of this study are remarkable because omega-3s are preferentially transported to the growing fetus during pregnancy, which can deplete fatty acid levels in mothers.

The beneficial effect of omega-3 fatty acids supplementation on depressive symptoms was also confirmed in elderly women (aged 66–95 years) residents in a nursing home [43,44]. Within a context of an eight-week double-blind RCT, 46 women who received a diagnosis of depression were randomly assigned to the intervention group (1.67 g/day of EPA plus 0.83 g/day of DHA) or the placebo group. Depressive symptoms, assessed with the Geriatric Depression Scale, quality of life assessed with the Short-Form 36-Item Health Survey and phospholipids fatty acids' profile improved. Nevertheless, the same authors in another study [45] measured some immunological parameters and cytokines in the same sample, but they did not find a significant amelioration of the immunological function in the intervention group.

Currently, there is not a general consensus concerning the efficacy of omega-3s in the treatment of depression. Rees and colleagues [46] found that omega-3 fatty acids were not superior over placebo in treating perinatal depressive symptoms. They administered 0.4 g/day of EPA plus 1.6 g/day of DHA as a monotherapy to 26 pregnant women for six weeks. Similar results were collected by Freeman and colleagues [47], who did not detect significant differences between omega-3 HUFAs (EPA 1.1 g/day plus DHA at the dose of 0.8 g/day) and placebo on perinatal depressive symptoms measured with the HDRS and the EPDS. All 59 women enrolled in this trial received also a supportive psychotherapy for eight weeks.

In a similar way, omega-3s were not found superior to placebo in treating depressive symptoms in three other studies. Marangell et al. [48], Silvers et al. [49] and Grenyer et al. [50] obtained no significant improvement in the symptoms of depression in patients who were treated with similar doses of EPA and/or DHA (ranging 2–3 g/day) as sole therapy or in addition to antidepressive drug. These studies were different for sample size, duration and instruments to assess depressive symptoms, but they drew the same conclusions.

Lespérance et al. (2011) [37] conducted an inclusive, double-blind, randomized controlled trial on 432 patients with a major depressive episode. They administered EPA (1.050 g/day) and DHA (150 mg/day) for eight weeks to a sample with a heterogeneous therapy (40.3% of the patients already received an antidepressant at the baseline). Omega-3 supplementation resulted in being superior over placebo only for the patients without comorbid anxiety disorders.

Two studies investigated the effectiveness of omega-3s on depression and on cognitive functions. Rogers et al. [51] in a 12-week trial tested the efficacy of EPA plus DHA (0.6 g/day + 0.85 g/day) on mood and cognition in 218 patients with mild to moderate depression. More recently, Antypa and colleagues [52] treated 71 depressed patients with omega-3 fatty acids or placebo for four weeks.

They evaluated cognitive reactivity with the Leiden Index of Depression Sensitivity-Revised (LEIDS-R) and the Profile of Mood States (POMS), and depressive symptoms were measured with the BDI. Both studies have not obtained favorable results on mood and cognition using omega-3s.

Two trials compared the effectiveness of different doses of EPA or DHA in the treatment of depressive disorders. Mischoulon and colleagues in 2008 [53] enrolled 35 depressed outpatients that were randomized into one of three double-blind dosing arms for 12 weeks: 1 g/day DHA; 2 g/day DHA; 4 g/day DHA. In this study, subjects who received 2 g/day or more DHA had a lower response rate (on the HDRS) compared to those who received 1 g/day. It is interesting to note that these findings are similar to Peet and Horrobin's results [35]: E-EPA, as well as DHA appear more effective at lower doses. In the same year (2008), Jazayeri and colleagues [38] compared EPA at the low dosage of 1 g/day with fluoxetine (20 mg/day) in 60 patients with major depressive disorder for eight weeks. The results showed that a low dose of EPA may have similar therapeutic effects as fluoxetine.

A recent and larger eight-week RCT [54] compared the potential therapeutic effects of three differing doses, (i) EPA (1 g/day), (ii) DHA (1 g/day) or (iii) placebo (containing 980 mg of soybean oil per cap; four capsules/day), in 196 depressed patients. The authors reported a significant improvement in depressive symptoms in all three groups; neither EPA nor DHA were superior to placebo.

Interesting results were obtained from one study that explored the association of omega-3 fatty acids and antidepressants in treating depressed patients [39]. The authors investigated the efficacy of combination therapy with citalopram plus omega-3 fatty acids (1.8 g/day of EPA + 0.4 g/day of DHA + 0.2 g/day of other omega-3s) vs. citalopram plus placebo in 42 patients with initial depression. Combined therapy showed grater improvements in depression symptoms assessed with HDRS, but did not enhance the speed of antidepressant response.

The effects of fish oil supplementation were also investigated in patients with major depression associated with coronary heart disease [55]. Carney and colleagues (2009) obtained negative results testing omega-3 in cardiopathic patients. They performed a 10-week RCT to evaluate the effects of ethyl-EPA (0.93 g/day) plus DHA (0.75 g/day) in addition to sertraline on symptoms of depression in 122 patients with major depressive disorder and coronary heart disease. The authors did not find any superiority of treatment over placebo.

In conclusion, supplementation with HUFA in patients with major depression seems useful in improving depressive symptoms, but the findings are not univocal. Systematic reviews and meta-analyses also provided controversial conclusions. Appleton and colleagues [56] reviewed 35 RCTs that included 329 adults and concluded that trials investigating the effects of HUFAs on depression are increasing, but it is difficult to evaluate their results because of data heterogeneity. Bloch and Hannestad [57] outlined the methodological limits of available studies that affect the validity of results. On the contrary, other meta-analyses [58–60] indicated a more encouraging prospective in this field and concluded that omega-3 fatty acids produce a significant antidepressant effect. In particular, EPA seems to be more efficacious than DHA in treating depression. A more recent comprehensive meta-analysis [61] of RCTs confirmed that the use of omega-3s as therapeutic agents was effective in patients with the diagnosis of major depression or depressive symptoms and suggested that patients with greater depressive severity and those meeting full criteria for a diagnosis of depressive disorder demonstrated greater treatment gains (Table 2).

Table 2. Double-blind controlled trials of HUFAs in the treatment of depressive disorders. HDRS, Hamilton Depression Rating Scale; MADRS, Montgomery-Åsberg Depression Rating Scale.

Study	Dose and Method	Sample	Treatment Duration	Results
Peet and Horrobin, 2002 [35]	ethyl-EPA 1, 2 or 4 g/day add-on standard antidepressant treatment	70 patients resistant to antidepressant treatment	12 weeks	↓ depressive symptoms measured with HDRS, MADRS and BDI in the group treated with 1 g/day of HUFAs
Nemets et al., 2002 [40]	ethyl-EPA 2 g/day	20 patients	4 weeks	↓ depressive symptoms measured with HDRS from the second week of treatment
Nemets et al., 2006 [41]	ethyl-EPA 0.4 g/day + DHA 0.2 g/day	20 patients 6–12 years-old	16 weeks	↓ depressive symptoms measured with CDRS, CDI and CGI
Su et al., 2003 [36]	ethyl-EPA 4.4 g/day + DHA 2.2 g/day add-on existing antidepressant treatment	22 patients	8 weeks	↓ depressive symptoms measured with HDRS
Su et al., 2008 [42]	ethyl-EPA 2.2 g/day + DHA 1.2 g/day	36 pregnant patients	8 weeks	↓ depressive symptoms measured with HDRS, EPDS and BDI
Rondanelli et al., 2010, 2011 [43,44]	EPA 1.67 g/day + DHA 0.83 g/day add-on existing antidepressant treatment	46 elderly female residents in a nursing home	8 weeks	↓ depressive symptoms assessed with GDS, improvement of phospholipids fatty acids' profile
Rees et al., 2008 [46]	ethyl-EPA 0.4 g/day + DHA 1.6 g/day	26 pregnant patients	6 weeks	no benefits on depressive symptoms
Freeman et al., 2008 [47]	EPA 1.1 g/day + DHA 0.8 g/day	59 women	8 weeks	no benefit on perinatal depressive symptoms
Lespérance et al., 2011 [37]	EPA 1.050 g/day + DHA 150 mg/day	432 patients with a major depressive episode	8 weeks	↓ depressive symptoms only for the patients without comorbid anxiety disorders
Mischoulon et al., 2008 [53]	DHA 1, 2, or 4 g/day	35 patients	12 weeks	measured in the group in treatment with 1 g/day of HUFAs
Jazayeri et al., 2008 [38]	EPA 1 g/day vs. fluoxetine 20 mg/day	60 patients	8 weeks	↓ depressive symptoms in both groups
Mischoulon et al., 2015 [54]	EPA 1 g/day or DHA 1 g/day	196 patients	8 weeks	EPA and DHA were not superior to placebo
Gertsik et al., 2012 [39]	EPA 1.8 g/day + DHA 0.4 g/day + other omega-3 fatty acids 0.2 g/day + citalopram vs. placebo + citalopram	42 patients	9 weeks	↓ depressive symptoms measured with HDRS
Carney et al., 2009 [55]	E-EPA (0.93 g/day) plus DHA (0.75 g/day) on depression in addition to sertraline	122 patients with major depression associated with coronary heart disease	10 weeks	EPA and DHA were not superior to placebo

Abbreviations: EPA = eicosapentaenoic acid; DHA = docosahexaenoic acid; ethyl-EPA = ethyl-eicosapentaenoic acid; CDRS = Childhood Depression Rating Scale; CDI = Childhood Depression Inventory; EPDS = Edinburgh Postnatal Depression Scale; GDS = Geriatric Depression Scale; ↓ = decrease of; ↑ = increase of.

2.3. Bipolar Disorders

In patients with a diagnosis of bipolar disorder, lower erythrocyte membrane levels of omega-3 fatty acids have been observed [62]. Based on this consideration, several investigators performed clinical trials to evaluate whether the implementation of these agents may impact the clinical features of this disorder. To date, only seven RCTs on omega-3 treatment for bipolar disorders have been published. Except for the first pioneering trial, they were all augmentation studies. Intervention length ranged from 6–16 weeks. Three of these [63–65] used EPA in addition to stable psychotropic medication. Two studies [66,67] explored the combination of EPA and DHA in addition to mood stabilizers or other usual treatments. In one trial [68], alpha-linolenic acid was administered in association with stable psychotropic medications. Finally, in one add-on RCT [69], omega-3 was associated with cytidine or not as augmentation to a stable medication. Doses ranged from 0.3–6.2 g/day of EPA and from 0.2–3.4 g/day of DHA. The dose of alpha-linolenic acid was 6.6 g/day.

In the first trial, Stoll and colleagues [66] administered a combination of EPA (6.2 g/day) and DHA (3.4 g/day) as a monotherapy to 14 patients, while 16 patients received placebo for 16 weeks. This study was affected by a large number (13 subjects) of drop-outs because of depression, mania, hypomania and mixed state. Outcomes revealed the efficacy of omega-3 in terms of the reduction and remission of depressive symptoms (HDRS), whereas no significant effects were registered on mania (Young Mania Rating Scale (YMRS)). These findings were replicated by Frangou and colleagues [63] in a 12-week controlled study including 75 patients treated with ethyl-EPA (1 or 2 g/day) as adjunctive treatment to stable psychotropic medications. The same authors [64] reported increased brain levels of N-acetyl-aspartate (NAA), a presumed marker of neuronal integrity, with 2 g/day of ethyl-EPA in 14 female patients with type I bipolar disorder that were treated with a stable dose of lithium. The study was controlled with placebo. The rise in NAA level provided the first evidence for a neurotrophic role of E-EPA treatment in bipolar disorder.

Concerning the manic phase, less encouraging findings were presented by Chiu et al. [67], who designed a four-week study to evaluate the efficacy of 4.4 g/day of EPA plus 2.4 g/day of DHA vs. placebo in addition to a fixed dose of valproate (20 mg/kg/day) in 15 patients with acute mania. The authors found a reduction in both groups of the YMRS scores from baseline, with no significant differences between omega-3 and placebo. Similar results were obtained in a larger RCT [65], which involved 121 patients with bipolar depression or rapid cycling bipolar disorder. The adjunction of 6 g/day of EPA to at least one mood stabilizer did not produce meaningful differences in reducing the severity of depressive or manic symptoms, assessed respectively with the Inventory for Depressive Symptomology total and the YMRS.

Gracious and colleagues [68] conducted a double-blind RCT of alpha-linoleic acid (ALA) as flax seed oil in children and adolescents with bipolar I or II disorder, assuming a stable psychotropic medication. In this study, there was a high rate of noncompliance with taking supplements because of the large number of capsules required (up to 12 per day). Those who were treated with an adequate amount of ALA, demonstrated a significant improvement of overall symptom severity in comparison with the placebo group. Nevertheless, depression and mania measures did not show significant differences between treatment and placebo groups. More recently, therapeutic properties of omega-3 fatty acids in bipolar disorder were further denied by Murphy et al. [69] in a four-month RCT. Forty-five patients with a diagnosis of type I bipolar disorder, who were already treated with a mood stabilizer, were randomly assigned to three different groups consisting of omega-3 fatty acids plus cytidine, omega-3 fatty acid plus placebo or only placebo. In this study, supplementation with omega-3 did not produce a significant improvement in affective symptoms over an extended period of treatment.

Overall, a moderate antidepressant effect was observed for adjunctive omega-3 agents compared to conventional therapy alone in the treatment of bipolar depression [66,67]. The small number of studies, the heterogeneity of HUFA doses and ratios and the small sample sizes were important limitations to obtain reliable data on this topic.

In summary, some beneficial effects of omega-3 HUFAs in bipolar disorders were observed. The conclusions of systematic reviews and meta-analyses [70–73] provided initial evidence that bipolar depressive symptoms, but not manic symptoms, may be improved by adjunctive administration of omega-3 fatty acids (Table 3).

Table 3. Double-blind controlled trials of HUFAs in the treatment of bipolar disorders (depressive and maniac phases).

Study	Dose and Method	Sample	Treatment Duration	Results
Stoll et al., 1999 [66]	EPA 6.2 g/day + DHA 3.4 g/day	30 patients	16 weeks	↓ depressive symptoms measured with HDRS
Frangou et al., 2006 [63]	ethyl-EPA 1 or 2 g/day add-on to stable psychotropic medications	75 patients	12 weeks	↓ depressive symptoms measured with HDRS
Chiu et al., 2003 [67]	EPA 4.4 g/day + DHA 2.4 g/day vs. placebo in addition to valproate 20 mg/kg/day	15 patients with acute mania	4 weeks	no significant differences between omega-3 fatty acids and placebo
Keck et al., 2006 [65]	EPA 6 g/day in addition to at least one mood stabilizer	121 patients with bipolar depression or rapid cycling bipolar disorder	4 months	no significant differences
Gracious et al., 2010 [68]	ALA in addition to psychotropic medication	children and adolescent with bipolar I or II disorder	16 weeks	significant improvement of overall symptom severity in comparison with placebo group
Murphy et al., 2012 [69]	omega-3 fatty acids plus cytidine, omega-3 fatty acid plus placebo or only placebo in addition to a mood stabilizer	45 patients with type I bipolar disorder	4 months	no benefits of omega-3 fatty acids on affective symptoms

Abbreviations: EPA = eicosapentaenoic acid; DHA = docosahexaenoic acid; ethyl-EPA = ethyl-eicosapentaenoic acid; ALA = α-linoleic acid; ↓ = decrease of; ↑ = increase of.

2.4. Anxiety Disorders

The hypothesis that omega-3s may have anxiolytic properties was formulated in the light of the frequent comorbidity between mood disorders and anxiety disorders and the effectiveness of some conventional pharmacotherapy on both disorders. Furthermore, low omega-3 erythrocyte membrane levels have been observed in patients with anxiety disorders [74–76]. Unfortunately, to our knowledge, there are no RCTs that have systematically investigated the effect of omega-3 PUFA in anxiety disorders. Only a small trial [77] showed a reduction in the levels of anxiety and tension in 24 substance abusers. Participants received 2.2 g of EPA/day plus 0.5 g of DHA/day vs. placebo (vegetable oil) for three months. Anxiety continued to be significantly decreased in the active treatment group after three months' discontinuation. In each case, the evidence supporting the use of omega-3 PUFAs as an anxiolytic is currently insufficient [78].

2.5. Obsessive-Compulsive Disorder

Only one RCT about obsessive-compulsive disorder was published by Fux and colleagues [79], who administered 2 g/day of EPA or placebo in augmentation of a stable dose of SSRIs to 11 patients (four of these received 40 mg; two received 30 mg; and two received 60 mg of paroxetine daily; one patient was on 250 mg of fluvoxamine daily; and two were on 40 mg of fluoxetine daily) for six weeks. The augmentation with HUFAs was not associated with significant improvement of anxious, obsessive-compulsive and depressive symptoms compared to placebo.

2.6. Attention Deficit Hyperactivity Disorder

Increasing attention has been given to the role of HUFAs in childhood developmental disorders. Since the 1980s, reduced HUFA levels have been reported in blood analysis of hyperactive children compared to healthy controls [80–83]. Recently, several double-blind placebo controlled trials have been conducted to assess the efficacy of omega-3 fatty acid in the treatment of children with ADHD [84–95], but results are still discordant and disputable. Due to the considerable heterogeneity of published investigations, additional large-cohort studies and well-designed clinical trials of ADHD patients are required. In particular, studies should be conducted with strict criteria concerning methodological issues, such as an accurate DSM-5 diagnosis of ADHD, a double-blind controlled design, the choice of reliable assessment instruments of symptoms and functioning, a clear definition of the doses and ratios of omega-3 fatty acids and of the possible association with conventional medications.

If we examine the available data, seven [84,85,87–90] of thirteen RCTs investigating the efficacy of omega-3 fatty acids had a positive effect on ADHD-related symptoms. The remaining studies did not obtain significant improvement in ADHD symptoms [81,91–95]. Only two of these thirteen RCTs aimed to determine whether taking omega-3 fatty acids confers any additional benefit to conventional patient treatment (stimulant and non-stimulant medications): one found negative results [91] and one positive [90].

In particular, not very encouraging findings have been presented by six RCTs comparing the association of EPA and DHA to placebo. In a double-blind study performed by Stevens and colleagues [81], fifty patients with ADHD-like symptoms received either placebo (olive oil) or HUFA supplementation (480 mg of DHA, 80 mg of EPA, 40 mg of arachidonic acid and 96 mg of gamma-linolenic acid/day) for four months. At baseline and at the end of the intervention period, both parents and teachers completed the Conners' Abbreviated Symptom Questionnaires (ASQ) and the Disruptive Behavior Disorders (DBD) Rating Scale. Other additional neuropsychological tests were administered: the Conners' Continuous Performance Test (CPT) and eight tests of cognitive ability of the Woodcock-Johnson Psycho-Educational Battery-Revised (WJ-R). No significant difference between active group and placebo was observed for any rating scale comparing patients who completed the trial. HUFAs supplementation led to a significant behavioral improvement over placebo on only two of the 16 outcome measures that were used (DBD-Conduct for Parents and the DBD-Attention for Teachers) and by intention-to-treat analysis only.

In 2004, Hirayama and colleagues [92] also reported no evidence of efficacy of omega-3 fatty acids compared to placebo in treating ADHD symptoms. In this double-blind placebo controlled trial, the majority of the 40 children did not receive ADHD medications (only six of them had been under conventional medications). They administered both DHA and EPA through fish oil-enriched food (the daily dose was approximately 100 mg of EPA and 500 mg of DHA) to twenty children with ADHD for two months. The control group ($n = 20$) took indistinguishable food without fish oil. The authors measured ADHD related symptoms according to the DSM-IV criteria, aggression, impatience and some cognitive features, but they did not find any significant changes in outcome measures.

In another study (Johnson and colleagues) [93], seventy-five children and adolescents 8–18 years old with ADHD were included and treated with 558 mg EPA, 174 mg DHA and 60 mg gamma linoleic acid daily, compared to placebo. Only one of the patients had been previously treated with a conventional drug for ADHD (methylphenidate). Investigators found that only a subgroup of patients characterized by the inattentive subtype of ADHD and associated neurodevelopmental disorders showed a meaningful clinical response to omega-3 and omega-6 treatment. They concluded the study results were essentially negative and did not support the superiority of HUFAs over placebo.

Milte [94] performed a double-blind RCT, including 90 children 7–12 years old with ADHD treated with EPA-rich oil (providing 1109 mg of EPA and 108 mg of DHA), DHA-rich oil (providing 264 mg of EPA and 1032 mg of DHA) vs. an omega-6 HUFA oil during a period of four months. Children were taking no other medication. Despite that this study demonstrated no statistically-significant differences between the two groups, the authors found that increased levels of erythrocyte DHA seemed associated with improved word reading and lower parent ratings of oppositional behavior. Interestingly, a subgroup of 17 patients with learning difficulties exhibited superior benefits from the supplementation with omega-3 fatty acids.

A more recent randomized, double-blind controlled trial (Widenhorn-Müller et al.) [95] was conducted in 95 ADHD patients aged between six and 12 years who received omega-3 fatty acids or placebo for 16 weeks, not treated with medications for ADHD. The authors found less negative results than those from previous studies, but not yet satisfactory. Supplementation with EPA and DHA (600 mg of EPA and 120 mg of DHA daily) improved working memory function, but had no effect on other cognitive measures or behavioral symptoms in the study population.

Only one study concerning the use of DHA has been reported: using a randomized, double-blind design, Voigt and colleagues [91] tested the effect of 345 mg/day of DHA for four months upon 63 children (6–12 years old) with ADHD, all receiving maintenance therapy with stimulant medication. Despite blood phospholipid DHA content being increased in the active treatment group, there was no statistically-significant improvement in any ADHD symptoms compared to placebo.

On the other hand, some investigations have provided more promising findings. In particular, interesting results have been obtained by the seven RCTs in which EPA and DHA were administered to ADHD patients and compared to placebo.

Richardson and colleagues [84] published a pilot double-blind RCT investigating the efficacy of the combination of omega-3 and omega-6 fatty acids (daily dose of 186 mg of EPA, 480 mg of DHA, 864 mg of linolenic acid and 42 mg of arachidonic acid) vs. placebo in 41 children with ADHD-related symptoms and specific learning disabilities. ADHD-type symptoms were assessed using the Conners's Teacher Rating Scale. After 12 weeks of treatment, mean scores for cognitive problems and general behavior improved more in the group treated with HUFAs than placebo. More recently, these findings were replicated by the same authors [85]. They conducted a larger double-blind placebo controlled RCT, including 117 children diagnosed with Developmental Coordination Disorder (DCD), which is characterized by deficit of motor functions and shows substantial overlap with ADHD in terms of difficulties with organizational skills and attention. The active treatment provided a high ratio of omega-3 and omega-6 fatty acids for three months. Despite no effects being reported on motor skills, HUFAs dietary supplementation led to improvement of reading, spelling and behavior in the treatment group compared to placebo. Subsequently, a one-way, uncontrolled crossover to active supplement followed for a further three months: similar changes were observed in the placebo-active group, while the original treatment group's scores continued to improve.

Sinn and Bryan (2008) on a large sample included 132 children aged 7–12 years with a diagnosis of ADHD [86]. Participants were enrolled in a 15-week double-blind controlled trial and were treated with 93 mg of EPA, 29 mg of DHA and 10 mg of gamma-linolenic acid daily, with or without a micronutrient supplement, and were compared to placebo. Children were not treated with ADHD medications. The results outlined that both groups treated with HUFAs improved more than placebo subjects in some core ADHD symptoms, such as inattention, hyperactivity and impulsivity. These results were confirmed by the same authors (Sinn and Bryan) [87] in a 15-week crossover study.

Bélanger et al. (2009), in a Canadian double-blind, one-way, crossover randomized trial [88], measured the impact on ADHD of omega-3 HUFAs, using equivalent quantities of omega-6 HUFAs (sunflower oil) as the control condition. Thirty seven subjects were enrolled, but only 26 children succeeded in completing the study. Participants did not receive any other medication. They were divided into two groups (A and B) and participated in a 16-week, double-blind, one-way, crossover randomized study. In the first phase, Group A received the n-3 HUFA supplement, and Group B received placebo. During the second phase, Group B received the active n-3 HUFA supplement that was continued in Group A. In the first phase of the study (Weeks 0–15), a meaningful improvement in inattention and global ADHD symptoms emerged in patients who received omega-3 treatment (20 mg/kg/day–25 mg/kg/day of EPA and 8.5 mg/kg/day–10.5 mg/kg/day of DHA). These positive results were maintained during the second phase (the treatment crossover, Weeks 16–30) but did not reach in this phase statistical significance.

Kirby et al. [89] have assessed the effects of the administration of 0.8 g/day fish oil (including 400 mg of DHA and 56 mg of EPA/day) on 450 healthy school-children. After a period of 16 weeks, the plasma ratio omega-6/omega-3 was measured, and patients were submitted to a series of cognitive tests to assess IQ, reading, language and writing skills, attention, working memory, impulsivity and hyperactivity. This RCT showed a significant improvement in impulsivity, evaluated with the Matching Familiar Figures Task (MFFT), handwriting and attentional capacity, evaluated with the Computerized Penmanship Evaluation Tool (COCOM) and a possible protective effect of omega-3s on behavioral dysregulation, compared to placebo.

In accordance with these findings, a six-month randomized double-blind controlled trial by Perera [90] indicated the efficacy of supplementation with a combined omega-3 and omega-6 preparation vs. placebo in 98 children with ADHD, refractory to methylphenidate treatment (all participants continued taking immediate-release methylphenidate during the study). In particular, omega-3 (600 mg/day) combined with omega-6 (360 mg/day) improved behavior and learning in restlessness, aggressiveness, completing work and academic performance, but not in inattention, impulsiveness and cooperation with parents and teachers.

A comprehensive meta-analysis conducted by Bloch et al. [96] of omega-3 fatty acids supplementation in children with ADHD found a small to modest effect size for EPA at high doses. Another recent meta-analysis conducted by Sonuga-Barke et al. [97] concluded that free fatty acids (omega-3 supplements, omega-6 supplements and both omega-3 and omega-6 supplements) produce small, but significant reductions in ADHD symptoms.

Besides, it provides evidence to justify the use of omega-3 fatty acids for ADHD as a supplement to other empirically-supported therapies. Gillies et al. [98] suggested that the efficacy of omega-3 fatty acids is supported only in combination with omega-6 fatty acids. A recent review [99] found that randomized clinical trials with omega-3 HUFAs have reported small-to-modest effects in reducing symptoms of ADHD in children and that available findings need to be replicated in future investigations of nonpharmacological interventions in clinical practice (Table 4).

Table 4. Double-blind controlled trials of HUFAs in the treatment of ADHD.

Study	Dose and Method	Sample	Treatment Duration	Results
Voigt et al., 2001 [91]	DHA 345 mg/day vs. placebo; with ADHD medication	63 children (6–12 years old) with ADHD	4 months	no statistically-significant improvement in any ADHD symptoms compared to placebo
Richardson et al., 2002 [84]	EPA 186 mg· g/day + DHA 480 mg/die + linolenic acid 864 mg/die + arachidonic acid 42 mg/die vs. placebo	41 children with ADHD-like symptoms	12 weeks	mean scores for cognitive problems and general behavior improved more in the group treated with HUFAs than placebo
Stevens et al., 2003 [81]	DHA 480 mg/day + EPA 80 mg/day + arachidonic acid 40 mg/day + gamma-linolenic acid 96 mg/day vs. placebo; no ADHD medications	50 children with ADHD-like symptoms	4 months	no significant difference between active group and placebo was observed for any rating scale comparing patients who completed the trial
Hirayama et al., 2004 [92]	EPA 100 mg/die + DHA 500 mg/die vs. placebo; mostly without ADHD medications (only six subjects had been under medications)	40 children with ADHD	2 months	no evidence of the efficacy of omega-3 fatty acids compared to placebo
Johnson et al., 2009 [93]	EPA 558 mg/die + DHA 174 mg/die + gamma linoleic acid 60 mg/die vs. placebo; only one patient with ADHD medication	75 children and adolescents 8–18 year old with ADHD	3 months	no evidence of the efficacy of omega-3 fatty acids compared to placebo
Bélanger et al., 2009 [88]	EPA 20–25 mg/kg/die + DHA 8.5–10.5 mg/kg/day vs. placebo; no ADHD medications	26 children	16-week	improvement in inattention and global ADHD symptoms only in the first phase of the study (Weeks 0–15)
Milte et al., 2012 [94]	EPA-rich oil (providing EPA 1109 mg and DHA 108 mg), DHA-rich oil (providing EPA 264 mg and DHA 1032 mg) vs. an omega-6 HUFAs oil; no ADHD medications	90 children (7–12 year old) with ADHD	4 months	no statistically-significant differences between the two groups

Table 4. *Cont.*

Study	Dose and Method	Sample	Treatment Duration	Results
Widenhorn-Müller et al., 2014 [95]	EPA 600 mg/die + DHA 120 mg/die; no ADHD medications	95 children (6–12 years) with ADHD	16 weeks	improved working memory function, but no effect on other cognitive measures or behavioral symptoms in the study population
Sinn and Bryan, 2008 [87]	EPA 93 mg/day + DHA 29 mg/day + gamma-linolenic acid 10 mg/day vs. placebo; no ADHD medications	132 children (7–12 years) with ADHD		improved in inattention, hyperactivity and impulsivity in most ADHD scales in parents' reports; no improvement in teacher reports; limits: no ADHD diagnosis (reported ADHD symptoms)
Perera et al., 2012 [90]	omega-3 + omega-6 vs. placebo; with ADHD medications	98 children (6–12 years) with ADHD diagnosis	6 months	improved behavior and learning in restlessness, aggressiveness, completing work and academic performance, but not in inattention, impulsiveness and cooperation with parents and teachers
Kirby et al. [89]	DHA 400 mg/day + EPA 56 mg/day; no ADHD medications	450 healthy school-children	16 weeks	significant improvement in impulsivity, handwriting and attentional capacity and a possible protective effect of omega-3 on behavioral dysregulation, compared to placebo

Abbreviations: EPA = eicosapentaenoic acid; DHA = docosahexaenoic acid.

2.7. Autism Spectrum Disorders

The efficacy of HUFAs as a treatment consideration has also been taken into account in other developmental disorders, such as autism spectrum disorder [100,101]. There is some evidence to suggest that autism may involve a cellular functional deficiency or imbalance of omega-3 [100–102]. Studies focused on the deficit in the concentration of HUFAs complexed to membrane phospholipids in children with autism showed controversial results. Vancassel and colleagues [102] examined the concentration of fatty acids in plasma in a population of children with autism and in another group of children with learning disabilities. This study reported a 23% reduction of DHA levels in the group with autism compared to the control group, a reduction in the erythrocytes membrane concentration of omega-3 and a concomitant increase in the levels of saturated fatty acids [100,101].

In addition, some evidence showed that omega-3 may improve the course of chronic inflammatory diseases [103], frequently associated with autism and potentially related to its pathophysiology [104].

Considering that data collected from uncontrolled studies are affected by severe limitations and that only three RCTs are available, evidence is insufficient at the moment to determine whether HUFAs are effective for autism spectrum disorder. Actually, only one study [105] supported HUFAs supplementation to treat autism-related symptoms, while the remaining did not find any positive effects [106,107].

The first RCT is a double-blind, randomized, placebo-controlled, pilot study, performed by Amminger in 13 children (aged 5–17 years) with autistic disorder [105]. After six weeks, the group treated with EPA (840 mg/day) and DHA (700 mg/day) showed an improvement of hyperactivity and stereotyped behaviors.

The second double-blind, placebo-controlled trial was conducted by Voigt [106] and presented different conclusions. In particular, the authors did not show any improvement in core symptoms of autism after a dietary DHA supplementation of 200 mg/day for six months in a group of 48 children with autism.

The third randomized, double-blind, placebo-controlled trial was conducted by Mankad et al. [107]. They designed a six-month trial of omega-3 fatty acid supplementation (1.5 g of EPA and DHA/day) in comparison with placebo in 38 children (2–5 years old) with autism. This study did not support the hypothesis that high dose supplementation of HUFAs in children with autism provides any efficacy in terms of improvement of core symptom domains or adaptive function.

Considering the scarcity of data in this field, we also reported the results from one case-report and one open-label study performed in patients with autism. The case report study [108] showed an improvement of symptoms in a child suffering from autism following treatment with EPA in the first time administered at a dose of 1 g/day, then at a dose of 3 g/day, for a period of four weeks. During the eight-month follow-up phase, the improvements were maintained. The open-label study [109] carried out on 20 autistic children reported a significant improvement of the disease after three months of treatment with omega-3, omega-6 and omega-9 at a dose of 1 g/day (1 g/day).

To date, one systematic review [110] about the efficacy of HUFAs in the treatment of autism spectrum disorders is available. The conclusions showed that the omega-6/omega-3 fatty acid ratio's alteration during early life can affect major processes in brain development and induces aberrant behavior. Thus, changes in dietary omega-6/omega-3 supplies may contribute to reducing the incidence of symptoms related to autism. So far, the studies are still few and provided limited results; therefore, further investigations on a larger population are required to draw conclusions in this field.

2.8. Aggression, Hostility and Impulsivity

In the last two decades, growing attention has been given to the potential role of omega-3 in clinical conditions characterized by high impulsivity, hostility and aggressive behaviors [5]. The discovery of low levels of EPA and DHA in the central nervous system of patients with impulsive-aggressive, self-harm and parasuicidal behaviors [111,112] has encouraged the investigators to perform trials on omega-3 implementation in this clinical population characterized by a high level of impulsivity and aggression with favorable results in terms of mood symptoms and control of impulsivity [113,114].

Two randomized, double-blind, placebo-controlled trials have been performed to analyze the effects of HUFA supplementation in populations without psychiatric diagnosis on aggression and impulsivity. Both showed positive results, but available data are limited by the heterogeneity of the study criteria. The first RCT [113] was conducted by Hamazaki in a group of 41 healthy controls (21–30 years old) monitoring the episodes of aggressive behaviors and cognitive functions during three months. Participants daily received 1.5–1.8 g of DHA or placebo. Aggression toward others significantly increased in the control group, while it decreased in the DHA supplement group. No significant differences were observed on cognitive functions. Another trial was conducted by Itomura et al. (2005) in 166 healthy school children 9–12 years old in order to investigate whether fatty acid nutrition may affect physical aggression [114]. Eighty-three children received a fish oil-fortified diet, providing a daily intake of 3.6 g of DHA and 0.84 of EPA for three months. Aggression against others and impulsivity were significantly decreased in the fish oil group, especially in girls.

In a six-week RCT, Bradbury and colleagues (2004) [115] investigated the possible role of DHA in improving adaptation to perceived stress in a group of 47 healthy controls (18–60 years). They found a significant reduction in stress for both the fish oil (1.5 g/day of DHA) and the placebo groups, but the stress reduction for the fish oil group was significantly superior to that in the no-treatment controls. The fish oil group obtained a more substantial stress reduction than the olive oil group, but the differences between treatments did not reach statistical significance.

2.9. Borderline Personality Disorder

The effects of omega-3 fatty acids supplementation has been studied in patients with personality disorders, who often show high levels of impulsive-behavioral dyscontrol and aggressiveness. Only two RCTs with a double-blind, randomized, placebo-controlled design have been conducted [116,117]. Both indicated the efficacy of HUFAs on borderline personality disorder (BPD) core symptoms, although they were different in diagnostic criteria, contemporary administration of conventional medications and the doses and ratios of omega-3 fatty acids.

Zanarini and Frankenburg [116] performed the first RCT in a group of 30 female patients with a diagnosis of BPD who were treated for eight weeks with 1 g/day of E-EPA or placebo and without any other psychotropic medication. The results showed a significant effect of E-EPA on aggressive behaviors measured with the Modified Overt Aggression Scale (MOAS) and on depressive symptoms assessed with the Montgomery-Åsberg Depression Rating Scale (MADRS) compared to placebo. In another study, published by Hallahan and colleagues [117], 49 patients with self-defeating behaviors (39 patients had received a diagnosis of BPD) were enrolled. Twenty-seven patients were randomly assigned to placebo, and 22 were treated with EPA at the dose of 1.2 g/day and DHA at the dose of 0.9 g/day for 12 weeks. Omega-3s were added to the standard psychiatric therapies. This RCT showed a significant improvement of affect (measured with the Beck Depression Inventory and the Hamilton for Depression Rating Scale (HDRS)), parasuicidal behaviors and stress reactivity in the treatment group. Aggressiveness, measured with the MOAS score, and impulsive behaviors, assessed with the Memory Delay Task, did not obtain a significant difference in the two groups.

On the basis of this background, our research group performed a RCT in order to assess the efficacy and tolerability of omega-3 fatty acids in combination with valproic acid in a group of 43 BPD patients [118] who were randomly assigned to two treatments for twelve weeks: (1) valproic acid (800–1300 mg/day) (plasma range: 50–100 μg/mL); (2) EPA (1.2 g/day) and DHA (0.6 g/day) in combination with the same dose of valproic acid. Results indicated that the association of omega-3 fatty acids and valproate was effective in reducing the severity of characteristic BPD symptoms, measured with the Borderline Personality Disorder Severity Index (BPDSI), impulsive behavioral dyscontrol, assessed with the Barratt Impulsiveness Scale (BIS-11), outbursts of anger, evaluated with the item "outburst of anger" of the BPDSI, and self-mutilating conduct, measured with the Self-Harm Inventory (SHI) (Table 5).

Table 5. Double-blind controlled trials of HUFAs in the treatment of impulsivity and borderline personality disorder.

Study	Drug and Dose	Sample	Treatment Duration	Results
Hamazaki et al., 1996 [113]	DHA 1.5–1.8 g/day	41 healthy controls (21–30 years)	3 months	↓ aggression
Bradbury et al. (2004) [115]	DHA 1.5 g/day	47 healthy controls (18–60 years)	6 weeks	↓ level of stress
Itomura et al. (2005) [114]	DHA 3.6 g/day + EPA 0.84 g/day	166 healthy controls (9–12 years)	3 months	↓ aggression, ↓ impulsivity
Zanarini and Frankenburg, 2003 [116]	EPA 1 g/day (with no standard psychiatric therapies)	30 BPD females	8 weeks	↓ aggression, ↓ depression
Hallahan et al., 2007 [117]	EPA 1.2 g/day + DHA 0.9 g/day (added to the standard psychiatric therapies)	49 patients with self-defeating behaviors (39 BPD patients)	12 weeks	↓ depression, ↓ parasuicidal behaviors, ↓ stress reactivity
Bellino et al., 2014 [118]	EPA (1.2 g/day) + DHA (0.6 g/day) in combination with valproic acid (800–1300 mg/day) vs. valproic acid (800–1300 mg/day) (plasma range: 50–100 μg/mL)	43 BPD patients	12 weeks	↓ severity of BPDSI, ↓ impulsive behavioral dyscontrol, ↓ anger, ↓ self-mutilating conduct

Abbreviations: EPA = eicosapentaenoic acid; DHA = docosahexaenoic acid; ethyl-EPA = ethyl-eicosapentaenoic acid; BPDSI = Borderline Personality Disorder Severity Index; ↓ = decrease of; ↑ = increase of.

2.10. Substance Dependence

According to research, proinflammatory cytokines are responsible for the physical and psychological symptoms concomitant to craving, and EPA can neutralize these molecules' toxic effects in the brain [75,119]. The neuroprotective effect of omega-3s on the production of serotonin and its action on the prefrontal cortex may also help with maintaining executive ability, both compromised during withdrawal and craving. Only two studies have been conducted to assess the efficacy of omega-3 fatty acid in the treatment of substance dependence [75,120]. The first study [75] evaluated the efficacy of EPA + DHA (3 g/day) for a period of three months on anxiety symptoms in addicted patients. The group treated with omega-3s showed a significant reduction in anxiety when compared to placebo. These results were replicated and confirmed by the following study performed by the same authors [120].

2.11. Anorexia Nervosa

Two studies, focused on the deficit in the concentration of HUFAs complexed to membrane phospholipids in patients with anorexia nervosa, showed similar results. Holman and colleagues [121] examined the concentration of fatty acids in plasma in a population of eight hospitalized anorexia nervosa fasting females compared to 19 healthy female adults <25 years old. Subjects with anorexia nervosa had deficiencies of essential fatty acids and showed decreased concentrations of total omega-6 and omega-3 acids, compared to the control group; this indicates compensatory changes in non-essential fatty acids and can lead to a consequent problem in terms of membrane structure and fluidity. Furthermore, Langan and Farrell [122] reported a concomitant significantly reduction of omega-3 and omega-6 in plasma phospholipids' concentration in a group of 17 patients (16 females, one male) hospitalized for anorexia nervosa compared to 11 normal females.

Only two trials have been conducted to assess the efficacy of omega-3 fatty acid in the treatment of anorexia nervosa. In the first pilot open label study, conducted by Ayton [123], seven patients between 13 and 22 years old with anorexia nervosa, restrictive subtype, received 1 g/day EPA in addition to standard treatment for three months. This small study showed a general improvement in sleep, mood, dry skin and constipation (measured with Weight 4 Height software, the Eating Disorder Inventory (EDI-2), the Morgan-Russell Average Outcome Scale (MRAOS), BDI-2, the Children's Global Assessment Scale (CGA-S) and CGI-S.

Negative results in this clinical population were reported by Barbarich and collaborators [124]. Twenty six subjects with anorexia nervosa (10 subjects were restricting-type; six subjects were restricting and purging only-type; and 10 subjects were binge eating/purging-type) participated in a six-month trial of fluoxetine (20–60 mg/die). Using a randomized, double-blind design, subjects were assigned to either nutritional supplements (600 mg of DHA and 180 mg of arachidonic acid daily, tryptophan, vitamins, minerals) or placebo. Patients were evaluated with: the Frost Multidimensional Perfectionism Scale (FMPS), the State-Trait Anxiety Inventory (STAI-Y) and Yale-Brown Obsessive Compulsive Scale (Y-BOCS). They were also weighed at weekly intervals for the first eight weeks, at two-week intervals for the following six weeks and at 4-week intervals for a further 12 weeks. There were no significant differences in weight gain per week between subjects treated with fluoxetine plus nutritional supplements vs. fluoxetine plus placebo. Moreover, there were no significant differences between groups in mean changes of anxiety or obsessive and compulsive symptoms.

3. Adverse Effects

Omega-3 fatty acids did not induce serious adverse effects and were generally well tolerated: most common side effects reported in clinical trials were nausea and a fishy aftertaste, but they were mild and rarely induced discontinuation [125]. The Panel of The European Food Safety Authority (EFSA) concluded that the available data are insufficient to establish a tolerable daily intake (UL) of DHA, EPA and DPA individually or in combination, but the supplementation with EPA and DHA up to 5 g/day is not dangerous for the general population [126]. In particular, EPA and DHA are generally recognized as safe and well tolerated at dose up to 5 g/day in terms of bleeding risk, as pointed out by Yokoyama et al. [127] and Tanaka et al. [128]. In addition, doses up to 5 g/day, consumed for a maximum period of 12–16 weeks, do not significantly affect glucose regulation in both healthy and diabetic subjects [119,129–131] and do not increase infection risk by the activation of inappropriate inflammatory responses [132]. The intake of EPA and DHA at the same dose and up to 16 weeks does not induce alteration of lipid peroxidation and does not increase cardiovascular risk [133]. Combined intake of EPA and DHA at the dose of 2–6 g/day and intake of DHA at the dose of 2–4 g/die are responsible for an LDL concentration increase (3%), but do not affect cardiovascular risk. At last, an intake of EPA at the maximum dose of 4 g/day does not induce significant changes in LDL plasma levels [134].

4. Conclusions

In the last decade, the role of long-chain HUFAs in the treatment of several psychiatric diseases has gradually increased, as confirmed by the growing number of randomized controlled trials testing the efficacy of essential fatty acid, especially omega-3 HUFA, supplementation. Nevertheless, an overall consensus about their efficacy is still lacking, and the findings of most of trials are controversial and inconclusive. Differences in methods, including sample size, selection criteria, choice and dosage of fatty acids (i.e., EPA, or DHA, or a combination of the two, or the addition of omega-6 HUFAs) and the duration of supplementation often make results not comparable.

The main evidence for the efficacy of EPA and DHA has been obtained in mood disorders. In particular, omega-3 fatty acids seem to be useful in preventing and improving depressive symptoms at a low dose of 1 g/day; EPA seems to be more efficacious than DHA; patients with more severe depression showed greater treatment gains. However, due to the considerable heterogeneity of the investigations, additional large cohort studies and well-designed clinical trials are warranted. Concerning bipolar disorder, the results of systematic reviews and meta-analyses suggested a potential beneficial role of omega-3 fatty acids in addition to stable medications in treating depressive symptom at the approximate dose of 1–2 g/day, but did not support their use in attenuating mania. Furthermore, studies using a combination of EPA and DHA reported a statistically-significant improvement in symptoms of bipolar depression, whereas trials using a single compound did not. In schizophrenia, little evidence of a meaningful clinical effect was reported, and current data do not allow us either to refuse or support the use of omega-3 fatty acids in psychotic patients. However, adverse effects of antipsychotics, in particular metabolic abnormalities and extrapyramidal symptoms, may benefit from the addition of EPA or a combination of EPA and DHA. In ADHD disorder, several RCTs have been performed, but the main findings have reported small-to-modest effects of omega-3 HUFAs in reducing ADHD symptoms in children. Most promising results in this field have been reached by studies using EPA at high doses or the association of omega-3 and omega-6 fatty acids. Anyway, the relative efficacy of these agents was modest compared to the currently available pharmacotherapies. To date, a small number of clinical trials have explored the impact of HUFAs on impulsive and aggressive behaviors and a growing number of studies has been conducted in order to test the efficacy of these agents in borderline personality disorder. Results are encouraging, although this area of psychopathology needs to be explored in depth by future investigations. In autism spectrum disorders, only two RCTs with opposite results are available, whereas there is a substantial lack of data about the use of omega-3 fatty acids in anxiety disorders and obsessive-compulsive disorder. The majority of trials assessing patients with mood disorders did not investigate changes in anxiety symptoms, although anxiety is frequently associated with depression or mania. HUFAs were not found efficacious in treating eating disorders and substance use disorders. Concerning tolerability, RCTs considered in this review share a common finding: omega-3 fatty acids did not induce serious adverse effects. A survey of studies concluded that omega-3 are generally recognized as safe and well tolerated at doses up to 5 g/day for a maximum period of 12–16 weeks. Several authors have assessed the effects of omega-3 HUFA administration in terms of bleeding risk, glucose metabolism, lipid profile, infection risk and cardiovascular function with a general consensus about their harmlessness.

In summary, preliminary findings on omega-3 fatty acids in psychiatric populations allow us to consider these naturally-derived and well-tolerated psychotropic agents as a promising therapeutic tool. However, their efficacy in treating specific mental disorders or clusters of psychiatric symptoms is not sufficiently proven, as the findings from studies and reviews are too divergent to draw any conclusion.

Acknowledgments: No funds or grants were received by the authors to support or cover the costs of publishing this work.

References

1. Ergas, D.; Eilat, E.; Mendlovic, S.; Sthoeger, Z.M. *n*-3 fatty acids and the immune system in autoimmunity. *Isr. Med. Assoc. J.* **2002**, *4*, 34–38. [PubMed]

2. Simopoulos, A.P. Essential fatty acids in health and chronic disease. *Am. J. Clin. Nutr.* **1999**, *70* (Suppl. 3), 560–569.

3. Lee, S.; Gura, K.M.; Kim, S.; Arsenault, D.A.; Bistrian, B.R.; Puder, M. Current clinical applications of omega-6 and omega-3 fatty acids. *Nutr. Clin. Pract.* **2006**, *21*, 323–341. [CrossRef] [PubMed]

4. Milte, C.M.; Sinn, N.; Buckley, J.D.; Coates, A.M.; Young, R.M.; Howe, P.R. Polyunsaturated fatty acids, cognition and literacy in children with ADHD with and without learning difficulties. *J. Child Health Care* **2011**, *15*, 299–311. [CrossRef] [PubMed]

5. Garland, M.R.; Hallahan, B. Essential fatty acids and their role in conditions characterised by impulsivity. *Int. Rev. Psychiatry* **2006**, *18*, 99–105. [CrossRef] [PubMed]

6. Ross, B.M.; Seguin, J.; Sieswerda, L.E. Omega-3 fatty acids as treatments for mental illness: Which disorder and which fatty acid? *Lipids Health Dis.* **2007**, *6*, 21. [CrossRef] [PubMed]

7. Hallahan, B.; Garland, M.R. Essential fatty acids and mental health. *Br. J. Psychiatry* **2005**, *186*, 275–277. [CrossRef] [PubMed]

8. Sinn, N.; Milte, C.; Howe, P.R. Oiling the brain: A review of randomized controlled trials of omega-3 fatty acids in psychopathology across the lifespan. *Nutrients* **2010**, *2*, 128–170. [CrossRef] [PubMed]

9. Assisi, A.; Banzi, R.; Buonocore, C.; Capasso, F.; Di Muzio, V.; Michelacci, F.; Renzo, D.; Tafuri, G.; Trotta, F.; Vitocolonna, M.; et al. Fish oil and mental health: The role of *n*-3 long-chain polyunsaturated fatty acids in cognitive development and neurological disorders. *Int. Clin. Psychopharmacol.* **2006**, *21*, 319–336. [CrossRef] [PubMed]

10. De la Pressa, O.S.; Innis, S.M. Docosahexanoic and arachidonic acid prevent a decrease in dopaminergic and serotoninergic neurotrasmitters in frontal cortex caused by a linoleic and alpha-linoleic acid deficient diet in formula-fed piglets. *J. Nutr.* **1999**, *129*, 2088–2093.

11. Hamazaki, K.; Maekawa, M. Fatty acid composition of the postmortem prefrontal cortex of patients with schizophrenia, bipolar disorder, and major depressive disorder. *Psychiatry Res.* **2015**, *227*, 353–359. [CrossRef] [PubMed]

12. Glen, A.I.; Glen, E.M.; Horrobin, D.F.; Vaddadi, K.S.; Spellman, M.; Morse-Fisher, N.; Ellis, K.; Skinner, F.S. A red cell membrane abnormality in a subgroup of schizophrenic patients: Evidence for two diseases. *Schizophr. Res.* **1994**, *12*, 53–61. [CrossRef]

13. Horrobin, D.F. The membrane phospholipid hypothesis as a biochemical basis for the neurodevelopmental concept of schizophrenia. *Schizophr. Res.* **1998**, *30*, 193–208. [CrossRef]

14. Schlögelhofer, M.; Amminger, G.P.; Schaefer, M.R.; Fusar-Poli, P.; Smesny, S.; McGorry, P.; Berger, G.; Mossaheb, N. Polyunsaturated fatty acids in emerging psychosis: A safer alternative? *Early Interv. Psychiatry* **2014**, *8*, 199–208. [CrossRef] [PubMed]

15. Amminger, G.P.; Schäfer, M.R.; Papageorgiou, K.; Klier, C.M.; Cotton, S.M.; Harrigan, S.M.; Mackinnon, A.; McGorry, P.D.; Berger, G.E. Long-chain omega-3 fatty acids for indicated prevention of psychotic disorders: A randomized, placebo-controlled trial. *Arch. Gen. Psychiatry* **2010**, *67*, 146–154. [CrossRef] [PubMed]

16. Markulev, C.; McGorry, P.D.; Nelson, B.; Yuen, H.P.; Schaefer, M.; Yung, A.R.; Thompson, A.; Berger, G.; Mossaheb, N.; Schlögelhofer, M.; et al. NEURAPRO-E study protocol: A multicentre randomized controlled trial of omega-3 fatty acids and cognitive-behavioural case management for patients at ultra high risk of schizophrenia and other psychotic disorders. *Early Interv. Psychiatry* **2015**. [CrossRef] [PubMed]

17. Peet, M.; Brind, J.; Ramchand, C.N.; Shah, S.; Vankar, G.K. Two double-blind placebo-controlled pilot studies of eicosapentaenoic acid in the treatment of schizophrenia. *Schizophr. Res.* **2001**, *49*, 243–251. [CrossRef]

18. Emsley, R.; Chiliza, B.; Asmal, L.; Emsley, R.; Chiliza, B.; Asmal, L.; du Plessis, S.; Phahladira, L.; van Niekerk, E.; van Rensburg, S.J.; et al. A randomized, controlled trial of omega-3 fatty acids plus an antioxidant for relapse prevention after antipsychotic discontinuation in first-episode schizophrenia. *Schizophr. Res.* **2014**, *158*, 230–235. [CrossRef] [PubMed]

19. Peet, M.; Horrobin, D.F.; Study Group. A dose-ranging exploratory study of the effects of ethyl-eicosapentaenoate in patients with persistent schizophrenic symptoms. *J. Psychiat. Res.* **2002**, *36*, 7–18. [CrossRef]

20. Jamilian, H.; Solhi, H.; Jamilian, M. Randomized, placebo-controlled clinical trial of omega-3 as supplemental treatment in schizophrenia. *Glob. J. Health Sci.* **2014**, *18*, 103–108. [CrossRef] [PubMed]

21. Pawełczyk, T.; Grancow-Grabka, M.; Kotlicka-Antczak, M.; Trafalska, E.; Pawełczyk, A. A randomized controlled study of the efficacy of six-month supplementation with concentrated fish oil rich in omega-3 polyunsaturated fatty acids in first episode schizophrenia. *J. Psychiat. Res.* **2016**, *73*, 34–44. [CrossRef] [PubMed]

22. Bentsen, H.; Osnes, K.; Refsum, H. A randomized placebo-controlled trial of an omega-3 fatty acid and vitamins E + C in schizophrenia. *Transl. Psychiatry* **2013**. [CrossRef] [PubMed]

23. Fenton, W.S.; Dickerson, F.; Boronow, J.; Hibbeln, J.R.; Knable, M. A placebo-controlled trial of omega-3 fatty acid (ethyl eicosapentaenoic acid) supplementation for residual symptoms and cognitive impairment in schizophrenia. *Am. J. Psychiatry* **2001**, *158*, 2071–2074. [CrossRef] [PubMed]

24. Berger, G.E.; Wood, S.J.; Wellard, R.M.; Proffitt, T.M.; McConchie, M.; Amminger, G.P.; Jackson, G.D.; Velakoulis, D.; Pantelis, C.; McGorry, P.D. Ethyl-eicosapentaenoic acid in first-episode psychosis. A 1H-MRS study. *Neuropsychopharmacology* **2007**, *33*, 2467–2473. [CrossRef] [PubMed]

25. Joy, C.B.; Mumby-Croft, R.; Joy, L.A. Polyunsaturated fatty acid supplementation for schizophrenia. *Cochrane Database Syst. Rev.* **2006**, *19*, CD001257.

26. Freeman, M.P.; Hibbeln, J.R.; Wisner, K.L.; Davis, J.M.; Mischoulon, D.; Peet, M.; Keck, P.E., Jr.; Marangell, L.B.; Richardson, A.J.; Lake, J.; et al. Omega-3 fatty acids: Evidence basis for treatment and future research in psychiatry. *J. Clin. Psychiatry* **2006**, *67*, 1954–1967. [CrossRef] [PubMed]

27. Fusar-Poli, P.; Berger, G. Eicosapentaenoic acid interventions in schizophrenia: Meta-analysis of randomized, placebo-controlled studies. *J. Clin. Psychopharmacol.* **2012**, *32*, 179–185. [CrossRef] [PubMed]

28. Akter, K.; Gallo, D.A.; Martin, S.A.; Myronyuk, N.; Roberts, R.T.; Stercula, K.; Raffa, R.B. A review of the possible role of the essential fatty acids and fish oils in the aetiology, prevention or pharmacotherapy of schizophrenia. *J. Clin. Pharm. Ther.* **2012**, *37*, 132–139. [CrossRef] [PubMed]

29. Emsley, R.; Myburgh, C.; Oosthuizen, P.; van Rensburg, S.J. Randomized, placebo-controlled study of ethyl-eicosapentaenoic acid as supplemental treatment in schizophrenia. *Am. J. Psychiatry* **2002**, *159*, 1596–1598. [CrossRef] [PubMed]

30. Emsley, R.; Niehaus, D.J.; Koen, L.; Oosthuizen, P.P.; Turner, H.J.; Carey, P.; Murck, H. The effects of eicosapentaenoic acid in tardive dyskinesia: A randomized, placebo-controlled trial. *Schizophr. Res.* **2006**, *84*, 112–120. [CrossRef] [PubMed]

31. Hibbeln, J.R.; Umhau, J.C.; Linnoila, M.; George, D.T.; Ragan, P.W.; Shoaf, S.E.; Vaughan, M.R.; Rawlings, R.; Salem, N., Jr. A replication study of violent and non-violent subjects: CSF metabolites of serotonin and dopamine are predicted by plasma essential fatty acids. *Biol. Psychiatry* **1998**, *44*, 243–249. [CrossRef]

32. Horrobin, D.F.; Bennett, C.N. Depression and bipolar disorder: Relationships to impaired fatty acid and phospholipid metabolism and to diabetes, cardiovascular disease, immunological abnormalities, cancer, ageing and osteoporosis. Possible candidate genes. *Prostaglandins Leukort. Essent. Fatty Acids* **1999**, *60*, 217–234. [CrossRef] [PubMed]

33. Tanskanen, A.; Hibbeln, J.R.; Hintikka, J.; Haatainen, K.; Honkalampi, K.; Viinamäki, H. Fish consumption, depression, and suicidality in a general population. *Arch. Gen. Psychiatry* **2001**, *58*, 512–513. [CrossRef] [PubMed]

34. Lin, P.Y.; Huang, S.Y.; Su, K.P. A meta-analytic review of polyunsaturated fatty acid compositions in patients with depression. *Biol. Psychiatry* **2010**, *68*, 140–147. [CrossRef] [PubMed]

35. Peet, M.; Horrobin, D.F. A dose-ranging study of the effects of ethyl-eicosapentaenoate in patients with ongoing depression despite apparently adequate treatment with standard drugs. *Arch. Gen. Psychiatry* **2002**, *59*, 913–919. [CrossRef] [PubMed]

36. Su, K.P.; Huang, S.Y.; Chiu, C.C.; Shen, W.W. Omega-3 fatty acids in major depressive disorder. A preliminary double-blind, placebo-controlled trial. *Eur. Neuropsychopharmacol.* **2003**, *13*, 267–271. [CrossRef]

37. Lespérance, F.; Frasure-Smith, N.; St-André, E.; Lespérance, F.; Frasure-Smith, N.; St-André, E.; Turecki, G.; Lespérance, P.; Wisniewski, S.R. The efficacy of omega-3 supplementation for major depression: A randomized controlled trial. *J. Clin. Psychiatry* **2011**, *72*, 1054–1062.

38. Jazayeri, S.; Tehrani-Doost, M.; Keshavarz, S.A.; Hosseini, M.; Djazayery, A.; Amini, H.; Jalali, M.; Peet, M. Comparison of therapeutic effects of omega-3 fatty acid eicosapentaenoic acid and fluoxetine, separately and in combination, in major depressive disorder. *Aust. N. Z. J. Psychiatry* **2008**, *42*, 192–198. [CrossRef] [PubMed]

39. Gertsik, L.; Poland, R.E.; Bresee, C.; Rapaport, M.H. Omega-3 fatty acid augmentation of citalopram treatment for patients with major depressive disorder. *J. Clin. Psychopharmacol.* **2012**, *32*, 61–64. [CrossRef] [PubMed]

40. Nemets, B.; Stahl, Z.; Belmaker, R.H. Addition of omega-3 fatty acid to maintenance medication treatment for recurrent unipolar depressive disorder. *Am. J. Psychiatry* **2002**, *159*, 477–479. [CrossRef] [PubMed]

41. Nemets, H.; Nemets, B.; Apter, A.; Bracha, Z.; Belmaker, R.H. Omega-3 treatment of childhood depression: A controlled, double-blind pilot study. *Am. J. Psychiatry* **2006**, *163*, 1098–1100. [CrossRef] [PubMed]

42. Su, K.P.; Huang, S.Y.; Chiu, T.H.; Huang, K.C.; Huang, C.L.; Chang, H.C.; Pariante, C.M. Omega-3 fatty acids for major depressive disorder during pregnancy: Results from a randomized, double-blind, placebo-controlled trial. *J. Clin. Psychiatry* **2008**, *69*, 644–651. [CrossRef] [PubMed]

43. Rondanelli, M.; Giacosa, A.; Opizzi, A.; Pelucchi, C.; La Vecchia, C.; Montorfano, G.; Negroni, M.; Berra, B.; Politi, P.; Rizzo, A.M. Long chain omega 3 polyunsaturated fatty acids supplementation in the treatment of elderly depression: Effects on depressive symptoms, on phospholipids fatty acids profile and on health-related quality of life. *J. Nutr. Health Aging* **2011**, *15*, 37–44. [CrossRef] [PubMed]

44. Rondanelli, M.; Giacosa, A.; Opizzi, A.; Pelucchi, C.; La Vecchia, C.; Montorfano, G.; Negroni, M.; Berra, B.; Politi, P.; Rizzo, A.M. Effect of omega-3 fatty acids supplementation on depressive symptoms and on health-related quality of life in the treatment of elderly women with depression: A double-blind, placebo-controlled, randomized clinical trial. *J. Am. Coll. Nutr.* **2010**, *29*, 55–64. [CrossRef] [PubMed]

45. Rizzo, A.M.; Corsetto, P.A.; Montorfano, G.; Opizzi, A.; Faliva, M.; Giacosa, A.; Ricevuti, G.; Pelucchi, C.; Berra, B.; Rondanelli, M. Comparison between the AA/EPA ratio in depressed and non depressed elderly females: Omega-3 fatty acid supplementation correlates with improved symptoms but does not change immunological parameters. *Nutr. J.* **2012**, *11*, 82. [CrossRef] [PubMed]

46. Rees, A.M.; Austin, M.P.; Parker, G.B. Omega-3 fatty acids as a treatment for perinatal depression: Randomized double-blind placebo-controlled trial. *Aust. N. Z. J. Psychiatry* **2008**, *42*, 199–205. [CrossRef] [PubMed]

47. Freeman, M.P.; Davis, M.; Sinha, P.; Wisner, K.L.; Hibbeln, J.R.; Gelenberg, A.J. Omega-3 fatty acids and supportive psychotherapy for perinatal depression: A randomized placebo-controlled study. *J. Affect Disord.* **2008**, *110*, 142–148. [CrossRef] [PubMed]

48. Marangell, L.B.; Martinez, J.M.; Zboyan, H.A.; Kertz, B.; Kim, H.F.; Puryear, L.J. A double-blind, placebo-controlled study of the omega-3 fatty acid docosahexaenoic acid in the treatment of major depression. *Am. J. Psychiatry* **2003**, *160*, 996–998. [CrossRef] [PubMed]

49. Silvers, K.M.; Woolley, C.C.; Hamilton, F.C.; Watts, P.M.; Watson, R.A. Randomised double-blind placebo-controlled trial of fish oil in the treatment of depression. *Prostaglandins Leukort. Essent. Fatty Acids* **2005**, *72*, 211–218. [CrossRef] [PubMed]

50. Grenyer, B.F.; Crowe, T.; Meyer, B.; Owen, A.J.; Grigonis-Deane, E.M.; Caputi, P.; Howe, P.R. Fish oil supplementation in the treatment of major depression: A randomised double-blind placebo-controlled trial. *Prog. Neuropsychopharmacol. Biol. Psychiatry* **2007**, *31*, 1393–1396. [CrossRef] [PubMed]

51. Rogers, P.J.; Appleton, K.M.; Kessler, D.; Peters, T.J.; Gunnell, D.; Hayward, R.C.; Heatherley, S.V.; Christian, L.M.; McNaughton, S.A.; Ness, A.R. No effect of *n*-3 long-chain polyunsaturated fatty acid (EPA and DHA) supplementation on depressed mood and cognitive function: A randomised controlled trial. *Br. J. Nutr.* **2008**, *99*, 421–431. [CrossRef] [PubMed]

52. Antypa, N.; Smelt, A.H.; Strengholt, A.; Van der Does, A.J. Effects of omega-3 fatty acid supplementation on mood and emotional information processing in recovered depressed individuals. *J. Psychopharmacol.* **2012**, *26*, 738–743. [CrossRef] [PubMed]

53. Mischoulon, D.; Best-Popescu, C.; Laposata, M.; Merens, W.; Murakami, J.L.; Wu, S.L.; Papakostas, G.I.; Dording, C.M.; Sonawalla, S.B.; Nierenberg, A.A.; et al. A double-blind dose-finding pilot study of docosahexaenoic acid (DHA) for major depressive disorder. *Eur. Neuropsychopharmacol.* **2008**, *18*, 639–645. [CrossRef] [PubMed]

54. Mischoulon, D.; Nierenberg, A.A.; Schettler, P.J.; Kinkead, B.L.; Fehling, K.; Martinson, M.A.; Hyman Rapaport, M. A double-blind, randomized controlled clinical trial comparing eicosapentaenoic acid *versus* docosahexaenoic acid for depression. *J. Clin. Psychiat.* **2015**, *76*, 54–61. [CrossRef] [PubMed]

55. Carney, R.M.; Freedland, K.E.; Rubin, E.H.; Rich, M.W.; Steinmeyer, B.C.; Harris, W.S. Omega-3 augmentation of sertraline in treatment of depression in patients with coronary heart disease: A randomized controlled trial. *JAMA* **2009**, *302*, 1651–1657. [CrossRef] [PubMed]

56. Appleton, K.M.; Rogers, P.J.; Ness, A.R. Updated systematic review and meta-analysis of the effects of *n*-3 long-chain polyunsaturated fatty acids on depressed mood. *Am. J. Clin. Nutr.* **2010**, *91*, 757–770. [CrossRef] [PubMed]

57. Bloch, M.H.; Hannestad, J. Omega-3 fatty acids for the treatment of depression: Systematic review and meta-analysis. *Mol. Psychiatry* **2012**, *17*, 1272–1282. [CrossRef] [PubMed]

58. Lin, P.Y.; Su, K.P. A meta-analytic review of double-blind, placebo-controlled trials of antidepressant efficacy of omega-3 fatty acids. *J. Clin. Psychiatry* **2007**, *68*, 1056–1061. [CrossRef] [PubMed]

59. Martins, J.G. EPA but not DHA appears to be responsible for the efficacy of omega-3 long chain polyunsaturated fatty acid supplementation in depression: Evidence from a meta-analysis of randomized controlled trials. *J. Am. Coll. Nutr.* **2009**, *28*, 525–542. [CrossRef] [PubMed]

60. Sublette, M.E.; Ellis, S.P.; Geant, A.L.; Mann, J.J. Meta-analysis of the effects of eicosapentaenoic acid (EPA) in clinical trials in depression. *J. Clin. Psychiatry* **2011**, *72*, 1577–1584. [CrossRef] [PubMed]

61. Grosso, G.; Pajak, A.; Marventano, S.; Castellano, S.; Galvano, F.; Bucolo, C.; Caraci, F. Role of omega-3 fatty acids in the treatment of depressive disorders: A comprehensive meta-analysis of randomized clinical trials. *PLoS ONE* **2014**, *9*, e96905. [CrossRef] [PubMed]

62. Chiu, C.C.; Huang, S.Y.; Su, K.P.; Lu, M.L.; Huang, M.C.; Chen, C.C.; Shen, W.W. Polyunsaturated fatty acid deficit in patients with bipolar mania. *Eur. Neuropsychopharmacol.* **2003**, *13*, 99–103. [CrossRef]

63. Frangou, S.; Lewis, M.; McCrone, P. Efficacy of ethyl-eicosapentaenoic acid in bipolar depression: Randomised double-blind placebo-controlled study. *Br. J. Psychiatry* **2006**, *188*, 46–50. [CrossRef] [PubMed]

64. Frangou, S.; Lewis, M.; Wollard, J.; Simmons, A. Preliminary in vivo evidence of increased *N*-acetyl-aspartate following eicosapentanoic acid treatment in patients with bipolar disorder. *J. Psychopharmacol.* **2007**, *21*, 435–439. [CrossRef] [PubMed]

65. Keck, P.E., Jr.; Mintz, J.; McElroy, S.L.; Freeman, M.P.; Suppes, T.; Frye, M.A.; Altshuler, L.L.; Kupka, R.; Nolen, W.A.; Leverich, G.S.; et al. Double-blind, randomized, placebo-controlled trials of ethyl-eicosapentanoate in the treatment of bipolar depression and rapid cycling bipolar disorder. *Biol. Psychiatry* **2006**, *60*, 1020–1022. [CrossRef] [PubMed]

66. Stoll, A.L.; Severus, W.E.; Freeman, M.P.; Rueter, S.; Zboyan, H.A.; Diamond, E.; Cress, K.K.; Marangell, L.B. Omega 3 fatty acids in bipolar disorder: A preliminary double-blind, placebo-controlled trial. *Arch. Gen. Psychiatry* **1999**, *56*, 407–412. [CrossRef] [PubMed]

67. Chiu, C.C.; Huang, S.Y.; Chen, C.C.; Su, K.P. Omega-3 fatty acids are more beneficial in the depressive phase than in the manic phase in patients with bipolar I disorder. *J. Clin. Psychiatry* **2005**, *66*, 1613–1614. [CrossRef] [PubMed]

68. Gracious, B.L.; Chirieac, M.C.; Costescu, S.; Finucane, T.L.; Youngstrom, E.A.; Hibbeln, J.R. Randomized, placebo-controlled trial of flax oil in pediatric bipolar disorder. *Bipolar Disord.* **2010**, *12*, 142–154. [CrossRef] [PubMed]

69. Murphy, B.L.; Stoll, A.L.; Harris, P.Q.; Ravichandran, C.; Babb, S.M.; Carlezon, W.A., Jr.; Cohen, B.M. Omega-3 fatty acid treatment, with or without cytidine, fails to show therapeutic properties in bipolar disorder: A double-blind, randomized add-on clinical trial. *J. Clin. Psychopharmacol.* **2012**, *32*, 699–703. [CrossRef] [PubMed]

70. Turnbull, T.; Cullen-Drill, M.; Smaldone, A. Efficacy of omega-3 fatty acid supplementation on improvement of bipolar symptoms: A systematic review. *Arch. Psychiat. Nurs.* **2008**, *22*, 305–311. [CrossRef] [PubMed]

71. Montgomery, P.; Richardson, A.J. Omega-3 fatty acids for bipolar disorder. *Cochrane Database Syst. Rev.* **2008**, *2*, CD005169. [CrossRef] [PubMed]

72. Kraguljac, N.V.; Montori, V.M.; Pavuluri, M.; Chai, H.S.; Wilson, B.S.; Unal, S.S. Efficacy of omega-3 fatty acids in mood disorders—A systematic review and metaanalysis. *Psychopharmacol. Bull.* **2009**, *42*, 39–54. [PubMed]

73. Sarris, J.; Mischoulon, D.; Schweitzer, I. Omega-3 for bipolar disorder: Meta-analyses of use in mania and bipolar depression. *J. Clin. Psychiatry* **2012**, *73*, 81–86. [CrossRef] [PubMed]

74. Ross, B.M. Omega-3 polyunsaturated fatty acids and anxiety disorders. *Prostaglandins Leukort. Essent. Fatty Acids* **2009**, *81*, 309–312. [CrossRef] [PubMed]

75. Green, P. Red cell membrane omega-3 fatty acids are decreased in nondepressed patients with social anxiety disorder. *Eur. Neuropsychopharmacol.* **2006**, *16*, 107–113. [CrossRef] [PubMed]

76. Liu, J.J. Omega-3 Polyunsaturated fatty acid status in major depression with comorbid anxiety disorders. *J. Clin. Psychiatry* **2013**, *74*, 732–738. [CrossRef] [PubMed]

77. Buydens-Branchey, L.; Branchey, M. *n*-3 polyunsaturated fatty acids decrease anxiety feelings in a population of substance abusers. *J. Clin. Psychopharmacol.* **2006**, *26*, 661–665. [CrossRef] [PubMed]

78. Ravindran, A.V.; da Silva, T.L. Complementary and alternative therapies as add-on to pharmacotherapy for mood and anxiety disorders: A systematic review. *J. Affect Disord.* **2013**, *150*, 707–719. [CrossRef] [PubMed]

79. Fux, M.; Benjamin, J.; Nemets, B. A placebo-controlled cross-over trial of adjunctive EPA in OCD. *J. Psychiat. Res.* **2004**, *38*, 323–325. [CrossRef]

80. Mitchell, E.A.; Aman, M.G.; Turbott, S.H.; Manku, M. Clinical characteristics and serum essential fatty acid levels in hyperactive children. *Clin. Pediatr. (Phila.)* **1987**, *26*, 406–411. [CrossRef] [PubMed]

81. Stevens, L.; Zhang, W.; Peck, L.; Kuczek, T.; Grevstad, N.; Mahon, A.; Zentall, S.S.; Arnold, L.E.; Burgess, J.R. EFA supplementation in children with inattention, hyperactivity, and other disruptive behaviors. *Lipids* **2003**, *38*, 1007–1021. [CrossRef] [PubMed]

82. Burgess, J.R.; Stevens, L.; Zhang, W.; Peck, L. Long-chain polyunsaturated fatty acids in children with attention-deficit hyperactivity disorder. *Am. J. Clin. Nutr.* **2000**, *71* (Suppl. 1), 327S–330S. [PubMed]

83. Hibbelna, J.R.; Gowb, R.V. Omega-3 fatty acid and nutrient deficits in adverse neurodevelopment and childhood behaviors. *Child Adolesc. Psychiatr. Clin. N. Am.* **2014**, *23*, 555–590.

84. Richardson, A.J.; Puri, B.K. A randomized double-blind, placebo-controlled study of the effects of supplementation with highly unsaturated fatty acids on ADHD-related symptoms in children with specific learning difficulties. *Prog. Neuropsychopharmacol. Biol. Psychiatry* **2002**, *26*, 233–239. [CrossRef]

85. Richardson, A.J.; Montgomery, P. The Oxford-Durham study: A randomized, controlled trial of dietary supplementation with fatty acids in children with developmental coordination disorder. *Pediatrics* **2005**, *115*, 1360–1366. [CrossRef] [PubMed]

86. Sinn, N.; Bryan, J. Effect of supplementation with polyunsaturated fatty acids and micronutrients on learning and behavior problems associated with child ADHD. *J. Dev. Behav. Pediatr.* **2007**, *28*, 82–91. [CrossRef] [PubMed]

87. Sinn, N.; Bryan, J.; Wilson, C. Cognitive effects of polyunsaturated fatty acids in children with attention deficit hyperactivity disorder symptoms: A randomised controlled trial. *Prostaglandins Leukort. Essent. Fatty Acids* **2008**, *78*, 311–326. [CrossRef] [PubMed]

88. Bélanger, S.A.; Vanasse, M.; Spahis, S.; Sylvestre, M.P.; Lippé, S.; L'heureux, F.; Ghadirian, P.; Vanasse, C.M.; Levy, E. Omega-3 fatty acid treatment of children with attention-deficit hyperactivity disorder: A randomized, double-blind, placebo-controlled study. *Paediatr. Child Health* **2009**, *14*, 89–98. [PubMed]

89. Kirby, A.; Woodward, A.; Jackson, S.; Wang, Y.; Crawford, M.A. A double-blind, placebo-controlled study investigating the effects of omega-3 supplementation in children aged 8–10 years from a mainstream school population. *Res. Dev. Disabil.* **2010**, *31*, 718–730. [CrossRef] [PubMed]

90. Perera, H.; Jeewandara, K.C.; Seneviratne, S.; Guruge, C. Combined $\omega 3$ and $\omega 6$ supplementation in children with attention-deficit hyperactivity disorder (ADHD) refractory to methylphenidate treatment: A double-blind, placebo-controlled study. *J. Child Neurol.* **2012**, *27*, 747–753. [CrossRef] [PubMed]

91. Voigt, R.G.; Llorente, A.M.; Jensen, C.L.; Fraley, J.K.; Berretta, M.C.; Heird, W.C. A randomized, double-blind, placebo-controlled trial of docosahexaenoic acid supplementation in children with attention-deficit/hyperactivity disorder. *J. Pediatr.* **2001**, *139*, 189–196. [CrossRef] [PubMed]

92. Hirayama, S.; Hamazaki, T.; Terasawa, K. Effect of docosahexaenoic acid-containing food administration on symptoms of attention-deficit/hyperactivity disorder—A placebo-controlled double-blind study. *Eur. J. Clin. Nutr.* **2004**, *58*, 467–473. [CrossRef] [PubMed]

93. Johnson, M.; Ostlund, S.; Fransson, G.; Kadesjö, B.; Gillberg, C. Omega-3/omega-6 fatty acids for attention deficit hyperactivity disorder: A randomized placebo-controlled trial in children and adolescents. *J. Atten. Disord.* **2009**, *12*, 394–401. [CrossRef] [PubMed]

94. Milte, C.M.; Parletta, N.; Buckley, J.D.; Coates, A.M.; Young, R.M.; Howe, P.R. Eicosapentaenoic and docosahexaenoic acids, cognition, and behavior in children with attention-deficit/hyperactivity disorder: A randomized controlled trial. *Nutrition* **2012**, *28*, 670–677. [CrossRef] [PubMed]

95. Widenhorn-Müller, K.; Schwanda, S.; Scholz, E.; Spitzer, M.; Bode, H. Effect of supplementation with long-chain ω-3 polyunsaturated fatty acids on behavior and cognition in children with attention deficit/hyperactivity disorder (ADHD): A randomized placebo-controlled intervention trial. *Prostaglandins Leukort. Essent. Fatty Acids* **2014**, *91*, 49–60. [CrossRef] [PubMed]

96. Bloch, M.H.; Qawasmi, A. Omega-3 fatty acid supplementation for the treatment of children with attention-deficit/hyperactivity disorder symptomatology: Systematic review and meta-analysis. *J. Am. Acad. Child Adolesc. Psychiatry* **2011**, *50*, 991–1000. [CrossRef] [PubMed]

97. Sonuga-Barke, E.J.S.; Brandeis, D.; Cortese, S.; Daley, D.; Ferrin, M.; Holtmann, M.; Stevenson, J.; Danckaerts, M.; van der Oord, S.; Döpfner, M.; et al. Nonpharmacological interventions for ADHD: Systematic review and metaanalyses of randomized controlled trials of dietary and psychological treatments. *Am. J. Psychiatry* **2013**, *170*, 275–289. [CrossRef] [PubMed]

98. Gillies, D.; Sinn, J.K.h.; Lad, S.S.; Leach, M.J.; Ross, M.J. Polyunsaturated fatty acids (PUFA) for attention deficit hyperactivity disorder (ADHD) in children and adolescents. *Cochrane Database Syst. Rev.* **2012**, *7*, CD007986. [PubMed]

99. Gow, R.V.; Hibbeln, J.R.; Parletta, N. Current evidence and future directions for research with omega-3 fatty acids and attention deficit hyperactivity disorder. *Curr. Opin. Clin. Nutr. Metab. Care* **2015**, *18*, 133–138. [CrossRef] [PubMed]

100. Bell, J.G.; Sargent, J.R.; Tocher, D.R.; Dick, J.R. Red blood cell fatty acid compositions in a patient with autistic spectrum disorder: A characteristic abnormality in neurodevelopmental disorders? *Prostaglandins Leukort. Essent. Fatty Acids* **2000**, *63*, 21–25. [CrossRef] [PubMed]

101. Bell, J.G.; MacKinlay, E.E.; Dick, J.R.; MacDonald, D.J.; Boyle, R.M.; Glen, A.C.A. Essential fatty acids and phospholipase A2 in autistic spectrum disorders. *Prostaglandins Leukort. Essent. Fatty Acids* **2004**, *71*, 201–204. [CrossRef] [PubMed]

102. Vancassel, S.; Durand, G.; Barthelemy, C. Plasma fatty acid levels in autistic children. *Prostaglandins Leukort. Essent. Fatty Acids* **2001**, *65*, 1–7. [CrossRef] [PubMed]

103. Belluzzi, A. *n*-3 fatty acids for the treatment of inflammatory bowel diseases. *Proc. Nutr. Soc.* **2002**, *61*, 391–395. [CrossRef] [PubMed]

104. Horvath, K.; Perman, J.A. Autism and gastrointestinal symptoms. *Curr. Gastroenterol. Rep.* **2002**, *4*, 251–258. [CrossRef] [PubMed]

105. Amminger, G.P.; Berger, G.E.; Schäfer, M.R.; Klier, C.; Friedrich, M.H.; Feucht, M. Omega-3 fatty acids supplementation in children with autism: A double-blind randomized, placebo controlled pilot study. *Biol. Psychiatry* **2007**, *61*, 551–553. [CrossRef] [PubMed]

106. Voigt, R.G.; Mellon, M.W.; Katusic, S.K.; Weaver, A.L.; Matern, D.; Mellon, B.; Jensen, C.L.; Barbaresi, W.J. Dietary docosahexaenoic acid supplementation in children with autism. *J. Pediatr. Gastroenterol. Nutr.* **2014**, *58*, 715–722. [PubMed]

107. Mankad, D.; Dupuis, A.; Smile, S.; Roberts, W.; Brian, J.; Lui, T.; Genore, L.; Zaghloul, D.; Iaboni, A.; Marcon, P.M.; et al. A randomized, placebo controlled trial of omega-3 fatty acids in the treatment of young children with autism. *Mol. Autism* **2015**. [CrossRef] [PubMed]

108. Johnson, S.M.; Hollander, E. Evidence that eicosapentaenoic acid is effective in treating autism. *J. Clin. Psychiatry* **2003**, *64*, 848–849. [CrossRef] [PubMed]

109. Patrick, L.; Salik, R. The effect of essential fatty acid supplementation on language development and learning skills in autism and Asperger's syndrome. *Autism Asperger's Dig.* Available online: http://omega-research.com/researchview.php?ID=672&catid=2 (accesssed on 21 June 2016).

110. Van Elst, K.; Bruining, H.; Birtoli, B.; Terreaux, C.; Buitelaar, J.K.; Kas, M.J. Food for thought: Dietary changes in essential fatty acid ratios and the increase in autism spectrum disorders. *Neurosci. Biobehav. Rev.* **2014**, *45*, 369–378. [CrossRef] [PubMed]

111. Stevens, L.J.; Zentall, S.S.; Abate, M.L.; Kuczek, T.; Burgess, J.R. Omega-3 fatty acids in boys with behavior, learning, and health problems. *Physiol. Behav.* **1996**, *59*, 915–920. [CrossRef]

112. Buydens-Branchey, L.; Branchey, M. Association between low plasma levels of cholesterol and relapse in cocaine addicts. *Psychosom. Med.* **2003**, *65*, 86–91. [CrossRef] [PubMed]

113. Hamazaki, T.; Sawazaki, S.; Itomura, M.; Asaoka, E.; Nagao, Y.; Nishimura, N.; Yazawa, K.; Kuwamori, T.; Kobayashi, M. The effect of docosahexaenoic acid on aggression in young adults. A placebo-controlled double-blind study. *J. Clin. Investig.* **1996**, *97*, 1129–1133. [CrossRef] [PubMed]

114. Itomura, M.; Hamazaki, K.; Sawazaki, S.; Kobayashi, M.; Terasawa, K.; Watanabe, S.; Hamazaki, T. The effect of fish oil on physical aggression in schoolchildren—A randomized, double-blind, placebo-controlled trial. *J. Nutr. Biochem.* **2005**, *16*, 163–171. [CrossRef] [PubMed]

115. Bradbury, J.; Myers, S.P.; Oliver, C. An adaptogenic role for omega-3 fatty acids in stress; a randomised placebo controlled double blind intervention study (pilot). *Nutr. J.* **2004**, *3*, 20. [CrossRef] [PubMed]

116. Zanarini, M.C.; Frankenburg, F.R. Omega-3 fatty acid treatment of women with borderline personality disorder: A double blind, placebo-controlled pilot study. *Am. J. Psychiatry* **2003**, *160*, 167–169. [CrossRef] [PubMed]

117. Hallahan, B.; Hibblen, J.R.; Davis, J.M.; Garland, M.R. Omega-3 fatty acids supplementation in patients with recurrent self-harm: Single center double bind randomized controlled trial. *Br. J. Psychiatry* **2007**, *190*, 118–122. [CrossRef] [PubMed]

118. Bellino, S.; Bozzatello, P.; Rocca, G.; Bogetto, F. Efficacy of omega-3 fatty acids in the treatment of borderline personality disorder: A study of the association with valproic acid. *J. Psychopharmacol.* **2014**, *28*, 125–132. [CrossRef] [PubMed]

119. Song, C.; Li, X.; Leonard, B.E.; Horrobin, D.F. Effects of dietary *n*-3 or *n*-6 fatty acids on interleukin-1beta-induced anxiety, stress, and inflammatory responses in rats. *J. Lipid Res.* **2003**, *44*, 1984–1991. [CrossRef] [PubMed]

120. Buydens-Branchey, L.; Branchey, M.; Hibbeln, J.R. Associations between increases in plasma *n*-3 polyunsaturated fatty acids following supplementation and decreases in anger and anxiety in substance abusers. *Prog. Neuropsychopharmacol. Biol. Psychiatry* **2008**, *32*, 568–575. [CrossRef] [PubMed]

121. Holman, R.T.; Adams, C.E.; Nelson, R.A.; Grater, S.J.; Jaskiewicz, J.A.; Johnson, S.B.; Erdman, J.W., Jr. Patients with anorexia nervosa demonstrate deficiencies of selected essential fatty acids, compensatory changes in nonessential fatty acids and decreased fluidity of plasma lipids. *J. Nutr.* **1995**, *125*, 901–907. [PubMed]

122. Langan, S.M.; Farrell, P.M. Vitamin E, vitamin A and essential fatty acid status of patients hospitalized for anorexia nervosa. *Am. J. Clin. Nutr.* **1985**, *41*, 1054–1056. [PubMed]

123. Ayton, A.K.; Azaz, A.; Horrobin, D.F. A pilot open case series of ethyl-EPA supplementation in the treatment of anorexia nervosa. *Prostaglandins Leukort. Essent. Fatty Acids* **2004**, *71*, 205–209. [CrossRef] [PubMed]

124. Barbarich, N.C.; McConaha, C.W.; Halmi, K.A.; Gendall, K.; Sunday, S.R.; Gaskill, J.; la Via, M.; Frank, G.K.; Brooks, S.; Plotnicov, K.H.; et al. Use of nutritional supplements to increase the efficacy of fluoxetine in the treatment of anorexia nervosa. *Int. J. Eat. Disord.* **2004**, *35*, 10–15. [CrossRef] [PubMed]

125. Freeman, M.P.; Fava, M.; Lake, J.; Trivedi, M.H.; Wisner, K.L.; Mischoulon, D. Complementary and alternative medicine in major depressive disorder: The American Psychiatric Association Task Force report. *J. Clin. Psychiatry* **2010**, *71*, 669–681. [CrossRef] [PubMed]

126. European Food Safety Authority (EFSA) Panel on Dietetic Products, Nutrition and Allergies (NDA). Scientific Opinion on the Tolerable Upper Intake Level of eicosapentaenoic acid (EPA), docosahexaenoic acid (DHA) and docosapentaenoic acid (DPA). *EFSA J.* **2012**, *10*, 2815.

127. Yokoyama, M.; Origasa, H.; Matsuzaki, M.; Matsuzawa, Y.; Saito, Y.; Ishikawa, Y.; Oikawa, S.; Sasaki, J.; Hishida, H.; Itakura, H.; et al. Effects of eicosapentaenoic acid on major coronary events in hypercholesterolaemic patients (JELIS): A randomised open-label, blinded endpoint analysis. *Lancet* **2007**, *369*, 1090–1098. [CrossRef]

128. Tanaka, K.; Ishikawa, Y.; Yokoyama, M.; Origasa, H.; Matsuzaki, M.; Saito, Y.; Matsuzawa, Y.; Sasaki, J.; Oikawa, S.; Hishida, H.; et al. Reduction in the recurrence of stroke by eicosapentaenoic acid for hypercholesterolemic patients: Subanalysis of the JELIS trial. *Stroke* **2008**, *39*, 2052–2058. [CrossRef] [PubMed]

129. Hartweg, J.; Perera, R.; Montori, V.; Dinneen, S.; Neil HA and Farmer, A. Omega-3 polyunsaturated fatty acids (HUFA) for type 2 diabetes mellitus. *Cochrane Database Syst. Rev.* **2008**. [CrossRef]

130. Hartweg, J.; Farmer, A.J.; Holman, R.R.; Neil, A. Potential impact of omega-3 treatment on cardiovascular disease in type 2 diabetes. *Curr. Opin. Lipidol.* **2009**, *20*, 30–38. [CrossRef] [PubMed]

131. MacLean, C.H.; Mojica, W.A.; Morton, S.C.; Pencharz, J.; Hasenfeld Garland, R. Effects of omega-3 fatty acids on lipids and glycemic control in type II diabetes and the metabolic syndrome and on inflammatory bowel disease, rheumatoid arthritis, renal disease, systemic lupus erythematosus, and osteoporosis. *Evid. Rep. Technol. Assess. (Summ.)* **2004**, *89*, 1–4. [PubMed]

132. Bloomer, R.J.; Larson, D.E.; Fisher-Wellman, K.H.; Galpin, A.J.; Schilling, B.K. Effect of eicosapentaenoic and docosahexaenoic acid on resting and exercise-induced inflammatory and oxidative stress biomarkers: A randomized, placebo controlled, cross-over study. *Lipids Health Dis.* **2009**. [CrossRef] [PubMed]

133. VKM (Norwegian Scientific Committee for Food Safety). *Opinion of the Steering Committee of the Norwegian Scientific Committee for Food Safety: Evaluation of Negative and Positive Health Effects of n-3 Fatty Acids as Constituents of Food Supplements and Fortified Foods.* Available online: http://english.vkm.no/dav/031c000d1a.pdf (accessed on 20 June 2016).

134. Farmer, A.; Montori, V.; Dinneen, S.; Clar, C. Fish oil in people with type 2 diabetes mellitus. *Cochrane Database Syst. Rev.* **2001**. [CrossRef]

12

Eicosopentaneoic Acid and Other Free Fatty Acid Receptor Agonists Inhibit Lysophosphatidic Acid- and Epidermal Growth Factor-Induced Proliferation of Human Breast Cancer Cells

Mandi M. Hopkins, Zhihong Zhang, Ze Liu and Kathryn E. Meier *

Department of Pharmaceutical Sciences, College of Pharmacy, Washington State University, Spokane, WA 99163, USA; mandi.hopkins@wsu.edu (M.M.H.); juliazhang2013@gmail.com (Z.Z.); zeliu1010@gmail.com (Z.L.)
* Correspondence: kmeier@wsu.edu

Academic Editors: Lindsay Brown, Bernhard Rauch and Hemant Poudyal

Abstract: Many key actions of ω-3 (*n*-3) fatty acids have recently been shown to be mediated by two G protein-coupled receptors (GPCRs) in the free fatty acid receptor (FFAR) family, FFA1 (GPR40) and FFA4 (GPR120). *n*-3 Fatty acids inhibit proliferation of human breast cancer cells in culture and in animals. In the current study, the roles of FFA1 and FFA4 were investigated. In addition, the role of cross-talk between GPCRs activated by lysophosphatidic acid (LPA), and the tyrosine kinase receptor activated by epidermal growth factor (EGF), was examined. In MCF-7 and MDA-MB-231 human breast cancer cell lines, both LPA and EGF stimulated proliferation, Erk activation, Akt activation, and CCN1 induction. LPA antagonists blocked effects of LPA and EGF on proliferation in MCF-7 and MDA-MB-231, and on cell migration in MCF-7. The *n*-3 fatty acid eicosopentaneoic acid inhibited LPA- and EGF-induced proliferation in both cell lines. Two synthetic FFAR agonists, GW9508 and TUG-891, likewise inhibited LPA- and EGF-induced proliferation. The data suggest a major role for FFA1, which was expressed by both cell lines. The results indicate that *n*-3 fatty acids inhibit breast cancer cell proliferation via FFARs, and suggest a mechanism involving negative cross-talk between FFARS, LPA receptors, and EGF receptor.

Keywords: breast cancer; lysophosphatidic acid; epidermal growth factor; ω-3 fatty acids; G protein-coupled receptors; free fatty acid receptors

---

1. Introduction

Our group recently demonstrated that the inhibitory effects of ω-3 fatty acids on prostate cancer cell proliferation are mediated by FFA4, a G protein-coupled receptor in the free fatty acid receptor (FFAR) family [1]. The purpose of the current study was to determine whether FFARs mediate similar inhibitory effects in human breast cancer cells.

The dietary polyunsaturated ω-3 fatty acids (*n*-3 FAs) are alpha-linolenic acid (ALA), docosahexaenoic acid (DHA) and eicosapentaneoic acid (EPA). Although effects of *n*-3 FAs in prostate cancer have been debated [2], there is relatively strong evidence supporting a preventative effect of *n*-3 FA consumption on many human cancers [3], including breast cancer [4]. Multiple reports show that *n*-3 fatty acids inhibit growth of breast cancer cells, either in cell culture [5,6], or in xenograft tumors [7–10].

The prevailing mechanistic paradigm has been that *n*-3 FAs exert anti-inflammatory and potentially anti-cancer effects by competitively reducing production of eicosanoids, and/or more directly by generating metabolites with anti-inflammatory activity (e.g., "resolvins") [11,12]. However, the direct effects of *n*-3 metabolites on cancer cells, as compared to their anti-inflammatory effects, are under-studied [13]. In one report, resolvin D2, a DHA metabolite, unexpectedly increased proliferation of MCF-7 breast cancer cells [14].

Alternatively, it was shown in the last decade that n-3 FAs are agonist ligands for free fatty acid receptors (FFARs) that were formerly "orphan receptors" [15]. Two G-protein-coupled receptors (GPCRs), FFA1 and FFA4, bind long-chain polyunsaturated fatty acids that include n-3 FAs. The "de-orphanization" discovery has led to the ongoing characterization of the roles of the FFARs in cellular regulation, and to the rapid development of selective FFAR agonists with therapeutic potential [16–19].

Several studies have specifically explored the mechanism of the inhibitory action of n-3 FAs on breast cancer cells. The pathways implicated in the response include decreased Akt activation [5], increased neutral sphingomyelinase activity [20], increased BRCA levels [21], and increased PTEN levels [22]. GPCR-independent mechanisms have been reviewed [23]. To date, there is little information available concerning the roles of FFARs in breast cancer. It has however been shown that FFA1 is expressed in MCF-7 cells [24], and that MCF-7 and MDA-MB-231 cells express both FFA1 and FFA4 [25,26].

One study investigated the role of FFA4 in breast cancer in a mouse model, focusing on the role of FFA4 in inhibiting inflammation [27]. In this study, n-3 FAs reduced tumor burden even when FFA4 was knocked out in the host mouse. The authors suggest that anti-inflammatory effects of n-3 FAs, mediated by FFA4, are not important for their anti-tumor effects. Using cultured cells derived from their mouse model, the investigators showed that DHA induced apoptosis in either wild-type or FFA4 knockdown cells when applied at high doses (40–100 μM). The role of the alternative n-3 FA receptor, FFA1, has not been examined in breast cancer cell, to our knowledge.

In this study, we utilized two commonly used human breast cancer cell lines: MCF-7 and MDA-MB-231, as experimental models. MCF-7 is a luminal A estrogen receptor positive cell line, while MDA-MB-231 is a highly metastatic triple negative cell line. These two cell lines were used to explore the role of FFARs in the mechanism of action of n-3 FAs in breast cancer.

2. Experimental Section

2.1. Materials

EPA (prepared in ethanol) was from Cayman Chemical (Ann Arbor, MI, USA). The FFAR agonists TUG-891 (4-[(4-fluoro-4′-methyl[1,1′-biphenyl]-2-yl)methoxy]-benzenepropanoic acid; prepared in dimethylsulfoxide (DMSO) and GW9508 (4-[[(3-phenoxyphenyl)methyl]amino]-benzenepropanoic acid; prepared in ethanol), were from Millipore (Billerica, MA, USA) and Cayman Chemical, respectively. AM966 (2-[4-[4-[4-[[(1R)-1-(2-chlorophenyl)ethoxy]carbonylamino]-3-methyl-1,2-oxazol-5-yl]phenyl] phenyl]acetic acid) was purchased pre-dissolved in DMSO from MedChem Express (Monmouth Junction, NJ, USA). Ki16425 (3-[[[4-[4-[[[1-(2-chlorophenyl)ethoxy]carbonyl]amino]-3-methyl-5-isoazoly]phenyl]methyl]thio]-propanoic acid; prepared in DMSO) was purchased from Cayman Chemical (Ann Arbor, MI, USA). Vehicle controls were included in all samples not receiving FFAR agonists or LPA receptor (LPAR) antagonists (final concentrations of 0.03% (v/v) ethanol or 0.01% DMSO). LPA (18:1; oleoyl) was obtained from Avanti Polar Lipids (Birmingham, UK), and was delivered to cells as a 1000X stock solution prepared in 4 mg/mL fatty acid-free bovine serum albumin (BSA). The vehicle control for LPA was a final concentration of 4 μg/mL BSA. EGF was from Sigma (St. Louis, MO, USA). Antibody recognizing CCN1 (lot # F0509; 1:1000 dilution) was obtained from Santa Cruz Biotechnology (Santa Cruz, CA, USA). Anti-actin, obtained from BD Transduction Laboratories (Lexington, KY, USA) (lot # 51711), was used at a 1:5000 dilution. Goat anti-rabbit secondary antibody (lot #083M4752) was purchased from Sigma (St Louis, MO, USA) and used at 1:20,000 dilution, while goat anti-mouse secondary antibody (lot #1124907A) was purchased from Invitrogen/Life Technologies (Grand Island, NE, USA) and used at a 1:5000 dilution.

2.2. Cell Culture

MCF-7 and MDA-MB-231 cells were obtained from the American Type Culture Collection (Manassas, VA, USA). The cells were grown in RPMI medium supplemented with 10% FBS (Hyclone/Thermo-Fisher Scientific, Waltham, MA, USA). Both cell lines were grown in an incubator at 37 °C in 5% CO_2 on standard tissue culture plastic.

2.3. Cell Proliferation Assays

Cells were seeded in 6-well plates at 3×10^5 cells/well in serum-containing medium. After 1 day, the medium was changed to RPMI 1640 without serum. On the next day, the medium was changed to RPMI 1640 with 10% FBS, 10 μM LPA, or 10 nM EGF, in the absence or presence of 100 nM AM966, 10 μM Ki16425, 20 μM EPA or 1 μM TUG-891. Control cells were incubated with the appropriate vehicle (0.03% ethanol, v/v; 0.01% DMSO, v/v; and/or 4 μg/mL BSA). Duplicate wells were prepared for each experimental condition. Cell numbers were evaluated after 24, 48, and 72 h by removing medium, incubating cells with trypsin/EDTA for 5 min, adding trypan blue, and counting the suspended live cells (excluding trypan blue) using a hemacytometer.

2.4. Cell Migration Assays

MCF-7 cell migration was assessed using a modified Boyden chamber method, as previously described [28]. Cells were serum starved for 24 h and then seeded in serum-free medium at 2.5×10^4 cells per insert in the upper chambers of 8-μm transwell inserts (BD Biosciences, San Jose, CA, USA). Cells were then treated with 10% FBS, 100 nM AM966, 20 μM EPA, 1 μM TUG-891, 10 μM LPA, or 10 nM EGF, either alone or in combination, with appropriate vehicle controls as described above. Serum-free medium was added to the lower wells. Following a 6-h migration, the insert membranes were fixed and stained using methanol and crystal violet. Cells that invaded the lower chambers were counted by microscopy.

2.5. Cell Incubations for Signal Transduction Assays

Cells were grown in DME medium supplemented with 10% FBS until ~80% confluent. Cells were serum-starved for 24 h in RPMI 1640 medium, then incubated with 10 μM LPA, 10 nM EGF, and/or 100 nM AM966 or 10 μM Ki16425 for 10 min. Cells were rinsed twice with ice-cold phosphate-buffered saline (PBS), harvested by scraping into 1 mL ice-cold PBS, collected by centrifugation at $10,000 \times g$ for 10 min at 4 °C, and resuspended in ice-cold lysis buffer (20 mM HEPES (pH = 7.4)), 1% Triton X-100, 50 mM NaCl, 2 mM EGTA, 5 mM β-glycerophosphate, 30 mM sodium pyrophosphate, 100 mM sodium orthovanadate, 1 mM phenylmethylsulfonyl fluoride, 10 μg/mL aprotinin, 10 μg/mL leupeptin). Insoluble debris was removed after centrifugation.

2.6. Reverse Transcription Polymerase Chain Reacton (RT-PCR)

For analysis of FFAR expression, total RNA was isolated using an RNeasy Mini kit (Qiagen, Valencia, Spain). First-strand complementary DNA (cDNA) was synthesized with SuperScript II Reverse Transcriptase (Invitrogen) following the manufacturer's instructions using 20 μL of reaction mixture containing 2 μg RNA. PCR was carried out using Platinum *Pfx* DNA Polymerase (Invitrogen) and Integrated DNA Technology (San Diego, CA, USA) primers: FFA4 (F: 5'-CCTGGAGAGATCTCGTGGGA-3'; and R: 5'-AGGAGGTGTTCCGAGGTCTG-3'); FFA1 (F: 5'-CTCCTTCGGCCTCTATGTGG-3'; and R: 5'-AGACCAGGCTAGGGGTGAGA-3'); RPLP0 (F: 5'-CGCTATCCGCGGTTTCTGAT-3'; and R: 5'-AGACGATGTCACTTCCACGA-3'). For each reaction, 5 μg cDNA template was used. Products were separated by ethidium bromide agarose gel electrophoresis, and were then imaged using a ChemiDoc with Image Lab software (Bio-Rad, Hercules, CA, USA). For analysis of LPA receptor expression, total RNA was extracted from harvested cells using TRIzol solution (Invitrogen, Carlsbad, CA, USA) according to the manufacturer's protocol. Reverse transcription was performed using iScriptTMcDNA synthesis kit (Bio-Rad, Hercules, CA) in a reaction volume of 20 μL under the conditions recommended by the manufacture. Total RNA (1 μg) was used as a template for cDNA synthesis. PCR was performed in a 50-μL reaction volume with a buffer consisting of $10 \times$ iTaq buffer, 50 mM MgCl$_2$, 10 mM dNTP mix, iTaq DNA polymerase;and 0.25 μmol/L each primer. The primers were: LPA1/Edg-2 (F: 5′-TGTCATGGCTGCCATCTC-3′; and R: 5′-CATCTCAGTTTCCGTTCTAA-3′); LPA2/Edg-4 (F: 5′-CCCAACCAACAGGACTGACT-3′; and R: 5′-GAGCCCTTATCTCTCCCCAC-3′); LPA3/Edg-7 (F: 5′-GGACACCCATGAAGCTAATG-3′; and R: 5′-TCTGGGTTCTCCTGAGAGAA-3′); β-actin (F: 5′-TGACGGGGTCACCCACACTGTGCCCATCTA-3′; and R: 5′-CTAGAAGCATTTGCGG TGGACGATGGAGGG-3′). RT-PCR products were separated on a 2% agarose gel by electrophoresis and visualized and imaged under UV illumination.

2.7. Immunoblotting

Whole-cell extracts containing equal amounts of protein (30 μg) were separated by SDS-PAGE on 10% Laemmli gels, transferred to nitrocellulose, and incubated with primary (overnight at 4 °C) and then secondary (one to two hours at room temperature) antibodies. Blots were developed using enhanced chemiluminescence (GE Healthcare, Pittsburgh, PA, USA), and imaged using a Gel Doc system (BioRad, Hercules, CA, USA). Protein expression was quantified by densitometry using Quantity One software (Bio-Rad). Results were normalized to the actin loading control, and then to the value obtained for untreated control cells.

2.8. Statistical Analysis

Data were analyzed by two-way ANOVA followed by Tukey's multiple comparisons test. The only exceptions were assays in which there was only one time point (e.g., migration assays); these data were analyzed by one-way ANOVA followed by Tukey's mutliple comparisons test. All analyses were done using Prism software (Graphpad, San Diego, CA, USA).

3. Results and Discussion

3.1. Effects of Lysophosphatidic Acid (LPA) and Epidermal Growth Factor (EGF) on Breast Cancer Cell Proliferation

Before testing for effects of FFAR agonists on breast cancer cells, we first established conditions for using growth factors to stimulate proliferation. Cells were serum-starved before treatments in order to remove confounding effects of LPA contained in serum, and to provide a baseline for testing effects of growth factors. The effects of serum, LPA, and EGF on proliferation of serum-starved MCF-7 and MDA-MB-231 cells are shown in Figure 1. All growth factors significantly increased cell number as compared to control. Serum was significantly more effective in inducing proliferation than LPA or EGF at all time points tested, in both cell lines; this result was expected since serum contains multiple mitogens including LPA. There was no significant difference between responses to LPA *versus* EGF at any time point.

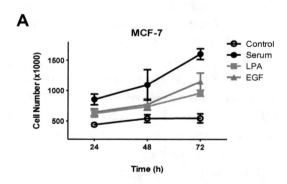

Figure 1. *Cont.*

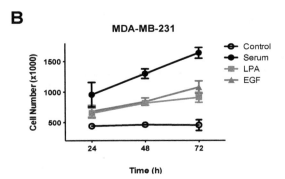

Figure 1. Effects of growth factors on proliferation of human breast cancer cells. Proliferation assays were conducted using serum-starved MCF-7 (**A**) or MDA-MB-231 (**B**) cells. Cells were incubated with or without 10% FBS (serum), 10 μM LPA, or 10 nM EGF for the indicated times (growth factors were added at time "0"). Each data point represents the mean ± SEM ($n = 4$) of values (number of live cells per well) from two separate experiments, each done in with two separate replicate wells of cells for each condition. Data analysis was performed using two-way ANOVA, followed by Tukey's multiple comparisons test. All growth factor values were significantly ($p < 0.05$) different from the control value at all time points shown, except for LPA at 24 h in MCF-7. Serum values were significantly different from lysophosphatidic acid (LPA) or epidermal growth factor (EGF) at all time points tested.

3.2. Signal Transduction Responses to LPA and EGF in Breast Cancer Cells

To further characterize responses to LPA and EGF in the breast cancer cell lines, we performed immunoblotting experiments to test for Erk and Akt activation (Figure 2). Both LPA and EGF increase activating phosphorylation of Erk and Akt in both MCF-7 and MDA-MB-231 cells (Figure 2A). These results are consistent with previous reports concerning the mitogenic activity of LPA and EGF in breast cancer cells [29,30].

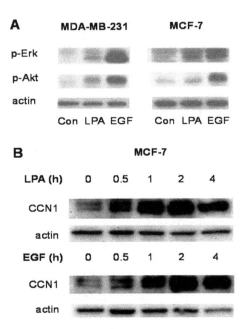

Figure 2. Effects of LPA and EGF on signal transduction events in human breast cancer cells. (**A**) Serum-starved MCF-7 and MDA-MB-231 cells were incubated with 10 μM LPA or 10 nM EGF for 5 min. Whole-cell extracts were immunoblotted using antibodies recognizing phosphorylated active Erk and Akt. An immunoblot for total actin was performed as a loading control; (**B**) Serum-starved MCF-7 cells were incubated for the indicated times with 10 μM LPA or 10 nM EGF. Whole-cell extracts were immunoblotted using antibody recognizing total CCN1. An immunoblot for total actin was performed as a loading control. Each experiment is representative of at least three separate experiments.

We also examined a more novel response to growth factors, CCN1 induction, in MCF-7 cells. CCN1 is an inducible matricellular protein whose expression is positively correlated with breast cancer progression [31,32]. As shown in Figure 2B, both LPA and EGF stimulate expression of CCN1 in MCF-7 cells. An increase in CCN1 protein levels was seen after only 30 min of treatment with either growth factor. Taken together, the results presented in Figure 2A,B confirm that both LPA and EGF activate pro-mitogenic signaling pathways in human breast cancer cell lines.

3.3. Effects of LPA Antagonists on Breast Cancer Cell Proliferation

Previous studies have shown that LPA receptors are expressed in breast cancer cell lines. One group performed a comprehensive analysis of LPA receptor expression in commonly-used breast cancer cell lines [33]. Their data show that MDA-MB-231 and MCF-7 cells, among other cell lines, express LPA_1, LPA_2, and LPA_3. LPA_1 has been determined to mediate many of the actions of LPA in breast cancer cells [34–37]. RT-PCR experiments conducted in our lab confirmed that LPA_1 was expressed in both MCF-7 and MDA-MB-231 cells under the conditions used herein (Figure 3A).

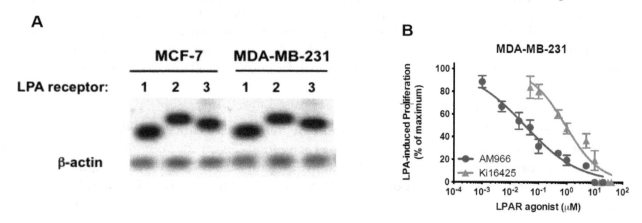

Figure 3. LPAR expression in breast cancer cell lines, and dose-response for the effects of LPA_1 antagonists on MDA-MB-231 cell proliferation. (**A**) Total RNA was extracted from MCF-7 and MDA-MB-231 breast cancer cells. RT-PCR was performed (separate gels for each cell line) using the cDNA primers described in the Methods. β-actin was amplified as loading control; (**B**) Serum-starved MDA-MB-231 cells were incubated for 48 h with and without 10 µM LPA in the absence and presence of the indicated concentrations of Ki16425 or AM966. The number of cells achieved in response to LPA alone was defined as 100% response; the number of cells in the absence of LPA was defined as 0% response. Each point represents mean ± SEM ($n \geq 4$) for values obtained from at least two experiments, each performed with two separate replicate wells of cells for each condition.

Two LPA receptor pharmacologic antagonists were used to further study the role of LPA_1 in breast cancer cells. Ki16425 is a selective inhibitor of LPA_1 and LPA_3 [38], while AM966 is an LPA_1-selective antagonist [39]. We used a dose-response study (Figure 3B) to test whether LPA_1 inhibitors inhibit LPA-induced proliferation in MDA-MB-231 breast cancer cells. As expected, based on their relative receptor affinities, the LPA_1-selective antagonist AM966 was more potent (IC_{50} = 32 nM) in inhibiting LPA-induced proliferation than was the pan-LPA inhibitor Ki16425 (IC_{50} = 904 nM). Interestingly, the amount of AM966 needed to completely inhibit MDA-MB-231 cell proliferation was 100-fold higher than in our previously published work using DU145 prostate cancer cells [1], although the amount of Ki16425 required was similar in both MDA-MB-231 and DU145. The dose-response curve for AM966 was very shallow, suggesting the involvement of multiple receptors. These results suggest that LPA_1 is not the only LPA receptor that mediates LPA-induced proliferation in these cells.

In Figure 4, we further tested the effects of LPA antagonists. We asked 1) whether the inhibitory effects of LPA antagonists extend to EGF-induced proliferation, and 2) whether LPA antagonists have similar effects in MCF-7 and MDA-MB-231 cells. The results of this series of experiments, which are presented in Figure 4, clearly demonstrate that the LPA receptor antagonists block proliferation in response to both LPA and EGF. This response was observed in both MCF-7 and MDA-MB-231 cells.

Taken together, these results are consistent with a crucial role for LPARs in EGF response, as has been noted in other cell types [1,40].

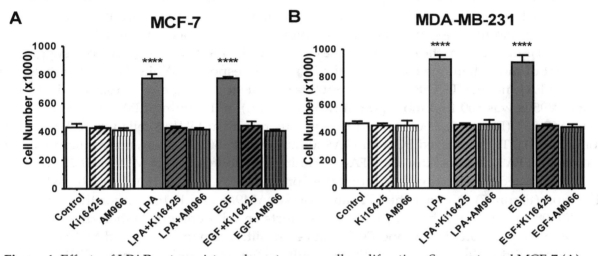

Figure 4. Effects of LPAR antagonists on breast cancer cell proliferation. Serum-starved MCF-7 (**A**) or MDA-MB-231 (**B**) cells were incubated with or without 10 μM LPA or 10 nM EGF in the absence and presence of 10 μM AM966 or 10 μM Ki16425. Each data point represents the mean ± SEM ($n = 4$) of values (number of live cells per well) from two separate experiments, each performed with two separate replicate wells of cells for each experimental condition (**** $p < 0.0001$ compared to control). The 48-h time is point shown; similar results were obtained at 24 and 72 h. Data analysis was performed using two-way ANOVA, followed by Tukey's multiple comparisons test.

3.4. Expression of Free Fatty Acid Receptors (FFARs) in Breast Cancer Cells

We next turned to the effects of *n*-3 FAs. We examined whether FFARs are expressed in MCF-7 and MDA-MB-231 cells. Both receptors have previously been reported to be present in MCF-7 cells, based on flow cytometry [25]. Using RT-PCR, we assessed mRNA levels for FFA4 and FFA1, the two receptors for long chain free fatty acid (Figure 5A). Both PCR products were detected, although the PCR product for FFA4 was present at such low levels that it was difficult to visualize. To confirm that FFA4 was expressed, we performed immunoblotting using an antibody previously validated in our laboratory [1], and did detect FFA4 protein (Figure 5B). We were unable to validate an appropriate antibody for FFA1, but our PCR results suggest that FFA1 is likely expressed at higher levels than FFA4 in the two breast cancer cell lines. These results indicate that the roles of both FFA1 and FFA4 need to be considered in breast cancer cells.

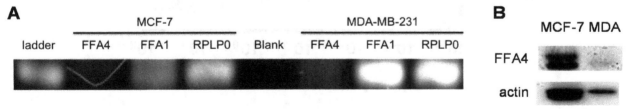

Figure 5. Expression of FFA1 and FFA4 in breast cancer cell lines. (**A**) RT-PCR reactions were carried out for human FFA4, FFA1, or RPLP0 (loading control) as described in Methods. Products were separated and visualized under UV light. Results shown are representative of two separate experiments, each done in triplicate. Faint signals for FFA4 were confirmed in additional experiments; (**B**) Whole-cell extracts, from MCF-7 and MDA-MB-231 cells growing in serum, were separated by SDS-PAGE and then immunoblotted for FFA4 and actin (loading control).

3.5. Effects of FFAR Agonists on Breast Cancer Cell Proliferation

We next performed a dose-response study (Figure 6) to test whether FFAR agonists inhibit proliferation of MDA-MB-231 cells. EPA, TUG-891, and GW9503 all inhibited proliferation of these cells. EPA was the least potent compound (IC_{50} 403 nM), which was expected based on results with other cell lines [1]. The IC_{50} for the FFA4-selective agonist, TUG-891, was 24 nM. However, a 100-fold higher dose of TUG-891 was required to completely inhibit LPA-induced proliferation in the breast cancer cell line (Figure 6) as compared to our previously published results with Du145 prostate cancer cells [1]. In addition, the dose-response curve for TUG-891 was very shallow, suggesting the involvement of more than one receptor in the inhibitory response. While TUG-891 is selective for FFA4 over FFA1, neither TUG-891 nor GW9508 is specific for a single receptor. The FFA1-specific agonist GW9508 was 100-fold more potent (IC_{50} = 16 nm) in inhibiting LPA-induced proliferation in MDA-MB-231 (Figure 6) as compared to previous results in DU145 cells where FFA4 response predominates [1]. The published EC_{50} for GW9508 at FFA1 is ~50 nM. Thus, our results are consistent with a role for FFA1, and possibly also FFA4, in inhibiting proliferation of MDA-MB-231 cells.

We next tested the effects of LPA_1 inhibitors on both LPA- and EGF-induced breast cancer cell proliferation (Figure 7). Neither the LPA antagonists AM966 and Ki16425, nor the FFAR agonists EPA, GW9508, and TUG891, had any significant effects on cell numbers on their own. However, all agents completely inhibited LPA- and EGF-induced proliferation in MCF-7 and MDA-MB-231 cells, when added individually, consistent with the results in Figures 4 and 6. Although EPA appeared to decrease cell numbers slightly below control values in the presence of LPA or EGF, the effect was not significant. There was no additional effect (e.g., cytotoxicity) on cell numbers when LPA antagonists were combined with FFAR agonists GW9508 or TUG891 (Figure 7). Thus, both LPA antagonists and FFAR agonists can block the effects of LPA and EGF on breast cancer cell proliferation.

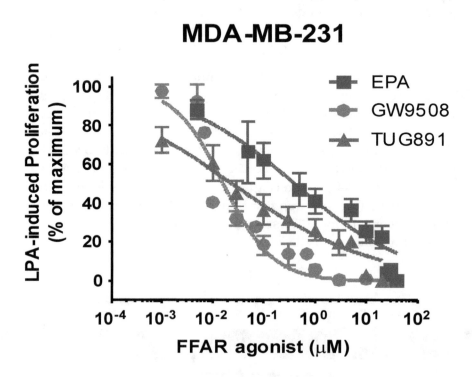

Figure 6. Dose-response for effects of FFAR agonists on breast cancer cell proliferation. Serum-starved MDA-MB-231 cells were incubated for 48 h with and without 10 μM LPA in the absence and presence of the indicated concentrations of EPA, GW9508, and TUG-891. The number of cells achieved in response to LPA alone was defined as 100% response; the number of cells present in the absence of LPA was defined as 0% response. Each point represents mean ± SEM ($n \geqslant 4$ for values obtained from at least two experiments, each performed with two separate replicate wells of cells for each experimental condition.

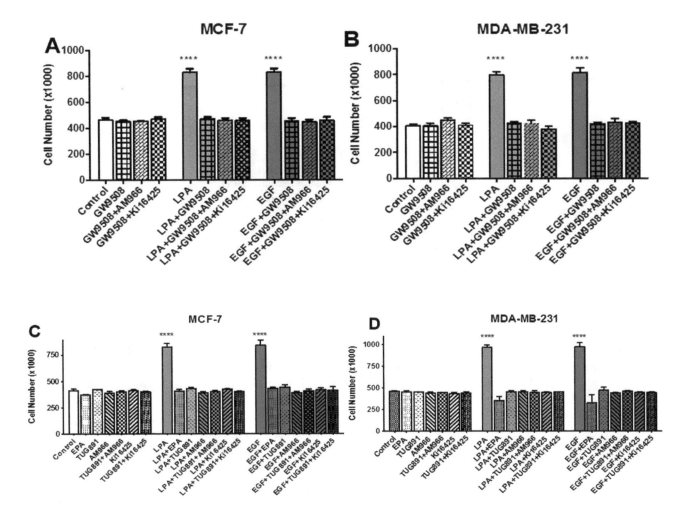

Figure 7. Effects of FFAR agonists on breast cancer cell proliferation. Serum-starved MCF-7 or MDA-MB-231 cells were incubated with or without 10 μM LPA or 10 nM EGF for 48 h in the absence and presence of 1 μM GW9508, 10 μM Ki16425, and/or 10 μM AM966 (Panels **A** and **B**), or (Panels **C** and **D**), 10 μM LPA or 10 nM EGF in the absence and presence of 10 μM TUG891, 10 μM Ki16425, and/or 10 μM AM966. In addition, Panels C and D show the effects of TUG-891 as compared to that of 25 μM EPA, and controls were included for the LPA antagonists alone. Some of the data points from Panels **C** and **D** were presented earlier in Figure 4, which was derived from the same series of experiments; panels (**A**) and (**B**) are from separate sets of experiments. Although only the 48-h time point is shown, similar inhibitory effects were observed at 24 and 72 h. Each value represents the mean ± SEM (*n* = 4) of values (number of live cells per well) obtained from two separate experiments, each of which used two separate replicate wells of cells for each experimental condition (**** *p* < 0.0001 compared to control). Data were analyzed done using two-way ANOVA, followed by Tukey's multiple comparisons test.

3.6. Effects of FFAR Agonists on Breast Cancer Cell Migration

Finally, we asked whether FFAR agonists inhibit migration of breast cancer cells. As shown in Figure 8, EPA and GW9508 both block LPA- and EGF-induced migration of MCF-7 cells. The LPAR antagonist Ki16425 has a similar effect. The combination of GW9508 and Ki16425 also yields complete inhibition; *i.e.*, there is no additional effect of the FFAR agonist in the presence of an LPA antagonist. We conclude that either activation of FFARs, or antagonism of LPARs, can inhibit migration in response to either LPA or EGF.

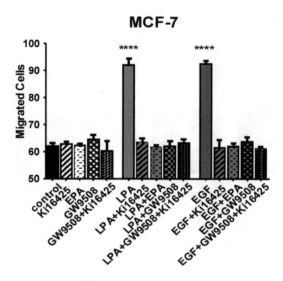

Figure 8. Effects of LPAR agonists on MCF-7 cell migration. Serum-starved MCF-7 cells were treated with 10 μM Ki16425, 20 μM EPA, 1 μM GW9508, 10 μM LPA, or 10 nM EGF, either alone or in combination. After a 6-h migration period, cells were analyzed as described in Methods. Each bar represents the mean $\pm$ SEM ($n = 4$) of values (total number of migrated cells/well) obtained from two separate experiments, each of which used two separate replicate wells of cells for each experimental condition (**** $p < 0.0001$ *vs.* control). Data were analyzed using one-way ANOVA, followed by Tukey's multiple comparisons test.

4. Conclusions

In extending our ongoing studies of FFAR activation to breast cancer cells, the intention was to expand our knowledge of the roles of FFARs in cancer. While others have examined the effects of *n*-3 FAs on breast cancer, to our knowledge no other studies have tested the roles of FFARs in human breast cancer cells.

The current study used LPA as one of the growth factors, based on our previous work implicating LPARs in the mechanism of FFAR-mediated inhibition of cancer cell proliferation. LPA has multiple actions that support breast cancer growth, migration, invasion, and survival [37,41–44]. An LPA antagonist was shown to induce regression of breast tumors in a mouse model [45]. Others reported that either an LPA$_1$ antagonist or LPA$_1$ knockdown decreases MDA-MB-231 cell metastasis, but not primary tumor size, in mice [46]. Together, these data have established a potential role for the LPA axis as a therapeutic target in breast cancer cells, as reviewed by Panupinthu and colleagues [29]. However, the overall roles of LPA and its receptors in breast cancer cell proliferation have not been fully delineated.

FFA1/GPR40 was first reported to be present in MCF-7 cells in 2004 [24]. This was later confirmed by another group using flow cytometry [25] and also in the current study by PCR (Figure 5). Soto-Guzman and colleagues also detected FFA4 expression in MCF-7 cells [25]. Our data demonstrate expression of FFA1 and FFA4 mRNA, and FFAR protein, in both MCF-7 and MDA-MB-231 cells. Interestingly, the results of dose-response studies using two selective FFAR agonists were consistent with a major role for FFA1 in MDA-MB-231 cells (Figure 6). While these results do not exclude a role for FFA4, this is the first demonstration in our lab that FFA1 and FFA4 may similarly mediate inhibition of cancer cell proliferation.

Figures 4 and 7 demonstrate that LPAR inhibition not only impedes LPA-induced proliferation, but also EGF-induced proliferation. This result suggests that, in MCF-7 and MDA-MB-231 cells, EGFR is reliant on one or more LPARs. This result is similar to those obtained with prostate cancer cells [1,40]. LPARs have been described as "masters" of EGFR signaling [47], as confirmed by studies in various cell types [1,48–53]. Further studies will be required to determine whether FFA1 or FFA4 act directly on both LPARs and EGFR to result in inhibition, or indirectly inhibit EGFR via effects on LPARs.

FFAR activation through EPA, GW9508, or TUG-891 abolishes LPA- and EGF-induced proliferation and migration in MCF-7 and MDA-MB-231 cells (Figures 6–8). GW9508 yields a classical dose-response curve with an IC_{50} consistent with action at FFA1. At the higher dose of TUG-891 used to achieve complete inhibition in breast cancer cells (10 μM), it is plausible that it is activating FFA1 in addition to, FFA4. Our results are consistent with other reports of inhibitory effects of n-3 FAs in breast cancer cells. In one study, low doses of n-3 FAs were shown to inhibit proliferation of MCF-7 cells, while high doses induced apoptosis [20]. This is consistent with our dose-response results for MDA-MB-231 cells, where inhibition of proliferation was achieved without cytotoxicity (Figure 6). The EPA concentration (25 μM) used in subsequent experiments was chosen as the dose that maximally inhibited proliferation but did not decrease viability, since our focus was on inhibition of growth factor response rather than toxic responses that may occur at high doses.

Although our results suggest that both FFAR agonists and LPAR antagonists inhibit proliferation in MCF-7 and MDA-MB-231 cells, more work is needed to fully elucidate the mechanism of action. It remains to be definitively determined which FFAR is responsible for the inhibition in breast cancer cells. It is also unclear at this point whether FFAR activation directly influences EGF-mediated signaling, or whether FFARs act indirectly via interference with LPAR activity as appears to be the case in prostate cancer cells [40]. Since the synthetic FFAR agonists used in the current study are not metabolized to resolvins, and are designed to act selectively at GPCRs, utilization of these agonist drugs is helpful in distinguishing receptor-mediated effects from effects of n-3 FAs on lipid metabolism. In addition, the emerging small-molecule FFAR agonists have therapeutic potential for the prevention and/or treatment of breast cancer. In summary, the results presented herein demonstrate for the first time that FFAR activation results in inhibition of breast cancer cell proliferation and migration. The inhibitory response mediated by FFARs needs to be taken into account when considering effects of n-3 fatty acids on breast cancer cells.

Acknowledgments: This work was supported by the College of Pharmacy at Washington State University. Mandi Hopkins, a member of the Graduate Program in Pharmaceutical Sciences in the College of Pharmacy, also received support from the NIH Protein Biotechnology Training Program at WSU [T32 GM008336]. Zhihong Zhang received support from NIH 1K05AA017149 (G. Meadows, principal investigator). The authors thank Renae Hamilton and Colin Kennedy for assistance in early phases of this project.

Author Contributions: Mandi Hopkins: wrote manuscript, designed and performed experiments; Zhihong Zhang: designed and performed experiments; Ze Liu: performed experiments; Kathryn Meier: edited manuscript, supervised the project.

References

1. Liu, Z.; Hopkins, M.M.; Zhang, Z.; Quisenberry, C.B.; Fix, L.C.; Galvan, B.M.; Meier, K.E. ω-3 Fatty acids and other FFA4 agonists inhibit growth factor signaling in human prostate cancer cells. *J. Pharm. Exp. Ther.* **2015**, *352*, 1–15. [CrossRef] [PubMed]

2. Hopkins, M.M.; Meier, K.E. ω-3 Fatty acids and their impact on prostate cancer risk. *Curr. Nutr. Rep.* **2015**. in press.

3. Hardman, W.E. ω-3 Fatty acids to augment cancer therapy. *J. Nutr.* **2002**, *132*, 3509S–3512S.

4. Zheng, J.S.; Hu, X.J.; Zao, Y.M.; Yang, J.; Li, D. Intake of fish and marine n-3 polyunsaturated fatty acids and risk of breast cancer: Meta-analysis of data from 21 Independent Prospective Cohort Studies. *Br. Med. J.* **2013**, *346*, f3706. [CrossRef] [PubMed]

5. Schley, P.D.; Jijon, H.B.; Robinson, L.E.; Field, C.J. Mechanisms of ω-3 fatty acid-induced growth inhibition in MDA-MB-231 human breast cancer cells. *Breast Cancer Res. Treat.* **2005**, *92*, 187–195. [CrossRef] [PubMed]

6. Pogash, T.J.; el-Bayoumy, K.; Amin, S.; Gowda, K.; de Cicco, R.L.; Barton, M.; Su, Y.; Russo, I.H.; Himmelberger, J.A.; Slifker, M.; *et al.* Oxidized derivative of docosahexaenoic acid preferentially inhibit cell proliferation in triple negative over luminal breas cancer cells. *Vitro Cell Dev. Biol. Anim.* **2015**, *52*, 121–127. [CrossRef] [PubMed]

7. Karmali, R.A.; Marsh, J.; Ruchs, C. Effect of ω-3 fatty acids on growth of a rat mammary tumor. *J. Natl. Cancer Inst.* **1984**, *73*, 457–461. [PubMed]

8. Rose, D.P.; Connolly, J.M. Effects of dietary ω-3 fatty acids on human breast cancer growth and metastases in nude mice. *J. Natl. Caner Inst.* **1993**, *85*, 1743–1747. [CrossRef]

9. Sauer, L.A.; Dauchy, R.T.; Blask, D.E.; Krause, J.A.; Davidson, L.K.; Dauchy, E.M. Eicosapenaenoic acid suppresses cell proliferation in MCF-7 human breast cancer xenografts in nude rats via a pertussis toxin-sensitive signal transduction pathway. *J. Nutr.* **2005**, *135*, 2124–2129. [PubMed]

10. Jiang, W.; Zhu, Z.; McGinley, J.N.; el Bayouny, K.; Manni, A.; Thompson, J.H. Identification of a molecular signature underlying inhibition of mammary carcinoma growth by dietary *n*-3 fatty acids. *Cancer Res.* **2012**, *72*, 3795–3806. [CrossRef] [PubMed]

11. Dwivedi, S.; Patel, S.; Jain, K. The what, where, and how of resolvins. *AsPac J. Mol. Biol. Biotechnol.* **2010**, *20*, 45–54.

12. Zhang, M.J.; Spite, M. Resolvins: Anti-inflammatory and pro-resolving mediators derived from ω-3 polyunsaturated fatty acids. *Annu. Rev. Nutr.* **2012**, *32*, 203–227. [CrossRef] [PubMed]

13. Janakiram, N.B.; Mohammed, A.; Rao, C.V. Role of lipoxins, resolvins, and other bioactive lipids in colon and pancreatic cancer. *Cancer Metastasis Rev.* **2011**, *30*, 507–523. [CrossRef] [PubMed]

14. Al-Zaubai, N.; Johnstone, C.N.; Leong, M.M.; Li, J.; Rizzacasa, M.; Stewart, A.G. Resolvin D2 supports MCF-7 cell proliferation via activation of estrogen receptor. *J. Pharmacol. Exp. Ther.* **2014**, *351*, 172–180. [CrossRef] [PubMed]

15. Oh, D.Y.; Talukdar, S.; Bae, E.J.; Imamura, T.; Morinaga, H.; Fan, W.Q.; Li, P.; Wendell, J.L.; Watkins, S.M.; Olefsky, J.M. GRP120 is an ω-3 fatty acid receptor mediating potent anti-inflammatory and insulin-sensitizing effects. *Cell* **2012**, *143*, 687–698.

16. Hara, T.; Hirasawa, A.; Ichimura, A.; Kimura, I.; Tsujimoto, G. Free fatty acid receptors FFAR1 and GPR120 as novel therapeutic targets for metabolic disorders. *J. Pharm. Sci.* **2011**, *100*, 3594–3601. [CrossRef] [PubMed]

17. Holliday, N.D.; Watson, S.J.; Brown, A.J.H. Drug discovery opportunities and challenges at G protein coupled receptors for long chain free fatty acids. *Front. Endocrinol.* **2011**, *2*, 1–12. [CrossRef] [PubMed]

18. Dranse, H.J.; Kelly, M.E.; Hudson, B.D. Drugs or diet? Developing novel therapeutic strategies targeting the free fatty acid family of GPCRs. *Br. J. Pharmacol.* **2013**, *170*, 695–711. [CrossRef] [PubMed]

19. Hudson, B.D.; Shimpukade, B.; Mackenzie, A.E.; Butcher, A.J.; Pediani, J.D.; Christiansen, E.; Heathcote, H.; Tobin, A.B.; Ulven, T.; Milligan, G. The pharmacology of TUG-891, a potent and selective agonist of the free fatty acid receptor 4 (FFA4/GPR120), demonstrates both potential opportunity and possible challenges to therapeutic agonism. *Mol. Pharmacol.* **2013**, *84*, 710–725. [CrossRef] [PubMed]

20. Wu, M.; Harvey, K.A.; Ruzmetov, N.; Welch, Z.R.; Sech, L.; Jackson, K.; Stillwell, W.; Zaloga, G.P. Siddiqui RA (2005) ω-3 polyunsaturated fatty acids attenuate breast cancer growth through activation of a neutral sphingomyelinase-mediated pathway. *Int. J. Cancer* **2015**, *117*, 340–348. [CrossRef] [PubMed]

21. Bernard-Gallon, D.J.; Vissac-Sabatier, C.; Antoine-Vincent, D.; Rio, P.G.; Maruizis, J.C.; Fustier, P.; Bignon, Y.J. Differential effects of *n*-3 and *n*-6 polyunsaturated fatty acids on *BRCA1* and *BRCA2* gene expression in breast cell lines. *Br. J. Nutr.* **2002**, *87*, 281–289. [CrossRef] [PubMed]

22. Ghosh-Choudhury, T.; Mandall, C.C.; Woodruff, K.; St. Clair, P.; Fernandes, G.; Chouhury, G.; Ghosh-Choudhury, N. Fish oil targets PTEN to regulate NFκB for downregulation of anti-apoptotic genes in breast tumor growth. *Breast Cancer Res. Treat.* **2009**, *118*, 213–228. [CrossRef] [PubMed]

23. Monk, J.M.; Turk, H.F.; Liddle, D.M.; de Boer, A.A.; Power, K.A.; Ma, D.W.; Robinson, L.E. *n*-3 Polyunsaturated fatty acids and mechanisms to mitigate inflammatory paracrine signaling in obesity—Associated breast cancer. *Nutrients* **2014**, *5*, 4760–4793. [CrossRef] [PubMed]

24. Yonezawa, T.; Katoh, K.; Obara, Y. Existence of GPR40 functioning in a human breast cancer cell line, MCF-7. *Biochem. Biophys. Res. Commun.* **2004**, *314*, 805–809. [CrossRef] [PubMed]

25. Soto-Guzman, A.; Tobledo, T.; Lopez-Perez, M.; Salazar, E.P. Oleic acid induces ERK1/2 activation and AP-1 DNA binding activity through a mechanism involving Src kinase and EGFR transactivation in breast cancer cells. *Mol. Cell. Endocrinol.* **2008**, *294*, 81–91. [CrossRef] [PubMed]

26. Navarro-Tito, N.; Robledo, T.; Salazar, E.P. Arachidonic acid promotes FAK activation and migration in MDA-MB-231 breast cancer cells. *Exp. Cell. Res.* **2008**, *314*, 3340–3355. [CrossRef] [PubMed]

27. Chung, H.; Lee, Y.S.; Mayoral, R.; Oh, D.Y.; Webster, N.J.; Sears, D.D.; Olefsky, J.M.; Ellies, L.G. ω-3 Fatty acids reduce obesity-induced tumor progression independent of GPR120 in a mouse model of postmenopausal breast cancer. *Oncogene* **2014**, *34*, 3504–3513. [CrossRef] [PubMed]

28. Zhang, Z.; Knoepp, S.M.; Sansbury, H.M.; Han, S.; Ku, H.; Xie, Y.; Hallman, M.; Meier, K.E. Differential expression of FAK and Pyk2 in phorbol ester-sensitive and -resistant EL4 thymoma cells. *Clin. Expt. Metastasis* **2011**, *28*, 551–565. [CrossRef] [PubMed]

29. Papupinthu, N.; Lee, H.Y.; Mills, G.B. Lysophosphatidic acid production and action: Critical new players in breast cancer initiation and progression. *Br. J. Cancer* **2010**, *102*, 941–946. [CrossRef] [PubMed]

30. Masuda, H.; Zhang, D.; Bartholomeusz, C.; Doihara, H.; Hortobagyi, G.N.; Ueno, N.T. Role of epidermal growth factor receptor in breast cancer. *Breast Cancer Res. Treat.* **2012**, *136*, 331–345. [CrossRef] [PubMed]

31. O'Kelly, J.; Chung, A.; Lemp, N.; Chumakova, K.; Yin, D.; Wang, H.J.; Said, J.; Gui, D.; Miller, C.W.; Karlan, B.Y.; et al. Functional domains of CCN1 (Cyr61) regulate breast cancer progression. *Int. J. Oncol.* **2008**, *33*, 59–67. [CrossRef] [PubMed]

32. Jun, J.I.; Lau, L.F. Taking aim at the extracellular matrix: CCN proteins as emerging therapeutic targets. *Nature Rev. Drug Discov.* **2011**, *10*, 945–963. [CrossRef] [PubMed]

33. Boucharaba, A.; Serre, C.M.; Gres, S.; Saulnier-Blache, J.S.; Bordet, J.C.; Guglielmi, J.; Clezardin, P.; Peyruchaud, O. Platelet-derived lysophosphatidic acid supports the progression of osteolytic bone metastases in breast cancer. *J. Clin. Invest.* **2004**, *114*, 1714–1725. [CrossRef] [PubMed]

34. Chen, M.; Towers, L.N.; O'Connor, K.L. LPA2 (EDG4) mediates Rho-dependent chemotaxis with lower efficacy than LPA1 (EDG2) in breast carcinoma cells. *Am. J. Physiol. Cell. Physiol.* **2007**, *292*, C1947–C1933. [CrossRef] [PubMed]

35. Li, T.T.; Alemayehu, M.; Aziziyeh, A.; Pape, C.; Pampilio, M.; Postovit, L.M.; Mills, G.B.; Babway, A.V.; Bhattacharya, M. Beta-arrestin/Ral signaling regulates lysophosphatidic acid-mediated migration and invasion of human breast tumor cells. *Mol. Cancer Res.* **2009**, *7*, 1064–1077. [CrossRef] [PubMed]

36. Swaney, J.S.; Chapman, C.; Correa, L.D.; Stebbins, K.J.; Bundey, R.A.; Prodanovich, P.C.; Fagan, P.; Baccei, C.S.; Santini, A.M.; Hutchinson, J.H.; et al. A novel, orally active LPA1 receptor antagonist inhibits lung fibrosis in the mouse bleomycin model. *Br. J. Pharmacol.* **2010**, *160*, 1699–1713. [CrossRef] [PubMed]

37. Alemayehu, M.; Dragan, M.; Pape, C.; Siddiqui, I.; Sacks, D.B.; di Guglielmo, G.M.; Babway, A.V.; Bhattacharya, M. β-Arrestin2 regulates lysophosphatidic acid-induced human breast tumor cell migration and invasion *via* Rap1 and IQGAP1. *PLoS ONE* **2013**, *8*, e56174. [CrossRef] [PubMed]

38. Sun, K.; Cai, H.; Duan, X.; Yang, Y.; Li, M.; Wu, J.; Zhang, X.; Wang, J. Aberrant expression and potential therapeutic target of lysophosphatidic acid receptor 3 in triple-negative breast cancers. *Clin. Exp. Med.* **2014**. [CrossRef] [PubMed]

39. Ohta, H.; Sata, K.; Murata, N.; Damirin, A.; Malchinkhuu, E.; Kon, J.; Kimura, T.; Tobo, M.; Yamazaki, Y.; Watanabe, T.; et al. Ki16425, a subtype-selective antagonist for EDG-family lysophosphatidic acid receptors. *Mol. Pharmacol.* **2003**, *64*, 994–1005. [CrossRef] [PubMed]

40. Hopkins, M.M.; Liu, Z.; Meier, K.E. Cross-talk between lysophosphatidic acid receptor a, free fatty acid receptor 4, and epidermal growth factor receptor in human prostate cancer cells. 2015, Submitted.

41. Boucharaba, A.; Guillet, B.; Menaa, F.; Hneino, M.; van Wijnen, A.J.; Clezardin, P.; Peyruchaud, O. Bioactive lipids lysophosphatidic acid and sphingosine 1-phosphate mediate breast cancer cell biological functions through distinct mechanisms. *Oncol. Res.* **2009**, *18*, 173–184. [CrossRef] [PubMed]

42. Du, S.; Sun, C.; Hu, Z.; Yang, Y.; Zhu, Y.; Zheng, D.; Gu, L.; Lu, X. Lysophosphatidic acid induces MDA-MB-231 breast cancer cells migration through activation of PI3K/PAK1/ERK signaling. *PLoS ONE* **2010**, *5*, e15940. [CrossRef] [PubMed]

43. Swamydas, M.; Nguyen, D.; Allen, L.D.; Eddy, J.; Dreau, D. Progranulin stimulated by LPA promotes the migration of aggressive breast cancer cells. *Cell. Commun. Adhes.* **2010**, *18*, 119–130. [CrossRef] [PubMed]

44. Sun, K.; Duan, X.; Cai, H.; Liu, X.; Yang, Y.; Li, M.; Zhang, X.; Wang, J. Curcumin inhibits LPA-induced invasion by attenuating RhoA/ROCK/MMPs pathway in MCF7 breast cancer cells. *Clin. Exp. Med.* **2015**, 1–11. [CrossRef] [PubMed]

45. Zhang, H.; Xu, X.; Gajewiak, J.; Tsukahara, R.; Fujiwara, Y.; Liu, J.; Fells, J.I.; Perygin, D.; Parrill, A.L.; Tigyi, G.; et al. Dual activity lysophosphatidic acid receptor pan-antagonist/autotaxin inhibitor reduces breast cancer cell migration *in vitro* and causes tumor regression. *Cancer Res.* **2009**, *69*, 5441–5449. [CrossRef] [PubMed]

46. Liu, S.; Umezu-Goto, M.; Murph, M.; Lu, Y.; Liu, W.; Zhang, F.; Yu, S.; Stephens, L.C.; Cui, X.; Murrow, G.; *et al.* Expression of autotaxin and lysophosphatidic acid receptors increases mammary tumorigenesis, invasion, and metastases. *Cancer Cell.* **2009**, *15*, 539–550. [CrossRef] [PubMed]

47. Daaka, Y. Mitogenic action of LPA in prostate. *Biochim. Biophys. Acta.* **2002**, *1582*, 265–269. [CrossRef]

48. Marshall, J.C.A.; Collins, J.W.; Nakayama, J.; Horak, C.E.; Liewehr, D.J.; Steinberg, S.M.; Albaugh, M.; Vidal-Vanaclocha, F.; Palmieri, D.; Marbier, M.; *et al.* Effects of inhibition of the lysophosphatidic acid receptor 1 on metastasis and metastatic dormancy in breast cancer. *J. Natl. Cancer Inst.* **2012**, *104*, 1306–1319. [CrossRef] [PubMed]

49. Kue, P.F.; Taub, J.S.; Harrington, L.B.; Polakiewicz, R.D.; Ullrich, A.; Daaka, Y. Lysophosphatidic acid-regulated mitogenic ERK signaling in androgen-insensitive prostate cancer PC-3 cells. *Int. J. Cancer* **2002**, *102*, 572–579. [CrossRef] [PubMed]

50. Bektas, M.; Payne, S.G.; Liu, H.; Goparaju, S.; Milstien, S.; Spiegel, S. A novel acylglycerol kinase that produces lysophophatidic modulates cross talk with EGFR in prostate cancer cells. *J. Cell. Biol.* **2005**, *169*, 801–811. [CrossRef] [PubMed]

51. Snider, A.J.; Zhang, Z.; Xie, Y.; Meier, K.E. Epidermal growth factor increases lysophosphatidic acid production in human ovarian cancer cells: Roles for phospholipase D2 and receptor transactivation. *Am. J. Physiol. Cell. Physiol.* **2009**, *298*, C163–C170. [CrossRef] [PubMed]

52. Mausbacher, N.; Schreiber, T.B.; Daub, H. Glycoprotein capture and quantitative phosphoproteomics indicate coordinated regulation of cell migration upon lysophosphatidic acid stimulation. *Mol. Cell. Proteom.* **2010**, *9*, 2337–2353. [CrossRef] [PubMed]

53. Colin-Santana, C.C.; Avendano-Vazquez, S.E.; Alcantara-Hernandez, R.; Garcia-Sainz, J.A. EGF and angiotensin II modulate lysophosphatidic acid LPA$_1$ receptor function and phosphorylation state. *Biochim. Biophys. Acta* **2011**, *1810*, 1170–1177. [CrossRef] [PubMed]

13

The Effect of Marine Derived *n*-3 Fatty Acids on Adipose Tissue Metabolism and Function

Marijana Todorčević and Leanne Hodson *

Academic Editors: Lindsay Brown, Hemant Poudyal and Bernhard Rauch

Oxford Centre for Diabetes, Endocrinology and Metabolism, University of Oxford, Churchill Hospital, OX3 7LE Oxford, UK; marijana.todorcevic@ocdem.ox.ac.uk
* Correspondence: leanne.hodson@ocdem.ox.ac.uk

Abstract: Adipose tissue function is key determinant of metabolic health, with specific nutrients being suggested to play a role in tissue metabolism. One such group of nutrients are the *n*-3 fatty acids, specifically eicosapentaenoic acid (EPA; 20:5*n*-3) and docosahexaenoic acid (DHA; 22:6*n*-3). Results from studies where human, animal and cellular models have been utilised to investigate the effects of EPA and/or DHA on white adipose tissue/adipocytes suggest anti-obesity and anti-inflammatory effects. We review here evidence for these effects, specifically focusing on studies that provide some insight into metabolic pathways or processes. Of note, limited work has been undertaken investigating the effects of EPA and DHA on white adipose tissue in humans whilst more work has been undertaken using animal and cellular models. Taken together it would appear that EPA and DHA have a positive effect on lowering lipogenesis, increasing lipolysis and decreasing inflammation, all of which would be beneficial for adipose tissue biology. What remains to be elucidated is the duration and dose required to see a favourable effect of EPA and DHA *in vivo* in humans, across a range of adiposity.

Keywords: *n*-3 fatty acids; subcutaneous; adipose tissue; marine

1. Introduction

Adipose tissue, the largest organ in the human body, was historically considered to be metabolically inert. However, white adipose tissue is now considered an endocrine organ as it secretes adipokines (and hormones) which act locally and distally through autocrine, paracrine and endocrine effects [1]. Although adipose tissue is comprised of several cell types, including pre-adipocytes, adipocytes, endothelial cells, fibroblasts, leukocytes and macrophages [2], all of which may impact on tissue function, one of the main functions of adipocytes/adipose tissue is to store fatty acids [3]. Adipose tissue acts to "buffer" the influx of dietary fat into the circulation [3,4], with excess dietary fat being stored in adipose tissue rather than "overflowing" to non-adipose organs. Ectopic fat deposition has been proposed to underlie obesity-associated metabolic diseases [5]. An increase in adipose tissue mass may alter the function of the tissue. For example, when adipose tissue starts to expand (such as with excess nutrition) macrophages infiltrate and orchestrate inflammatory responses via molecules such as tumor necrosis factor α (TNFα), interleukin 6 (IL-6) and monocyte chemoattractant protein-1 (MCP-1), all of which have been implicated in the development of pathological changes in adipose tissue physiology [6–9]. Intriguingly, a proportion of overweight/obese individuals remain metabolically healthy even with further weight gain, whilst others do not; it has recently been suggested this is due to an increased capacity of adipose tissue for lipogenesis [10]. Multiple factors have been suggested to impact on the function of adipose tissue, however as the tissue is the primary site for dietary fat storage and reflects dietary fat intakes [11] it is reasonable to suggest that the composition or type of fat that the tissue is exposed to may also influence the function.

A class of fatty acids that has received a lot of attention over the last 30 years is the *n*-3 (or ω-3) fatty acids, specifically those derived from marine sources. *n*-3 fatty acids have been suggested to lower the risk of a number of non-communicable metabolic diseases including cardiovascular disease, obesity and diabetes [12–14]. Here we review the effect of long chain *n*-3 polyunsaturated fatty acids (LCPUFA), specifically eicosapentaenoic acid (EPA, 20:5*n*-3) and docosahexaenoic acid (DHA, 22:6*n*-3) on white adipose tissue metabolism and function. Although other *n*-3 fatty acids such as α-linolenic acid (ALA, 18:3*n*-3) and docosapentanoic acid (DPA, 22:5*n*-3) are of potential interest, data are limited. A number of reviews on the effect of fish oil or *n*-3 fatty acids on adipose tissue have previously been undertaken [15–20], therefore we have chosen to review the evidence from human, animal (rodent and fish) and *in vitro* cellular studies regarding the specific effects EPA and DHA have on the metabolism and function of white adipose tissue from different depots. Specifically, we will discuss the mechanisms by which EPA and DHA are proposed to reduce adiposity along with discussion regarding how *n*-3 fatty acids may influence markers of adipose tissue inflammation and cytokine production.

2. Dietary Sources of Eicosapentaenoic Acid (EPA) and Docosahexaenoic Acid (DHA)

EPA and DHA, commonly referred to as fish oil fatty acids, are not synthesized *de novo* by fish. Fish accumulate them through consumption of water plants, such as plankton and algae, which are part of the marine food chain [21]. Therefore, if plankton and algae are not a dietary component or if fish oil is replaced by other feed sources, such as in fish farming where a vegetable-oil based diet rich in linoleic acid (18:2*n*-6) and oleic acid (18:1*n*-9) may be given, the EPA and DHA content of the fish will decrease [22,23]. Marine fish tend to have higher amounts of EPA and DHA than freshwater fish. Fish typically store EPA and DHA mainly as triacylglycerol, at the middle position (sn-2) of the glycerol backbone however, in krill, a shrimp-like crustacean that feed off algae in deep ocean waters, 30%–65% of EPA and DHA is in phospholipids [24].

Within the human diet, EPA and DHA can be produced from ALA but the capacity of conversion is low in humans, although higher in women of child-bearing age than men [25]. Thus, it is likely that the majority of EPA and DHA within the body, for most individuals are derived from fish and fish oil intakes. Fish oil is often considered to be the best source of EPA and DHA however, as mentioned above, the amount of EPA and DHA varies amongst species and within a species according to environmental variables such as diet, temperature and salinity of the water.

3. Fatty Acid Composition of Adipose Tissue

As the fatty acid composition of adipose tissue has a half-life between 6 months and 2 years, it reflects long-term dietary intake along with endogenous metabolism [11]. The abundance of EPA and DHA in human subcutaneous adipose tissue is low, typically less than 0.2 for EPA and up to 1.0 mol% for DHA [11]. The amount of EPA and DHA in adipose tissue has been reported to increase or remain unchanged with increasing age [26–28], which is suggested to be an age-dependent effect independent of dietary intake [28].

Studies measuring the change in adipose tissue fatty acid composition, as a marker of compliance to *n*-3 supplementation are limited and findings inconsistent with some [29–32] but not all [33,34] noting small but significant increases in the abundance of adipose tissue EPA and DHA after varying periods of fish oil supplementation (Table 1). The inconsistency in findings may in part be explained by differences in: duration of supplementation, amount of EPA and DHA consumed, participant age, sex and adiposity, or site where the adipose biopsy was taken. Elegant work by Katan *et al.* [30] clearly demonstrated that the levels of DHA rose more rapidly in subcutaneous abdominal compared to gluteal adipose tissue depots whilst differences between the depots for EPA were not as obvious (Table 1). The difference in the appearance of DHA in subcutaneous abdominal compared to gluteal adipose tissue, may be explained by the fact that dietary fat extraction (from chylomicron-triacylglycerol) occurs to a greater extent in subcutaneous abdominal than gluteal adipose tissue [35]. Of note, Katan *et al.* [30] found that the proportion of EPA and DHA in subcutaneous abdominal and gluteal adipose tissue was approximately one-sixth and one-third respectively of dietary intake. It would be of interest to determine the extent to which the fatty acid composition of visceral (intra-abdominal) adipose tissue changed with n-3 fatty acid supplementation. However, as visceral adipose tissue samples are often obtained during elective surgery, it would be challenging to undertake a well-controlled study. Taken together, the data presented in Table 1 clearly demonstrate that even with supplementation the abundance of EPA and DHA in adipose tissue does not increase notably. This suggests that EPA and DHA are not preferentially stored in adipose tissue triacylglycerol long-term, rather they may be partitioned to oxidation pathways or to storage in other lipid fractions, such as phospholipids; red blood cell and plasma phospholipids have a notably higher abundance of both EPA and DHA than adipose tissue [11]. However, a change in adipose tissue fat mass and therefore dilution of EPA and DHA abundance cannot be ruled out as the majority of studies do not indicate if there were changes in participants' body weight over the course of the study. Changes in fatty acid composition of adipose tissue have been reported with weight loss, notably there was not change in EPA abundance but an increase in DHA abundance, without a reported change in n-3 fatty acid intake, over the weight maintenance period [36]. These changes highlight the importance of weight/fat mass stability in subjects participating in intervention studies where adipose tissue fatty acid composition is being measured as a marker of compliance.

Table 1. Overview of human studies investigating change in eicosapentaenoic acid (EPA) and docosahexaenoic acid (DHA) abundance in subcutaneous adipose tissue.

Reference	Study Design	Subjects	Dose	Length	SCAT Biopsy Site	Abundance in AT EPA and DHA
[33]	Randomized double-blind, placebo controlled, parallel groups	Control: n = 25 (12 M/13 F) Age 55.4 y; BMI 29.5 kg/m²	Control: 2 g olive oil	6 wk	Gluteal	Control (baseline vs. 6 wk): EPA—0.11% to 0.11%; DHA—0.29% to 0.29%
		n-3 PUFA: n = 25 (12M/13F) Age 58.0 y; BMI 30.8 kg/m²	n-3 PUFA: 2 g fish oil/d (640 mg EPA and 480 mg DHA)			n-3 PUFA: EPA—0.12% to 0.13%; DHA—0.27% to 0.30%
[34]	Randomized double-blind, placebo controlled	Control: Pre-menopausal: n = 22 Age 44 y, BMI 24.6 kg/m²; Post-menopausal: n = 23 Age 55.6 y, BMI 23.1 kg/m²	Control: 4 g thistle oil	12 wk	Gluteal	Control (baseline vs. 12 wk): Pre-menopausal: EPA 0.1% to 0.1%; DHA 0.2% to 0.3%; Post-menopausal: EPA 0.1% to 0.1%; DHA 0.3% to 0.3%
		Fish oil: Pre-menopausal: n = 23 Age 41.6 y, BMI 24.5 kg/m²; Post-menopausal: n = 22, Age 56.0 y; BMI 24.5 kg/m²	Fish oil: 4 g fish oil (38.5% EPA and 25.9% DHA)			Fish oil: Pre-menopausal: EPA 0.1% to 0.1%; DHA 0.2% to 0.2%; Post-menopausal: EPA 0.1% to 0.2%; DHA 0.3% to 0.4%
[31]	Observational	Eight control; Seven patients attending lipid disorder clinic	Control: low fish/no fish oil supplementation; Patients (fish oil): 10–15 g MaxEPA (17% EPA, 10.6% DHA)	12 m	Not reported	Control Group: EPA 0.003% (total FA); DHA 0.1%; Fish oil Group: EPA 0.4%; DHA 0.7%
[32]	Randomised placebo controlled parallel	Control: n = 14 (6M/8F) Age‡ 62 y, BMI‡ 29.2 kg/m² all had T2D	Control: 20 g/d corn oil	9 wk	Gluteal	Control (0 vs. 9 wk); EPA 0.16% to 0.15%; DHA 0.39% to 0.39%
		Fish oil: n = 12 (7M/5F) Age‡ 57 y, BMI‡ 30.1 kg/m² all had T2D	Fish oil: 20 g/d fish oil (13% EPA, 21% DHA)			Fish oil (0 vs. 9 wk); EPA 0.18% to 0.23%; DHA 0.49% to 0.55% *

Table 1. *Cont.*

Reference	Study Design	Subjects	Dose	Length	SCAT Biopsy Site	Abundance in AT EPA and DHA
[30]	Parallel study 4 groups (0, 3, 6 or 9 g fish oil/d)	58 months; Age 56.2 y	0 g/d = olive + palm oil; 3 g/d = 0.81 g EPA, 0.16 g DHA; 6 g/d = 1.62 g EPA, 0.33 g DHA; 9 g/d = 2.43 g EPA, 0.49 g DHA	12 m	Abdominal Gluteal	Average change/g FA/d; EPA: Abdo = ↑0.12 wt %; Gluteal = ↑0.11 wt % DHA: Abdo = ↑0.24 wt %; Gluteal = ↑0.14 wt %
[29]	Parallel study 5 groups (received capsules to be equal to one portion of oily fish for 0, 1, 2 or 4 d/wk)	M and F 20–80 y; BMI >18 or <35 kg/m^2	0 = high oleic sunflower oil; 1 = 1.5 g EPA, 1.77 g DHA/wk; 2 = 3.0 g EPA, 3.54 g DHA /wk; 4 = 6.0 g EPA, 7.08 g DHA/wk	12 m	Abdominal	Average change (% total FAs) compared to 0 portions; EPA: 0 portions = 0.18 % total; 1 portion = ↑0.05 % total; 2 portions = ↑0.04 % total; 4 portions = ↑0.11 % total ** DHA: 0 portions = 0.22 % total; 1 portion = ↑0.05 % total; 2 portions = ↑0.06 % total; 4 portions = ↑0.13 % total **

Abbreviations: Ref, reference; M, males; F, females; y, years; BMI, body mass index; m, months; d, day; wk, week; T2D, type 2 diabetes; PUFA, polyunsaturated fatty acids; EPA, eicosapentaenoic acid; DHA, docosahexaenoic acid; SCAT, subcutaneous adipose tissue; FA, fatty acid; abdo, abdominal. Mean reported unless otherwise stated; ‡ median reported

* $p < 0.05$ between baseline and end of study; ** $p < 0.001$ increase across groups.

4. The "Anti-Obesity" Effect of EPA and DHA

Measuring an anti-obesity effect of increased EPA and DHA consumption in humans is challenging, not least as there are many other factors to control for (e.g., exercise and other dietary components) and methodology sensitive to small changes in adipose tissue mass needs to be used. In 2009, Buckley and Howe [37] reviewed the available evidence for an anti-obesity effect of EPA and DHA. They suggested from the limited human studies, that increased consumption of EPA and DHA may reduce body fat; the majority of these studies were short-term, with a small number of subjects. It remains unclear if similar conclusions can be drawn from longer-term studies. A recent meta-analysis by Du and colleagues [38] identified randomised, placebo controlled trials where adults were assigned to either fish oil/marine group for a period of greater than 4 weeks and had reported at least one anthropometric measure of body composition (*i.e.*, body weight, BMI, waist circumference or waist to hip ratio). From the 21 studies (a total of 1329 individuals) they found no evidence to support an anti-obesity role of *n*-3 LCPUFA [38]. It is plausible that changes were not detected due to the non-specific and insensitive methods used to assess changes in body fat. By using computed tomography Sato *et al.* [39] noted that 6 months supplementation with EPA only (1800 mg/day) resulted in a significant decrease in epicardial and visceral adipose tissue mass, with no change in subcutaneous abdominal adipose tissue, in individuals with confirmed coronary artery disease. It is possible that subcutaneous abdominal adipose tissue mass did decrease however it was only measured in a single slice at the level of the umbilicus, thus changes in other depots would not have been detected. Results from some, but not all animal studies have suggested EPA and DHA consumption to have an anti-obesity effect with a lack of increase in fat mass even when an obesogenic diet is consumed [40], as well as a reduction in body weight if already obese [41]. Moreover, these studies, along with cellular studies have been used to tease out the mechanisms involved in this process, as discussed below with data from human [42–48], animal [40,41,49–55] and cellular [56–69] studies provided in Tables 2–4.

4.1. Suppression of Fat Deposition and Adipogenesis

A decrease in fatty acid deposition within adipose tissue may occur due to a decrease in triacylglycerol synthesis via decreased *de novo* lipogenesis or re-esterification of fatty acids within the tissue; alternatively it may occur due to a lower flux of fatty acids to the tissue. In the latter situation, fatty acids could be repartitioned to other tissues (such as muscle) for disposal, rather than going to adipose tissue for storage. In humans, the absolute contribution of *de novo* synthesized fatty acids to adipose tissue triacylglycerol is potentially small [70] and measuring adipose tissue *de novo* lipogenesis (or fatty acid esterification/re-esterification) *in vivo* in humans is challenging. Therefore, it is not surprising that studies have not been undertaken investigating how EPA and DHA supplementation influence these processes in humans. Although not a direct measure of fatty acid synthesis or esterification/re-esterification within the tissue, the measurement of the expression of genes related to these processes provides some insight to the effect of EPA and DHA on these processes. Camargo *et al.* [42] reported that consumption of 4 g/day of fish oil (containing a total of 1.24 g EPA and DHA) for 12 weeks significantly decreased the expression of genes related to fatty acid uptake and storage in subcutaneous obese adipose tissue (Table 2).

Work in animal models has typically found EPA and DHA to limit lipid accumulation in adipose tissue (Table 3). The majority of studies have reported lower fad pad mass and adipocytes number and size which was suggested to occur via suppression of lipogenic genes and, in some studies, a concomitant activation of lipolytic genes after supplementation with EPA and DHA (Table 3). Despite reporting a significant decrease in inguinal retroperitoneal fat pad mass Hainault *et al.* [52] did not find any significant change in fatty acid synthase (FAS) activity or mRNA expression in these depots. Of note, one study reported that EPA and DHA consumption resulted in higher total and perigonadal fat mass than control group [55]. This discrepancy in findings maybe in part explained that this study used an LDL receptor deficient (LDLR$^{-/-}$) mouse model whilst others have typically used C57Bl/6 mice or Wistar rats.

Table 2. Overview of human studies investigating the effect of EPA and DHA supplementation on markers of adipose tissue metabolism and function.

Reference	Study Design	Subjects	Dose	Length	Measured	Adipose Tissue Outcome
[42]	Parallel (LIPGENE) study) 4 Groups	Group 1. high SFA ($n = 8$, Age 57.8 y; BMI 36 kg/m^2)	Group 1. No n-3	12 wk	SCAT abdo; mRNA expression of genes related to fatty acid uptake and storage	n-3 Supplementation group only had a significant decreased expression of PLIN1 and FABP4
		Group 2. high MUFA ($n = 9$, Age 57.1 y; BMI 34.5 kg/m^2)	Group 2. No n-3			
		Group 3.LFHCC (plus 4×1 g/d sunflower oil) ($n = 12$, Age 56.5 y; BMI 35.7 kg/m^2)	Group 3. supplement 4×1 g sunflower oil			
		Group 4. LFHCC plus 4×1 g/d FO ($n = 10$, Age 54.8 y; BMI 35.0 kg/m^2)	Group 4. supplement 4×1 g FO (1.24 g n-3 fatty acids in ratio 1.4 EPA:1 DHA)			
[45]	Parallel (LIPGENE study) 4 Groups	See Reference [42] (Table 2) for participant characteristics and dietary groups	Group 1. No n-3	12 wk	SCAT abdo mRNA and protein expression of genes related to insulin signaling and carbohydrate metabolism	n-3 Supplementation for 12 wk increased expression of IRS-1 protein and CAP and decreased the expression of JNK, pAKT, EHD2, GAPDH, PEPCK1 and Anxa2. There was no change in PDK1
			Group 2. no n-3			
			Group 3. supplement 4×1 g sunflower oil			
			Group 4. supplement 4×1 g FO (1.24 g n-3 fatty acids in ratio 1.4 EPA:1 DHA)			
[47]	Parallel (LIPGENE study) 4 Groups	See Reference [42] (Table 2) for participant characteristics and dietary groups	Group 1. No n-3	12 wk	SCAT abdo mRNA expression of genes related to antioxidant processes; Postprandial = 4 h after high fat meal consumption	Postprandial increase in AT NADPH oxidase subunit p40^{phox} after 12 wk consumption n-3 fatty acids; Compared to SFA diet postprandial expression of SOD2, GPX4, TXN and KEAP1 were significantly lower whilst GPX3 and TXNRD1 were significantly higher
			Group 2. no n-3			
			Group 3. supplement 4×1 g sunflower oil			
			Group 4. supplement 4×1 g FO (1.24 g n-3 fatty acids in ratio 1.4 EPA:1 DHA)			

Table 2. *Cont.*

Reference	Study Design	Subjects	Dose	Length	Measured	Adipose Tissue Outcome
[46]	Parallel	Control (n = 13 (5M/8F) 37.8 y; BMI 30.1 kg/m²); n-3 PUFA (n = 11 (3M/8M) 40.5 y; BMI 30.4 kg/m²)	Control: n-3 fatty acids %TE intake = 0; n-3 PUFA: EPA—0.68% TE and DHA—0.47% TE	14 wk (2 wk isocaloric, 12 wk *ad libitum*)	SCAT abdo; mRNa expression of gene related to inflammation	No change in the mRNA expression of genes encoding mediators of inflammation after consumption of n-3 fatty acids or when compared to control group.
[44]	Parallel	Control (n = 28 (15M/23F) 38 y; BMI 44.6 kg/m²); n-3 PUFA (n = 27 (14M/23F) 39 y; BMI 48.7 kg/m²)	Control: butter fat (5g/d) on control diet; n-3 PUFA: 4 g/d n-3 as ethyl esters (46% EPA and 38% DHA)	8 wk	VAT and SCAT abdo biopsies taken at end of intervention only. Expression of inflammatory related genes. Production of anti-inflammatory n-3 PUFA-derived eicosanoids.	Compared to control significant decreases in SCAT abdo on n-3 PUFA group for CCL2, CCL3, IL6, HIF-1A, TGFB1, CD40 and an increase in ADIPOQ. No differences in inflammatory genes in VAT. DHA-derived lipid mediators were more increased in VAT than in SAT.
[43]	Parallel (2 doses)	Group A: n = 6 (4 M) age 50.5 ± 10.8 y; BMI < 27 kg/m2 with CKD; Group B: n = 6 (2 M) age 50.2 ± 6.7 y; BMI < 27 kg/m2 with CKD	Group A: 6 MaxEPA capsule/d (180 mg and 120 mg DHA per capsule); Group B: 12 MaxEPA capsule/d (180 mg and 120 mg DHA/capsule)	10 wk	SCAT Abdo mRNA expression of genes related to inflammation	Group A: decreased mRNA expression of MMP9 and CD68 (baseline vs. 10 wk); Group B: non-significant increase in MMP9 and CD68 (baseline vs. 10 wk)
[48]	Parallel	Placebo: n = 14 (5M) 53.3 ± 2.2 y; BMI 33.4 (27–43) kg/m2 with IR; Fish oil: n = 19 (6 M), 48.8 ± 2.3 (sem) y; BMI 33.4 (27–43) kg/m2 with IR	Placebo: 4 g/d corn oil; Fish oil (FO): 4 g/d EPA and DHA (Lovaza/Omacor)	12 wk	SCAT Abdo FAC, macrophages, capillaries, expression of inflammatory genes	Baseline vs. 12 weeks: Abundance of EPA and DHA in SCAT Abdo increased in FO group only; Significant decrease in macrophages and crown like structures in tissue of FO group only; Significant decrease in mRNA expression of tissue MCP-1 and CD68 in FO group only

Data for age and BMI where data was available presented as mean ± sem. Abbreviations: Ref, reference number; M, males; F, females; y, years; BMI, body mass index; CKD, chronic kidney disease; CAD, coronary artery disease; SFA, saturated fat rich diet (16% total energy (TE)); MUFA, monounsaturated fat rich diet (20%TE); LFHCC, low-fat, high complex carbohydrate diet; PUFA, polyunsaturated fatty acids; FO, fish oil; EPA, eicosapentaenoic acid; DHA, docosahexaenoic acid; SCAT, white subcutaneous adipose tissue; Abdo, abdominal; VAT, visceral adipose tissue; AT, adipose tissue, IR, insulin resistance; MMP9, metalloprotease; CD68 phagocytic activity; FAC, fatty acid composition; MCP-1, macrophage chemoattractant protein 1; PLIN1, perilipin; FABP4, fatty acid binding protein-4; CAV1, caveolin; IRS-1, insulin receptor substrate-1; CAP, cbl-associated protein; JNK, jun N-terminal kinase; pAKT, phosphorylated v-akt murine thymoma viral oncogene homolog; EHD2, EH-domain containin-2; PDK1, 3-phosphoinositide-dependent protein kinase-1; GAPDH, glyceraldehyde-3-phosphate dehydrogenase; PEPCK1, phosphenolpyruvate carboxykinase-1; SOD2, superoxide dismutase 2; GPX, glutathione peroxidase; TXN, thioredoxine; TXNRD1, thioredoxin reductase 1; CCL2, chemokine (C-C motif) ligand 2; CCL3, chemokine (C-C motif) ligand 3; IL6, interleukin 6; HIF-1A, hypoxia-inducible factor 1-α; TGFB1, transforming growth factor β1; CD40, Cluster of differentiation 40; ADIPOQ: adiponectin.

Table 3. Overview of animal studies investigating the effect of EPA and DHA supplementation on markers of adipose tissue metabolism and function.

Reference	Study Design/Diet	Model	Dose	Duration	Measured	Adipose Tissue Outcome
[41]	Weight gain HF diet	C57BL/6J mice	EPA and DHA combined increasing from 1% to 12% (wt/wt) dietary lipids	7–8 wk	Adiposity	AT accumulation limited when the amount of EPA/DHA increased on high fat diet. Epididymal fat decreased by 30%–50% of tissue cellularity.
[51]	HF diet with different combination of fatty acids added: 4 groups	4 m C57BL/6J male mice	Group 1: HF-F high fat with 20% (wt/wt) flaxseed oil. Group 2: HF-F2: 44% dietary lipids—6% EPA and 51% DHA (EPAX1050). Group 3: cHF-HF low n-3 PUFA content. Group 4: HF-F1 high fat 15% EPAX1050	4–5 wk	Adiposity	The EPA/DHA group (HF-F2) decreased body weight and had lowest increase in epididymal fat. Epididymal mRNA expression of genes related to OXPHOS and fatty acid uptake increased and those related to lipogenesis decreased.
[50]	HF diets comparing MaxEPA oil, herring oil, olive oil + beef tallow	50 d Wistar rats	MaxEPA—n-3 fatty acids ~41% diet; Herring oil—n-3 fatty acids-3 ~19% diet; Olive oil + beef tallow: n-3 fatty acids ~1% diet	4 wk	Adiposity	MaxEPA group has significantly lower lipid mass and fat cell size (but no change in number) in retroperitoneal fat compared to the low n-3 (olive oil + beef tallow) and herring oil diets. MaxEPA group had significantly lower epididymal fat mass and fat cell number compared to olive oil + beef tallow group.
[52]	HF (50% TE) diets. Three groups: Group 1. high lard / Group 2: high lard plus FO / Group 3: high lard plus corn oil	6 wk male Wistar rats	Not described	16–20 d	Adiposity	High lard and high lard plus corn oil significantly increased retroperitoneal fat whilst high lard plus FO had significant decrease in weight of inguinal, retroperitoneal and epididymal AT. No change in any group in FAS activity or expression in inguinal and retroperitoneal fat depots.
[49]	HF feeding with corn oil or FO	Male Fisher 344 rats	40% diet FO or 40% diet corn oil	6 wk	Adiposity	FO group had significantly lower epididymal fat pads than the corn oil group.
[53]	HF feeding with or without FO	Male C57Bl/6 (WT) or GPR120 knockout mice—15 wk	With or without 27% menhaden FO (wt/wt menhanden FO 16% EPA and 9% DHA)	5 wk	AT inflammation	Wild-type animals: FO group had decreased mRNA expression of genes related to inflammation and macrophage infiltration in AT. FO supplementation had no effect in GPR120 knockout.

Table 3. *Cont.*

Reference	Study Design/Diet	Model	Dose	Duration	Measured	Adipose Tissue Outcome
[55]	HF diets (39% energy) comparison of olive oil and FO.	LDL receptor deficient (LDLR−/−) mice on C57BL/6J background. Females 2–3 m old.	Olive oil group: 6% energy olive FO group: 6% energy menhaden oil (140 mg EPA and 95 mg DHA/g oil)	12 wk	Adiposity and inflammation	Compared to olive oil group the FO group had: - significantly higher total and perigonadal fat mass than olive oil group. - significantly higher distribution of larger adipocytes. - significantly increased AT cholesterol content and decreased gene expression in WAT related to inflammation and insulin sensitivity compared to olive oil group.
[54]	Control (FO 6% fat dry wt) and cafeteria (HF 62% fat dry wt) and	Male Wistar rats	Control and cafeteria groups: EPA 1 g/1kg/per day	5 wk	Adiposity, apoptosis and inflammation	Cafeteria + EPA group had lower fat mass gain, reduced retroperitoneal fat mass, decreased food intake and increased leptin production compared to cafeteria only fed rats. Control + EPA group had marked increase in markers of adipocyte apoptosis compared to control only. No different in cafeteria fed groups. TNFα expression significantly decreased in cafeteria + EPA compared to cafeteria only.
[40]	High and low dietary levels of EPA and DHA	Atlantic salmon	Control (rapeseed oil 10% of total fatty acids), FO (20% of total fatty acids), DHA enriched oil diet (42% DHA and 9% EPA), EPA enriched oil diet (43% EPA and 12% DHA)	21 wk	Lipid accumulation, β-oxidation, apoptosis	FO in decrease fat percentage of WAT and increase the FA β-oxidation capacity. High levels of DHA and EPA in DHA and E PA enriched oil diets lead to, loss of mitochondrial functions, and induction of caspase-3, indicating an onset of apoptosis.

Abbreviations: Ref, reference number; EPA, eicosapentanoeic acid; DHA, docosahexanoic acid; wk, weeks, m, months; AT, adipose tissue; WAT, white adipose tissue; HF, high fat; FO, fish oil; FAS, fatty acid synthase; WT, wild-type; GPR120. G-couple protein receptor 120; LDL, low density lipoprotein; wt, weight; TNFα, tumor necrosis factor α.

Studies investigating the effects of dietary EPA and DHA on adipose tissue function have also been undertaken in fish (Table 3). Todorcevic *et al.* [40] demonstrated that a diet supplemented with EPA and DHA (20% of total fatty acids) for 21 weeks repressed the development of adiposity, regulating triacylglycerol accumulation in visceral adipose tissue of Atlantic salmon. A positive influence of dietary EPA and DHA on lipid accumulation in adipose tissue was also reported in grass carp [71]. Diet containing EPA and DHA, (12% of total fatty acids for 75 days), suppressed lipid accumulation in intraperitoneal adipose tissue and significantly up-regulated the expression lipolytic genes including: lipoprotein lipase (LPL), stearoyl-CoA desaturase 1 (SCD1) and peroxisome proliferator activated receptor α (PPARα) [71]. Furthermore, similar results were reported by Liu *et al.* [72] in grass carp treated with dietary EPA and DHA (11% of total fatty acids) for 95 days.

The process of adipogenesis (or an increase in fat mass) involves the differentiation of preadipocytes to mature adipocytes, is a complex and tightly regulated process involving a cascade of transcription factors which are sensitive to the nutritional environment [73]. In a comprehensive review by McMillen and Robinson [74] the role of the nutritional environment an individual is exposed to before birth and in early infancy impacts on risk of obesity and obesity-related diseases later in life was discussed. Evidence from animal studies shows that offspring of mothers fed a diet high in calories or high in fat before birth are heavier and have a higher percentage body fat throughout life [75,76]. Findings from human studies are compelling; children born to mothers who are obese during their pregnancy have an increased incidence of obesity over the life course [75]. Therefore, it has been suggested that targeting maternal nutrition during pregnancy may reduce risk of obesity in subsequent generations [77]; *n*-3 fatty acids may decrease adipogenesis and lipogenesis and thus exposure in utero to these fatty acids may lower the risk of obesity in offspring. In 2011 Muhlhausler and colleagues [77] reviewed animal studies to determine the effects of *n*-3 LCPUFA supplementation during pregnancy and lactation on postnatal body composition of offspring. Although 13 potential studies were identified, only four met the inclusion criteria and the authors found from albeit limited data that there was a suggestion that the offspring from *n*-3 LCPUFA supplemented dams had a lower fat mass [77]. In contrast, supplementation of dams with a high DHA diet (5% fat of which DHA was 0.95% total fatty acids) during pregnancy and lactation resulted in offspring that had significantly higher total and subcutaneous fat mass (as percentage of total body weight) at 6 weeks of age, compared to control animals fed a diet containing the same amount of fat but devoid of *n*-3 LCPUFA [78]. Thus it remains unclear if increased exposure in utero to *n*-3 fatty acids decreases adipogenesis and lipogenesis and is an area that warrants further investigation.

To date, the majority of *in vitro* evidence regarding the mechanistic effects of EPA and DHA on triacylglycerol accumulation/lipid deposition comes from the clonal murine cell line, 3T3-L1 (Table 4). This cell line offers advantages over primary cells, as they are homogenous with regards to cellular population and stage of differentiation; however, their ability to reflect human adipose tissue function and metabolism remains to be clarified. Primary pre-adipocyte cultures have been shown to better reflect *in vivo* adipose function, than cell lines because they can be isolated from different species and fat depots. The latter is of interest as there are distinct molecular and biochemical hallmarks between different adipose tissue depots and at a cellular level; pre-adipocytes isolated from different adipose tissue depots and cultured *in vitro* retain depot-specific functional properties [79–81]. Unlike cell lines, the function and metabolism of primary cells will be influenced by the age, sex, and genetics of the donor and therefore consideration is needed when comparing across studies.

Results from *in vitro* cellular studies that have added EPA and DHA to media for periods of 24 h to 3 weeks are mixed; some suggest EPA and DHA to be anti-adipogenic whilst others find a pro-adipogenic response. EPA and DHA have been found to inhibit, promote or have no effect on the differentiation of pre-adipocytes (Table 4). Typically the markers of adipocytes adipogenesis that have been measured include: the accumulation of triacylglycerol, lipid droplet formation, expression of master adipogenic transcription factors, and lipid genes. Using 3T3-L1 pre-adipocytes, Kim *et al.* [59] investigated the effects of DHA alone (6 days) on lipogenesis and lipolysis and found mean lipid droplet size, percent lipid area, as well as glycerol-3-phosphate dehydrogenase (GPDH) activity all significantly decreased whilst basal lipolysis increased in fully differentiated adipocytes. The results from this work demonstrate the anti-adipogenic effects of DHA via inhibition of triacylglycerol accumulation and increased lipolysis [59]. When comparing the effects of EPA and DHA on lipid droplet formation in 3T3-L1 cells it was found that although both fatty acids reduced the presence of lipid droplets, DHA was more potent than EPA [56]. In addition to the decreased lipid droplet formation, there were notable reductions in the expression of key protein involved in this process, including perilipin A, caveolin-1 and Cidea [56], however there was no effect of DHA on PPARγ expression [56]. In contrast, Murali et al. [62] reported that incubating 3T3-L1 with EPA and DHA induced adipogenesis; DHA being more potent than EPA in inducing the differentiation process. The authors suggested the differential effects of EPA and DHA on adipognesis could be due to differential accumulation of n-3 fatty acids in membrane phospholipids [62]. In line with Murali et al. [62], Wojcik et al. [69] reported increased accumulation of neutral lipids in mature 3T3-L1 adipocytes; however, others have reported no effect on triacylglycerol accumulation at any stage of maturation in 3T3-L1 adipocytes [65]. A reduced expression of both adipogenic and lipogenic genes, including sterol regulatory element-binding protein 1 (SREBP1), FAS, and peroxisome proliferator-activated receptor γ (PPARγ) after EPA and DHA treatment of mature adipocytes has been report by some [69] but not by others [67]. Using human breast adipocytes as a cell model, Wang et al. [68] demonstrated exposure of DHA for 24 h decreased the expression of lipogenic genes, including FAS, LPL and PPARγ, whilst expression of lipolytic genes was increased. Lee et al. [82] found EPA to stimulate glycerol and free fatty acids release which was associated with induction of lipolytic gene expression and suppression of adipogenic gene expression in 3T3-L1 adipocytes. Treatment of fish primary adipocytes with EPA and DHA (for 3 weeks) resulted in decreased triacylglycerol accumulation in mature adipocytes [83]. In an acute study, using mature adipocytes isolated from grass carp Liu et al. [72] found that 6 h of incubation with EPA and DHA was sufficient to notably decreased triacylglycerol accumulation, significantly increased glycerol release and the expression of genes involved in lipolysis (e.g., adipose triglyceride lipase (ATGL), hormone-sensitive lipase (HSL)). The findings from in vitro cellular studies, notably those using primary adipocytes demonstrate that EPA and DHA inhibit triacylglycerol accumulation, which may be the result of effects mediated through genes related to lipogenesis and lipolysis.

Overall, the effects of EPA and DHA as well as EPA versus DHA in modifying adipogensis and lipid accumulation, in particular in humans, and to a lesser extent in murine models, remain unclear. Plausible reasons the discrepancies in findings between in vitro cellular studies are likely to be in part due to the use of different in vitro models, i.e., using primary cells versus immortalized cell lines, studying the cells at different developmental stages, differences in the concentrations of fatty acid(s) the cells were exposed to, along with the duration of exposure.

Table 4. Overview of cellular studies investigating the effect of EPA and DHA supplementation on markers of adipocytes metabolism and function.

Reference	Cell Type	Cell Stage	Control Cells *	EPA/DHA Dose	Culture Duration	Measured	Outcome
[59]	3T3-L1	Pre-confluent pre-adipocytes; Post confluent pre-adipocytes; Early and fully differentiated adipocytes	BSA	DHA: 25, 50, and 200 μM	4, 24, 48 h, and 6 d	DNA denaturation; lipid accumulation; GPDH and LDH activity; glycerol secretion in media	DHA had anti-adipogenic effect with decreased mean lipid droplet size and % of lipid area but increased basal lipolysis and apoptosis
[69]	3T3-L1	Different stages of differentiation	NI	EPA, DHA: 100 μM	24-48 h	Lipid accumulation; UPS activity; MTT cytotoxicity assay; expression of NFκB, TNFα, adiponectin, SREBP1, FAS, PPARγ	EPA and DHA reduced expression of adipogenic genes, decreased activity of UPS, increased accumulation of neutral fats and induced TNFα mRNA level
[67]	3T3-L1	Fully differentiated adipocytes	BSA	EPA, DHA: 100 μM	48 h	Expression of PPARγ, ACC1, SCD1, adiponectin	DHA did not affect expression of any measured genes. EPA only increased mRNA expression of SCD1
[61]	3T3-L1	Fully differentiated	DMSO and/or Ethanol	EPA: 100, 200 μM	24 h	Apelin secretion and gene expression	EPA stimulated apelin secretion and apelin gene expression
[57]	3T3-L1	Fully differentiated	TZD	EPA, DHA: 100 μM	48 h	Adiponectin secretion	EPA and DHA increased adiponectin secretion
[56]	3T3-L1	Fully differentiated	2% BSA + 100% ethanol	EPA, DHA: 100 μM	7 d	Lipid accumulation, glycerol release in media and mRNA expression of adipogenic, lipolytic and LD markers	EPA and DHA reduced lipid droplet formation and SCD1 expression compared to cells treated with stearic acid. DHA increased lipolysis, ATGL gene and protein expression and reduced gene expression of perilipin, caveolin-1, Cidea
[60]	3T3-L1	Differentiated adipocytes	BSA	EPA, DHA: 100 μM	24 h	mRNA and protein levels of anti-oxidative enzyme HO-1, gene expression of SOD, CAT and GPX	EPA and DHA prevented oxidative stress induced HO-1 and activation of Nrf-2
[58]	3T3-L1	Differentiated adipocytes	NI	EPA: 100 μM	24 h	CPT-1—Activity, protein level and mRNA expression	EPA increased β-oxidation but did not inhibit lipogenesis

Table 4. *Cont.*

Reference	Cell Type	Cell Stage	Control Cells *	EPA/DHA Dose	Culture Duration	Measured	Outcome
[62]	3T3-L1	Fully differentiated	Differentiation media no FA added	EPA, DHA: 50 μM	7 d	mRNA expression of PPARγ, C/EBPα, aP2; oil red O staining; adiponectin secretion; pro-inflammatory signalling pathways	DHA but not EPA significantly increased differentiation markers. DHA more effective than EPA at increasing adiponectin secretion. DHA only inhibited activation of ERK 1/2 and P38 MAPK
[65]	3T3-L1	Different stages of differentiation	Albumin	EPA: 100 μM; DHA: 50 μM	48 h	Lipid accumulation and glycerol release. Secretion of IL-6, leptin, adiponectin	EPA and DHA did not affect lipid accumulation or lipolysis. EPA and DHA increased secretion of adiponectin in early differentiated adipocytes. EPA and DHA had an opposite effect on IL-6 secretion: EPA increased secretion at all stages, DHA decreased it. EPA only had an impact on leptin secretion in early stage of differentiation
[64]	3T3-L1	Fully differentiated	Albumin	EPA, DHA: 125 μM	24 h	Adiponectin secretion and adiponectin cellular protein	EPA and DHA increased the secreted adiponectin concentration but did not affect cellular adiponectin protein content
[68]	Human breast adipocytes	Fully differentiated	NI	DHA: 50, 100 μM	24 h	mRNA expression of IL-6, TNFα, PPARγ, PPARα, HSL, perilipin, LPL, FAS, glycerol release	DHA decreased the expression of PPARγ and other lipogenic genes and increased the expression of lipolytic genes and glycerol release
[63]	Human primary adipocytes	Fully differentiated	Differentiation media or BSA	EPA, DHA: 5 and 10 μM	6 and 12 h	IL-6,TNFα, MCP1 secretion before and after LPS treatment	EPA and DHA reduced the secretion of LPS induced cytokine secretion
[66]	Human primary adipocytes	Fully differentiated	BSA	EPA, DHA: 100 μM	48 h	Adiponectin secretion and adiponectin cellular protein	EPA and DHA increased adiponectin secretion. EPA but not DHA increased cellular adiponectin protein

* Control or comparison cells. Abbreviations: EPA, eicosapentaenoic acid; DHA, docosahexaenoic acid; BSA, bovine serum albumin; h, hour; d, day; NI, not indicated; FA, fatty acid; GPDH, glycerol-3-phosphate dehydrogenase; LDH; lactate dehydrogenase; UPS, ubiquitin–proteasome system: NFκB, nuclear factor kappa-light-chain-enhancer of activated B cells; TNFα, tumor necrosis factor α; SREBP1, sterol regulatory element-binding protein 1; FAS, fatty acid synthase; PPARγ, peroxisome proliferator-activated receptor γ; TZD, troglitazone; SCD1, steroyl-CoA desaturase 1; ATGL, adipose triglyceride lipase; HO-1, heme oxygenase 1; Nef-2, Nucleotide Excision Repair Factor 2; LD, lipid droplet; SOD, Superoxide dismutase; CAT, catalyse; GPX, glutathione peroxidase; CPT-1, carnitine palmitoyltransferase 1; aP2, adipocyte protein 2; IL6, interleukin 6; HSL, hormone sensitive lipase; LPL, lipoprotein lipase; MCP-1, monocyte chemoattractant protein-1; LPS, Lipopolysaccharide; ERK1/2, extracellular-signal-regulated kinases; MAPK, Mitogen-activated protein kinases; MTT, colorimetric assay for assessing cell metabolic activity: ACC1, Acetyl-CoA carboxylase; DMSO, dimethyl sulfoxide.

4.2. Adipocyte Apoptosis

To our knowledge, there have been no studies in humans investigating the effect of *n*-3 fatty acids on adipocyte apoptosis and only limited work has been undertaken in animal and *in vitro* cellular models. Although outside the scope of this review, there have been a large number of studies investigating the effect of *n*-3 fatty acids and cancer in relation to apoptosis, as reviewed by Wendel and Heller [84].

Limiting findings from human *in vitro* and *in vivo* studies have reported apoptosis in white adipose tissue along with alternations in adipose tissue mass. Thus consideration is required when looking at adipose tissue mass in relation to cell number as they might be partly regulated by pre-adipocyte/adipocyte apoptosis [85,86]. Nelson-Dooley *et al.* [87] have suggested targeting apoptotic pathways in adipocytes as a novel way of treating obesity. Apoptosis is often assessed by cytomorphological alterations, DNA fragmentation and condensation, detection of caspases, protein cleavage at specific locations, cell membrane alterations and and increased mitochondrial membrane permeability [88]. In 2004 Ruszickova *et al.* [41] were the first to suggest the concept of *n*-3 fatty acids and regulation of cellularity in adipose tissue. Using a rodent model the authors suggested that increased intakes of EPA and DHA (Table 3) reduced high-fat diet-induced obesity by decreasing the number of adipocytes in adipose tissue, which could be interpreted as evidence of a pro-apoptotic effect. Perez-Matute *et al.* [54] demonstrated increased levels of histone-associated DNA oligonucleosomal fragments, classical markers of apoptosis in the white adipose tissue of rats fed a standard diet with additional oral administration EPA ethyl ester (1 g/kg per day) daily for 5 weeks. Moreover, they found a cafeteria diet strongly impaired the apoptotic action induced by EPA and suggested that EPA-induced apoptosis depends on the nutritional and metabolic status of the animals [54]. High dietary-*n*-3 fatty acid levels are at increased susceptibility to fatty acid peroxidation which has been reported to occur in different tissues within a fish model [89] including adipose tissue [40]. Fish contain a greater amount of more highly unsaturated fatty acids than mammals which makes them more prone to fatty acid peroxidation leading to apoptosis [90]. Todorcevic *et al.* [40] were the first to demonstrate that high dietary intakes of EPA and DHA induced oxidative stress and apoptosis in the visceral adipose tissue in Atlantic salmon. Salmon was fed with diets containing 50% EPA and 55% DHA of total fatty acid for 21 weeks and found increased activity of caspase-3, indicative of apoptosis occurring in white adipose tissue. The authors concluded that decreased adipocytes cell number due to apoptosis, may be one factor explaining the lower triacylglycerol accumulation occurring in fish white adipose tissue when diets enriched with EPA and DHA are fed [40]. On the basis of these finding, it would be prudent to suggest the measurement of adipose tissue apoptotic markers when EPA and DHA, notably at high dietary doses, are given.

Even though there is a growing literature on the studying the mechanisms for the inhibitory effects of *n*-3 fatty acids on proliferation of various tumor cells (reviewed by [91]) but also on non-cancerous cells [92], there are surprisingly very few *in vitro* studies that have investigated the effect of EPA and DHA on adipocyte apoptosis. Kim *et al.* [59] reported significant DHA-induced apoptosis in 3T3-L1 post-confluent pre-adipocytes after 48 h incubation with 200 µM/L compared to 100 µM/L DHA, demonstrating the inhibitory effects of DHA on adipocyte differentiation. Todorcevic *et al.* [93] treated primary antioxidant glutathione (GSH) depleted salmon adipocytes with high doses of EPA and DHA (600 µM for 6 days) in present or absence of α tocopherol and showed increased expression of genes encoding a set of well-known apoptotic markers in the groups with no added α tocopherol, suggesting that the induction of adipocyte cell death by EPA and DHA likely plays an important part in the adipose tissue homeostasis especially in animals exposed to high dietary *n*-3 fatty acids.

Taken together, the available data from animal and *in vitro* studies suggests that high doses of EPA and DHA may induce adipocyte apoptosis. How targeting the apoptotic pathway in white adipose tissue would decrease obesity and influence adipose tissue function and overall metabolic health in humans remains to be elucidated.

4.3. Increased Fatty acid Oxidation (Energy Expenditure)

Although an increase in fatty acid oxidation, via β-oxidation has been suggested to play a role in a reduction of triacylglycerol accumulation in adipocytes, evidence for this in white adipose tissue is limited; fatty acid oxidation and mitochondrial function has been studied more often in brown adipose tissue. The number and activity of mitochondria within adipocytes has been suggested to contribute to insulin resistance and type 2 diabetes [94]. Changes in the expression of genes related to insulin-signaling have been reported to increase, whilst the expression of genes related to glycolysis, gluconeogenesis and glyceroneogenesis decreased in subcutaneous abdominal adipose tissue after 12 weeks supplementation with *n*-3 fatty acids [45] (Table 2). On the basis of these changes, the authors suggested that a low-fat (fat 28% total energy (TE)) high complex carbohydrate diet supplemented with 1.24 g/day *n*-3 fatty acids (EPA and DHA) improved adipose tissue insulin sensitivity compared to diets high saturated or monounsaturated fat in individuals with the metabolic syndrome [45]. To lower the risk of obesity-mediated diseases such as the metabolic syndrome, weight loss is often encouraged to decrease fat mass; weight loss by calorie restriction has been suggested to increase subcutaneous abdominal adipose tissue capacity for lipid oxidation [95]. Whether similar changes occur in subcutaneous gluteal or visceral adipose tissue remains to be determined. Moreover, it would be of interest to determine if calorie restriction in combination with EPA and DHA supplementation has an additive effect on up-regulating adipose tissue fatty acid oxidation in different adipose tissue depots. The amount of EPA and DHA has varied between studies, with higher doses tending to be used in animal and *in vitro* studies, translation to the appropriate dose, along with duration required to see an effect in humans needs to be elucidated.

In vivo or *in vitro* cellular studies investigating the effects of EPA and DHA on adipose tissue fatty acid oxidation and/or mitochondrial function are sparse. Specifically measuring markers of adipose tissue fatty acid oxidation *in vivo* in humans has not, to our knowledge, been undertaken. This is most likely to be due to the challenges associated with assessing adipose tissue fatty acid β-oxidation directly. Surprisingly no study in humans has yet investigated changes in the expression of relevant genes in adipose tissue before and after supplementation with EPA and DHA. Fasting whole-body fatty acid oxidation (assessed by indirect calorimetry) has been reported to increase in young, healthy men (*n* = 5) after 3 weeks of supplementation with fish oil (6 g/day) when compared to a control diet containing equal amounts of total dietary fat [96]. Only a few animal studies have investigated the effect of EPA and DHA on fatty acid β-oxidation in white adipose tissue (Table 3). Flachs *et al.* [51] reported that feeding mice for 4 weeks with diet containing increasing amounts of EPA and DHA, preferentially up-regulated several mitochondrial regulatory genes, increased β-oxidation and suppressed lipogenesis in white abdominal fat. Using a fish model, Atlantic salmon, Todorcevic *et al.* [40] reported an increase in adipose tissue fatty acid β-oxidation after fish consumed fish oil rich in EPA and DHA for 21 weeks.

In vitro cellular studies have found increased β-oxidation in 3T3-L1 adipocytes after incubation with 100 μM of EPA for 24 h [58]. The increase in β-oxidation was associated with increased carnitine palmitoyltransferase 1 (CPT-1) activity but mRNA and protein expression did not change [58]. As EPA treatment increased the proportion of EPA in mitochondrial membrane lipids, the authors concluded that the activity of CPT-1 and β-oxidation was due to changes in the structure or dynamics of the mitochondrial membranes [58]. EPA and DHA are reported to activate AMP-activated protein kinase (AMPK) in 3T3-L1 adipocytes, which could be a mechanism for their effect on fatty acid oxidation [97]. Todorcevic *et al.* [83] demonstrated that EPA and DHA increased β-oxidation in salmon primary adipocytes, which may in part explain the concomitant reduction in adipocyte triacylglycerol. A possible mechanism, by which EPA and DHA may result in increased fatty acid oxidation and therefore less body fat accumulation, is through induction of thermogenesis mediated by mitochondrial uncoupling protein-1 (UCP1); the thermogenic capacity of brown adipose tissue (BAT) is associated with uncoupling whereas white adipose tissue is typically not [98]. In 2013 Flach *et al.* [98] reviewed the effect of *n*-3 fatty acids on mitochondrial oxidative phosphorylation (OXPHOS) and fatty acid oxidation in white adipose tissue. In this comprehensive review they reported that in a murine model, supplementation with n-3 fatty acids in combination with mild calorie restriction induced mitochondrial OXPHOS in epididymal white adipose tissue only, independent of UCP1 induction; other studies in rodents have reported increased levels of UCP1 mRNA and/or protein in BAT in response to n-3 fatty acid supplementation [98]. Recently, Zhao and Chen [99] using an *in vitro* cellular model of isolated stromal-vascular (SV) cells from inguinal adipose tissue of suggested that EPA enhanced energy dissipation capacity by recruiting brite adipocytes to stimulate oxidative metabolism. From the limited data available it appears that EPA and DHA increase fatty acid β-oxidation in adipocytes, however the mechanisms responsible and the effect on mitochondrial OXPHOS and thermogenesis in human adipose tissue remains to be elucidated.

5. The "Anti-Inflammatory" Effects of EPA and DHA on Adipose Tissue

An expansion of adipose tissue mass, is often associated with macrophage infiltration which may lead to inflammatory responses, which have been implicated in the development of pathological changes in adipose tissue physiology [6–9]. These changes potentially move the tissue toward a pro-inflammatory phenotype and there is accumulating evidence suggesting pro-inflammatory processes in adipose tissue increase the risk of obesity-related disorders, such as insulin resistance [100–103]. For example, several studies reported positive associations between degree of obesity and the expression of genes related to inflammation in adipose tissue [7,9]. A number of studies have investigated the "anti-inflammatory" effect of EPA and DHA in white adipose tissue.

Suppression of Pro-Inflammatory Cytokine Production

Studies investigating the effect of n-3 fatty acid supplementation, for periods between 8 weeks up to 6 months, on the expression of genes related to inflammation in human subcutaneous white adipose tissue have been undertaken. Overall results are variable, with some suggesting consumption of EPA and DHA decreases the expression of genes related to inflammation, whilst other report no change (Table 2). For example, Guebre-Egziabher *et al.* [43] noted decreased expression of metalloprotease 9 (MMP9) and CD68 in subcutaneous abdominal adipose tissue on a low not high dose of MaxEPA in a small number ($n = 12$) of individuals with chronic kidney disease (CKD) who were randomised to take either a low ($n = 6$) or high ($n = 6$) dose of MaxEPA for 10 weeks. In contrast, Itariu *et al.* [44] found that high doses of EPA and DHA (total 4 g/day) for 8 weeks significantly decreased the expression of genes related to inflammation in subcutaneous obese adipose tissue and increased production of anti-inflammatory eicosanoids in visceral adipose tissue (Table 2).

Work in murine models has found consumption of n-3 fatty acids decreased inflammatory gene expression in white adipose tissue depots (Table 3). Todoric *et al.* [104] investigated the effect of an n-3 fatty acid diet on macrophage infiltration in white adipose tissue of obese, diabetic mice, as well as on gene expression of several immune genes. They found that consumption of 25.1 mg of n-3 fatty acids (containing EPA and DHA) per gram of fat for 6 weeks resulted in a reduction in macrophage infiltration in combination with decreased expression of inflammatory genes in white adipose tissue [104]. Sarawathi *et al.* [55] used LDLR$^{-/-}$ mice and showed similar results to Todoric *et al.* [104] despite a gain in white adipose tissue mass. They reported a diet supplemented with fish oil containing 140 mg EPA and 95 mg DHA/day for 12 weeks reduced expression of macrophage markers such as MAC-1 and CD68 as well as inflammatory markers such as TNFα, metalloprotease 3 (MMP3), and serum amyloid A3 (SAA3) in white adipose tissue [55]. Taken together these data demonstrate that consumption of n-3 fatty acids have the potential to modulate immune response in adipose tissue.

In vitro studies, using cell-lines and human primary cells, have been utilised to investigate the potential cellular mechanisms and pathways involved in an n-3 fatty acid mediated alteration in immune response (Table 4). Adiponectin, an adipocyte-specific protein, is often suggested to be anti-inflammatory cytokine and it has been postulated that a change in secretion may be associated with visceral obesity [105]. *In vitro* cellular work has found that incubation of primary human adipocytes isolated from subcutaneous adipose tissue with either with EPA or DHA significantly increased the concentration of secreted adiponectin [106], which is in agreement with several studies performed using primary cultured rat adipocytes [107], 3T3-L1 adipocytes [64] and human adipocyte cell lines [66]. From the work of Oster *et al.* [64] it appears that EPA and DHA have differential effects on adiponectin secretion, which may be influenced by the cell model used. They found DHA increased adiponectin mRNA expression and secreted adiponectin protein to a greater extent than the same dose of EPA in 3T3-L1 adipocyte after 24 h incubation [64]. In contrast, Tishinsky *et al.* [99] found using a commercial line of human adipocytes that EPA significantly increased cellular adiponectin protein content after 48 h of treatment while DHA did not affect cellular adiponectin protein.

The effects of *n*-3 fatty acids on the adipokine leptin, have been investigated *in vitro* however results show conflicting effects of *n*-3 fatty acids on leptin mRNA expression and secretion. EPA has been shown to have a stimulatory effect on leptin gene expression and secretion in 3T3-L1 adipocytes [108] and primary cultured rat adipocytes [109]. Reseland *et al.* [110] reported an opposite effect to the work of Murata *et al.* [108] and Perez-Matute *et al.* [109], where exposure to both EPA and DHA reduced leptin mRNA expression in 3T3-L1 adipocytes. Furthermore, the effect of EPA and DHA on leptin expression has been shown to vary depending on the stage of adipocyte maturation [65]. Thus, the discrepancy in reported results could be related to differences in different cell models used (primary cells *vs.* cell lines) or in measuring the effects of *n*-3 fatty acids on leptin at different stages of adipogenesis. Culturing human primary adipocytes in either EPA or DHA resulted in a down-regulation of IL6 and TNFα secretion [63]. In contrast, differential effects of EPA and DHA were found for IL6 secretion in 3T3-L1 cells with EPA increasing and DHA decreasing secretion [65]; the underlying mechanisms for these responses were unable to be clarified by the authors. Another divergent finding is that from Wojcik *et al.* [69] who noted culturing 3T3-L1 cells in either EPA or DHA increased TNFα mRNA expression; it is unclear if this lead to increased secretion as it was not measured. The authors speculated that their finding would not be replicated in adipose tissue *in vivo*, as the anti-inflammatory effects of EPA and DHA on TNFα expression would be modulated through the direct effect of these fatty acids on macrophages; cells that were not present in their *in vitro* culture [69]. It remains unclear if EPA and DHA have a differential effect on anti-inflammatory markers in human and animal models as typically these fatty acids have been given together and not directly compared.

6. Conclusions

In recent years evidence demonstrating that an increased consumption of EPA and DHA may have a beneficial effect on white adipose tissue function and metabolism is starting to emerge. Although current literature cannot support an exact mechanistic role of EPA and DHA on adipose tissue biology it is apparent that these fatty acids have the potential to be potent modulators of adipose tissue and adipocyte function. More work has been undertaken using animal and cell models therefore consideration is required regarding the dose and duration of EPA and DHA, the animal and cell model used (e.g., primary *vs.* cell-lines). Moreover, *in vitro* cellular cells often investigate the effects of EPA and DHA on adipocytes and it is plausible a different response may be found in whole adipose tissue due to the presence of other cell types (e.g., macrophages, endothelial cells) and their interaction with adipocytes. Although the effects of *n*-3 fatty acid supplementation on the fatty acid composition of subcutaneous abdominal and gluteal adipose tissue have been investigated, mechanistic studies (*in vivo* and *in vitro*) appears to be limited to primarily subcutaneous abdominal adipose tissue and/or adipocytes. Evidence for an effect of *n*-3 fatty acids in human visceral adipose tissue is sparse and therefore not well understood. Evidence for a reduction in fat accumulation in animal models, along with an anti-inflammatory effect appears to be consistent when intakes of EPA and DHA are high (up to 20% of total fatty acids); however recommendations for human intakes are between 0.5% and

2% of total energy intake [111]. Thus, the duration and amount of dietary EPA or DHA required for beneficial effects in human subcutaneous adipose tissue depots remains to be elucidated.

Acknowledgments: Leanne Hodson is a British Heart Foundation Intermediate Fellow.

Author Contributions: Marijana Todorčević and Leanne Hodson wrote the manuscript.

References

1. Mohamed-Ali, V.; Pinkney, J.H.; Coppack, S.W. Adipose tissue as an endocrine and paracrine organ. *Int. J. Obes. Relat. Metab. Disord.* **1998**, *22*, 1145–1158. [CrossRef] [PubMed]
2. Trayhurn, P. Adipocyte biology. *Obes. Rev.* **2007**, *8*, 41–44. [CrossRef] [PubMed]
3. Frayn, K.N. Adipose tissue as a buffer for daily lipid flux. *Diabetologia* **2002**, *45*, 1201–1210. [CrossRef] [PubMed]
4. Lewis, G.F.; Carpentier, A.; Adeli, K.; Giacca, A. Disordered fat storage and mobilization in the pathogenesis of insulin resistance and type 2 diabetes. *Endocr. Rev.* **2002**, *23*, 201–229. [CrossRef] [PubMed]
5. Unger, R.H.; Orci, L. Lipotoxic diseases of nonadipose tissues in obesity. *Int. J. Obes. Relat. Metab. Disord.* **2000**, *24*, S28–S32. [CrossRef] [PubMed]
6. Sun, K.; Kusminski, C.M.; Scherer, P.E. Adipose tissue remodeling and obesity. *J. Clin. Investig.* **2011**, *121*, 2094–2101. [CrossRef] [PubMed]
7. Weisberg, S.P.; McCann, D.; Desai, M.; Rosenbaum, M.; Leibel, R.L.; Ferrante, A.W., Jr. Obesity is associated with macrophage accumulation in adipose tissue. *J. Clin. Investig.* **2003**, *112*, 1796–1808. [CrossRef] [PubMed]
8. Wellen, K.E.; Hotamisligil, G.S. Obesity-induced inflammatory changes in adipose tissue. *J. Clin. Investig.* **2003**, *112*, 1785–1788. [CrossRef] [PubMed]
9. Xu, H.; Barnes, G.T.; Yang, Q.; Tan, G.; Yang, D.; Chou, C.J.; Sole, J.; Nichols, A.; Ross, J.S.; Tartaglia, L.A.; et al. Chronic inflammation in fat plays a crucial role in the development of obesity-related insulin resistance. *J. Clin Investig.* **2003**, *112*, 1821–1830. [CrossRef] [PubMed]
10. Fabbrini, E.; Yoshino, J.; Yoshino, M.; Magkos, F.; Tiemann Luecking, C.; Samovski, D.; Fraterrigo, G.; Okunade, A.L.; Patterson, B.W.; Klein, S. Metabolically normal obese people are protected from adverse effects following weight gain. *J. Clin. Investig.* **2015**, *125*, 787–795. [CrossRef] [PubMed]
11. Hodson, L.; Skeaff, C.M.; Fielding, B.A. Fatty acid composition of adipose tissue and blood in humans and its use as a biomarker of dietary intake. *Prog. Lipid Res.* **2008**, *47*, 348–380. [CrossRef] [PubMed]
12. Marik, P.E.; Varon, J. ω-3 Dietary supplements and the risk of cardiovascular events: A systematic review. *Clin. Cardiol.* **2009**, *32*, 365–372. [CrossRef] [PubMed]
13. Delarue, J.; LeFoll, C.; Corporeau, C.; Lucas, D. *n*-3 Long chain polyunsaturated fatty acids: A nutritional tool to prevent insulin resistance associated to type 2 diabetes and obesity? *Reprod. Nutr. Dev.* **2004**, *44*, 289–299. [CrossRef] [PubMed]
14. Buckley, J.D.; Howe, P.R. Long-chain ω-3 polyunsaturated fatty acids may be beneficial for reducing obesity-a review. *Nutrients* **2010**, *2*, 1212–1230. [CrossRef] [PubMed]
15. Flachs, P.; Rossmeisl, M.; Bryhn, M.; Kopecky, J. Cellular and molecular effects of *n*-3 polyunsaturated fatty acids on adipose tissue biology and metabolism. *Clin. Sci.* **2009**, *116*. [CrossRef] [PubMed]
16. Torres-Fuentes, C.; Schellekens, H.; Dinan, T.G.; Cryan, J.F. A natural solution for obesity: Bioactives for the prevention and treatment of weight gain. A review. *Nutr. Neurosci.* **2015**, *18*, 49–65. [CrossRef] [PubMed]
17. Puglisi, M.J.; Hasty, A.H.; Saraswathi, V. The role of adipose tissue in mediating the beneficial effects of dietary fish oil. *J. Nutr. Biochem.* **2011**, *22*, 101–108. [CrossRef] [PubMed]
18. Kalupahana, N.S.; Claycombe, K.J.; Moustaid-Moussa, N. *n*-3 Fatty acids alleviate adipose tissue inflammation and insulin resistance: Mechanistic insights. *Adv. Nutr.* **2011**, *2*, 304–316. [CrossRef] [PubMed]
19. Pinel, A.; Morio-Liondore, B.; Capel, F. *n*-3 Polyunsaturated fatty acids modulate metabolism of insulin-sensitive tissues: Implication for the prevention of type 2 diabetes. *J. Physiol. Biochem.* **2014**, *70*, 647–658. [CrossRef] [PubMed]
20. Martinez-Fernandez, L.; Laiglesia, L.M.; Huerta, A.E.; Martinez, J.A.; Moreno-Aliaga, M.J. ω-3 Fatty acids and adipose tissue function in obesity and metabolic syndrome. *Prostaglandins Other Lipid Mediat.* **2015**. [CrossRef] [PubMed]

21. Berge, J.P.; Barnathan, G. Fatty acids from lipids of marine organisms: Molecular biodiversity, roles as biomarkers, biologically active compounds, and economical aspects. *Adv. Biochem. Eng. Biotechnol.* **2005**, *96*, 49–125. [PubMed]

22. Rørå, A.M.B.; Ruyter, B.; Skorve, J.; Berge, R.; Slinning, K.-E. Influence of high content of dietary soybean oil on quality of large fresh, smoked and frozen atlantic salmon (*Salmo salar*). *Aquac. Int.* **2005**, *13*, 217–231. [CrossRef]

23. Torstensen, B.E.; Bell, J.G.; Rosenlund, G.; Henderson, R.J.; Graff, I.E.; Tocher, D.R.; Lie, O.; Sargent, J.R. Tailoring of atlantic salmon (*Salmo salar* L.) flesh lipid composition and sensory quality by replacing fish oil with a vegetable oil blend. *J. Agric. Food Chem.* **2005**, *53*, 10166–10178. [CrossRef] [PubMed]

24. Schuchardt, J.P.; Hahn, A. Bioavailability of long-chain ω-3 fatty acids. *Prostaglandins Leukot. Essent. Fat. Acids* **2013**, *89*. [CrossRef] [PubMed]

25. Burdge, G.C.; Finnegan, Y.E.; Minihane, A.M.; Williams, C.M.; Wootton, S.A. Effect of altered dietary *n*-3 fatty acid intake upon plasma lipid fatty acid composition, conversion of [^{13}C]α-linolenic acid to longer-chain fatty acids and partitioning towards β-oxidation in older men. *Br. J. Nutr.* **2003**, *90*, 311–321. [CrossRef] [PubMed]

26. Bolton-Smith, C.; Woodward, M.; Tavendale, R. Evidence for age-related differences in the fatty acid composition of human adipose tissue, independent of diet. *Eur. J. Clin. Nutr.* **1997**, *51*, 619–624. [CrossRef] [PubMed]

27. Ogura, T.; Takada, H.; Okuno, M.; Kitade, H.; Matsuura, T.; Kwon, M.; Arita, S.; Hamazaki, K.; Itomura, M.; Hamazaki, T. Fatty acid composition of plasma, erythrocytes and adipose: Their correlations and effects of age and sex. *Lipids* **2010**, *45*, 137–144. [CrossRef] [PubMed]

28. Walker, C.G.; Browning, L.M.; Mander, A.P.; Madden, J.; West, A.L.; Calder, P.C.; Jebb, S.A. Age and sex differences in the incorporation of EPA and DHA into plasma fractions, cells and adipose tissue in humans. *Br. J. Nutr.* **2014**, *111*, 679–689. [CrossRef] [PubMed]

29. Browning, L.M.; Walker, C.G.; Mander, A.P.; West, A.L.; Madden, J.; Gambell, J.M.; Young, S.; Wang, L.; Jebb, S.A.; Calder, P.C. Incorporation of eicosapentaenoic and docosahexaenoic acids into lipid pools when given as supplements providing doses equivalent to typical intakes of oily fish. *Am. J. Clin. Nutr.* **2012**, *96*, 748–758. [CrossRef] [PubMed]

30. Katan, M.B.; Deslypere, J.P.; van Birgelen, A.P.; Penders, M.; Zegwaard, M. Kinetics of the incorporation of dietary fatty acids into serum cholesteryl esters, erythrocyte membranes, and adipose tissue: An 18-month controlled study. *J. Lipid Res.* **1997**, *38*, 2012–2022. [PubMed]

31. Leaf, D.A.; Connor, W.E.; Barstad, L.; Sexton, G. Incorporation of dietary *n*-3 fatty acids into the fatty acids of human adipose tissue and plasma lipid classes. *Am. J. Clin. Nutr.* **1995**, *62*, 68–73. [PubMed]

32. Mostad, I.L.; Bjerve, K.S.; Bjorgaas, M.R.; Lydersen, S.; Grill, V. Effects of *n*-3 fatty acids in subjects with type 2 diabetes: Reduction of insulin sensitivity and time-dependent alteration from carbohydrate to fat oxidation. *Am. J. Clin. Nutr.* **2006**, *84*, 540–550. [PubMed]

33. Gammelmark, A.; Madsen, T.; Varming, K.; Lundbye-Christensen, S.; Schmidt, E.B. Low-dose fish oil supplementation increases serum adiponectin without affecting inflammatory markers in overweight subjects. *Nutr. Res.* **2012**, *32*, 15–23. [CrossRef] [PubMed]

34. Witt, P.M.; Christensen, J.H.; Ewertz, M.; Aardestrup, I.V.; Schmidt, E.B. The incorporation of marine *n*-3 PUFA into platelets and adipose tissue in pre- and postmenopausal women: A randomised, double-blind, placebo-controlled trial. *Br. J. Nutr.* **2010**, *104*, 318–325. [CrossRef] [PubMed]

35. McQuaid, S.E.; Humphreys, S.M.; Hodson, L.; Fielding, B.A.; Karpe, F.; Frayn, K.N. Femoral adipose tissue may accumulate the fat that has been recycled as VLDL and nonesterified fatty acids. *Diabetes* **2010**, *59*, 2465–2473. [CrossRef] [PubMed]

36. Kunesova, M.; Hlavaty, P.; Tvrzicka, E.; Stankova, B.; Kalouskova, P.; Viguerie, N.; Larsen, T.M.; van Baak, M.A.; Jebb, S.A.; Martinez, J.A.; *et al.* Fatty acid composition of adipose tissue triglycerides after weight loss and weight maintenance: The diogenes study. *Physiol. Res.* **2012**, *61*, 597–607. [PubMed]

37. Buckley, J.D.; Howe, P.R. Anti-obesity effects of long-chain ω-3 polyunsaturated fatty acids. *Obes. Rev.* **2009**, *10*, 648–659. [CrossRef] [PubMed]

38. Du, S.; Jin, J.; Fang, W.; Su, Q. Does fish oil have an anti-obesity effect in overweight/obese adults? A meta-analysis of randomized controlled trials. *PLoS ONE* **2015**, *10*, e0142652. [CrossRef] [PubMed]

39. Sato, T.; Kameyama, T.; Ohori, T.; Matsuki, A.; Inoue, H. Effects of eicosapentaenoic acid treatment on epicardial and abdominal visceral adipose tissue volumes in patients with coronary artery disease. *J. Atheroscler. Thromb.* **2014**, *21*, 1031–1043. [CrossRef] [PubMed]

40. Todorcevic, M.; Kjaer, M.A.; Djakovic, N.; Vegusdal, A.; Torstensen, B.E.; Ruyter, B. *n*-3 HUFAs affect fat deposition, susceptibility to oxidative stress, and apoptosis in Atlantic salmon visceral adipose tissue. *Comp. Biochem. Physiol. B Biochem. Mol. Biol.* **2009**, *152*, 135–143. [CrossRef] [PubMed]

41. Ruzickova, J.; Rossmeisl, M.; Prazak, T.; Flachs, P.; Sponarova, J.; Veck, M.; Tvrzicka, E.; Bryhn, M.; Kopecky, J. ω-3 PUFA of marine origin limit diet-induced obesity in mice by reducing cellularity of adipose tissue. *Lipids* **2004**, *39*, 1177–1185. [CrossRef] [PubMed]

42. Camargo, A.; Meneses, M.E.; Perez-Martinez, P.; Delgado-Lista, J.; Jimenez-Gomez, Y.; Cruz-Teno, C.; Tinahones, F.J.; Paniagua, J.A.; Perez-Jimenez, F.; Roche, H.M.; *et al.* Dietary fat differentially influences the lipids storage on the adipose tissue in metabolic syndrome patients. *Eur. J. Nutr.* **2014**, *53*, 617–626. [CrossRef] [PubMed]

43. Guebre-Egziabher, F.; Debard, C.; Drai, J.; Denis, L.; Pesenti, S.; Bienvenu, J.; Vidal, H.; Laville, M.; Fouque, D. Differential dose effect of fish oil on inflammation and adipose tissue gene expression in chronic kidney disease patients. *Nutrition* **2013**, *29*, 730–736. [CrossRef] [PubMed]

44. Itariu, B.K.; Zeyda, M.; Hochbrugger, E.E.; Neuhofer, A.; Prager, G.; Schindler, K.; Bohdjalian, A.; Mascher, D.; Vangala, S.; Schranz, M.; *et al.* Long-chain *n*-3 pufas reduce adipose tissue and systemic inflammation in severely obese nondiabetic patients: A randomized controlled trial. *Am. J. Clin. Nutr.* **2012**, *96*, 1137–1149. [CrossRef] [PubMed]

45. Jimenez-Gomez, Y.; Cruz-Teno, C.; Rangel-Zuniga, O.A.; Peinado, J.R.; Perez-Martinez, P.; Delgado-Lista, J.; Garcia-Rios, A.; Camargo, A.; Vazquez-Martinez, R.; Ortega-Bellido, M.; *et al.* Effect of dietary fat modification on subcutaneous white adipose tissue insulin sensitivity in patients with metabolic syndrome. *Mol. Nutr. Food Res.* **2014**, *58*, 2177–2188. [CrossRef] [PubMed]

46. Kratz, M.; Kuzma, J.N.; Hagman, D.K.; van Yserloo, B.; Matthys, C.C.; Callahan, H.S.; Weigle, D.S. N3 PUFAs do not affect adipose tissue inflammation in overweight to moderately obese men and women. *J. Nutr.* **2013**, *143*, 1340–1347. [CrossRef] [PubMed]

47. Pena-Orihuela, P.; Camargo, A.; Rangel-Zuniga, O.A.; Perez-Martinez, P.; Cruz-Teno, C.; Delgado-Lista, J.; Yubero-Serrano, E.M.; Paniagua, J.A.; Tinahones, F.J.; Malagon, M.M.; *et al.* Antioxidant system response is modified by dietary fat in adipose tissue of metabolic syndrome patients. *J. Nutr. Biochem.* **2013**, *24*, 1717–1723. [CrossRef] [PubMed]

48. Spencer, M.; Finlin, B.S.; Unal, R.; Zhu, B.; Morris, A.J.; Shipp, L.R.; Lee, J.; Walton, R.G.; Adu, A.; Erfani, R.; *et al.* ω-3 Fatty acids reduce adipose tissue macrophages in human subjects with insulin resistance. *Diabetes* **2013**, *62*, 1709–1717. [CrossRef] [PubMed]

49. Baillie, R.A.; Takada, R.; Nakamura, M.; Clarke, S.D. Coordinate induction of peroxisomal acyl-coa oxidase and UCP-3 by dietary fish oil: A mechanism for decreased body fat deposition. *Prostaglandins Leukot. Essent. Fat. Acids* **1999**, *60*, 351–356. [CrossRef]

50. Belzung, F.; Raclot, T.; Groscolas, R. Fish oil *n*-3 fatty acids selectively limit the hypertrophy of abdominal fat depots in growing rats fed high-fat diets. *Am. J. Physiol.* **1993**, *264*, R1111–R1118. [PubMed]

51. Flachs, P.; Horakova, O.; Brauner, P.; Rossmeisl, M.; Pecina, P.; Franssen-van Hal, N.; Ruzickova, J.; Sponarova, J.; Drahota, Z.; Vlcek, C.; *et al.* Polyunsaturated fatty acids of marine origin upregulate mitochondrial biogenesis and induce β-oxidation in white fat. *Diabetologia* **2005**, *48*, 2365–2375. [CrossRef] [PubMed]

52. Hainault, I.; Carolotti, M.; Hajduch, E.; Guichard, C.; Lavau, M. Fish oil in a high lard diet prevents obesity, hyperlipemia, and adipocyte insulin resistance in rats. *Ann. N. Y. Acad. Sci.* **1993**, *683*, 98–101. [CrossRef] [PubMed]

53. Oh, D.Y.; Talukdar, S.; Bae, E.J.; Imamura, T.; Morinaga, H.; Fan, W.; Li, P.; Lu, W.J.; Watkins, S.M.; Olefsky, J.M. GPR120 is an ω-3 fatty acid receptor mediating potent anti-inflammatory and insulin-sensitizing effects. *Cell* **2010**, *142*, 687–698. [CrossRef] [PubMed]

54. Perez-Matute, P.; Perez-Echarri, N.; Martinez, J.A.; Marti, A.; Moreno-Aliaga, M.J. Eicosapentaenoic acid actions on adiposity and insulin resistance in control and high-fat-fed rats: Role of apoptosis, adiponectin and tumour necrosis factor-α. *Br. J. Nutr.* **2007**, *97*, 389–398. [CrossRef] [PubMed]

55. Saraswathi, V.; Gao, L.; Morrow, J.D.; Chait, A.; Niswender, K.D.; Hasty, A.H. Fish oil increases cholesterol storage in white adipose tissue with concomitant decreases in inflammation, hepatic steatosis, and atherosclerosis in mice. *J. Nutr.* **2007**, *137*, 1776–1782. [PubMed]

56. Barber, E.; Sinclair, A.J.; Cameron-Smith, D. Comparative actions of ω-3 fatty acids on *in-vitro* lipid droplet formation. *Prostaglandins Leukot. Essent. Fat. Acids* **2013**, *89*, 359–366. [CrossRef] [PubMed]

57. DeClercq, V.; d'Eon, B.; McLeod, R.S. Fatty acids increase adiponectin secretion through both classical and exosome pathways. *Biochim. Biophys. Acta* **2015**, *1851*, 1123–1133. [CrossRef] [PubMed]

58. Guo, W.; Xie, W.; Lei, T.; Hamilton, J.A. Eicosapentaenoic acid, but not oleic acid, stimulates β-oxidation in adipocytes. *Lipids* **2005**, *40*, 815–821. [CrossRef] [PubMed]

59. Kim, H.K.; Della-Fera, M.; Lin, J.; Baile, C.A. Docosahexaenoic acid inhibits adipocyte differentiation and induces apoptosis in 3T3-L1 preadipocytes. *J. Nutr.* **2006**, *136*, 2965–2969. [PubMed]

60. Kusunoki, C.; Yang, L.; Yoshizaki, T.; Nakagawa, F.; Ishikado, A.; Kondo, M.; Morino, K.; Sekine, O.; Ugi, S.; Nishio, Y.; *et al.* ω-3 Polyunsaturated fatty acid has an anti-oxidant effect via the Nrf-2/HO-1 pathway in 3T3-L1 adipocytes. *Biochem. Biophys. Res. Commun.* **2013**, *430*, 225–230. [CrossRef] [PubMed]

61. Lorente-Cebrian, S.; Bustos, M.; Marti, A.; Martinez, J.A.; Moreno-Aliaga, M.J. Eicosapentaenoic acid up-regulates apelin secretion and gene expression in 3T3-L1 adipocytes. *Mol. Nutr. Food Res.* **2010**, *54*, S104–S111. [CrossRef] [PubMed]

62. Murali, G.; Desouza, C.V.; Clevenger, M.E.; Ramalingam, R.; Saraswathi, V. Differential effects of eicosapentaenoic acid and docosahexaenoic acid in promoting the differentiation of 3T3-L1 preadipocytes. *Prostaglandins Leukot. Essent. Fat. Acids* **2014**, *90*, 13–21. [CrossRef] [PubMed]

63. Murumalla, R.K.; Gunasekaran, M.K.; Padhan, J.K.; Bencharif, K.; Gence, L.; Festy, F.; Cesari, M.; Roche, R.; Hoareau, L. Fatty acids do not pay the toll: Effect of SFA and PUFA on human adipose tissue and mature adipocytes inflammation. *Lipids Health Dis.* **2012**, *11*, 175. [CrossRef] [PubMed]

64. Oster, R.T.; Tishinsky, J.M.; Yuan, Z.; Robinson, L.E. Docosahexaenoic acid increases cellular adiponectin mRNA and secreted adiponectin protein, as well as PPARγ mRNA, in 3T3-L1 adipocytes. *Appl. Physiol. Nutr. Metab.* **2010**, *35*, 783–789. [CrossRef] [PubMed]

65. Prostek, A.; Gajewska, M.; Kamola, D.; Balasinska, B. The influence of EPA and DHA on markers of inflammation in 3T3-L1 cells at different stages of cellular maturation. *Lipids Health Dis.* **2014**, *13*, 3. [CrossRef] [PubMed]

66. Tishinsky, J.M.; Ma, D.W.; Robinson, L.E. Eicosapentaenoic acid and rosiglitazone increase adiponectin in an additive and PPARγ-dependent manner in human adipocytes. *Obesity* **2011**, *19*, 262–268. [CrossRef] [PubMed]

67. Vaidya, H.; Cheema, S.K. Arachidonic acid has a dominant effect to regulate lipogenic genes in 3T3-L1 adipocytes compared to ω-3 fatty acids. *Food Nutr. Res.* **2015**, *59*, 25866. [CrossRef] [PubMed]

68. Wang, Y.C.; Kuo, W.H.; Chen, C.Y.; Lin, H.Y.; Wu, H.T.; Liu, B.H.; Chen, C.H.; Mersmann, H.J.; Chang, K.J.; Ding, S.T. Docosahexaenoic acid regulates serum amyloid a protein to promote lipolysis through down regulation of perilipin. *J. Nutr. Biochem.* **2010**, *21*, 317–324. [CrossRef] [PubMed]

69. Wojcik, C.; Lohe, K.; Kuang, C.; Xiao, Y.; Jouni, Z.; Poels, E. Modulation of adipocyte differentiation by ω-3 polyunsaturated fatty acids involves the ubiquitin-proteasome system. *J. Cell. Mol. Med.* **2014**, *18*, 590–599. [CrossRef] [PubMed]

70. Hodson, L.; Humphreys, S.M.; Karpe, F.; Frayn, K.N. Metabolic signatures of human adipose tissue hypoxia in obesity. *Diabetes* **2013**, *62*, 1417–1425. [CrossRef] [PubMed]

71. Ji, H.; Li, J.; Liu, P. Regulation of growth performance and lipid metabolism by dietary n-3 highly unsaturated fatty acids in juvenile grass carp, ctenopharyngodon idellus. *Comp. Biochem. Physiol. B Biochem. Mol. Biol.* **2011**, *159*, 49–56. [CrossRef] [PubMed]

72. Liu, P.; Li, C.; Huang, J.; Ji, H. Regulation of adipocytes lipolysis by n-3 HUFA in grass carp (*Ctenopharyngodon idellus*) *in vitro* and *in vivo*. *Fish. Physiol. Biochem.* **2014**, *40*, 1447–1460. [CrossRef] [PubMed]

73. Desai, M.; Beall, M.; Ross, M.G. Developmental origins of obesity: Programmed adipogenesis. *Curr. Diab. Rep.* **2013**, *13*, 27–33. [CrossRef] [PubMed]

74. McMillen, I.C.; Robinson, J.S. Developmental origins of the metabolic syndrome: Prediction, plasticity, and programming. *Physiol. Rev.* **2005**, *85*, 571–633. [CrossRef] [PubMed]

75. Catalano, P.M.; Ehrenberg, H.M. The short- and long-term implications of maternal obesity on the mother and her offspring. *BJOG* **2006**, *113*, 1126–1133. [CrossRef] [PubMed]

76. Sewell, M.F.; Huston-Presley, L.; Super, D.M.; Catalano, P. Increased neonatal fat mass, not lean body mass, is associated with maternal obesity. *Am. J. Obstet. Gynecol.* **2006**, *195*, 1100–1103. [CrossRef] [PubMed]

77. Muhlhausler, B.S.; Gibson, R.A.; Makrides, M. The effect of maternal ω-3 long-chain polyunsaturated fatty acid (*n*-3 LCPUFA) supplementation during pregnancy and/or lactation on body fat mass in the offspring: A systematic review of animal studies. *Prostaglandins Leukot. Essent. Fat. Acids* **2011**, *85*, 83–88. [CrossRef] [PubMed]

78. Muhlhausler, B.S.; Miljkovic, D.; Fong, L.; Xian, C.J.; Duthoit, E.; Gibson, R.A. Maternal ω-3 supplementation increases fat mass in male and female rat offspring. *Front. Genet.* **2011**, *2*, 48. [CrossRef] [PubMed]

79. Hilton, C.; Karpe, F.; Pinnick, K.E. Role of developmental transcription factors in white, brown and beige adipose tissues. *Biochim. Biophys. Acta* **2015**, *1851*, 686–696. [CrossRef] [PubMed]

80. Pinnick, K.E.; Neville, M.J.; Fielding, B.A.; Frayn, K.N.; Karpe, F.; Hodson, L. Gluteofemoral adipose tissue plays a major role in production of the lipokine palmitoleate in humans. *Diabetes* **2012**, *61*, 1399–1403. [CrossRef] [PubMed]

81. Pinnick, K.E.; Nicholson, G.; Manolopoulos, K.N.; McQuaid, S.E.; Valet, P.; Frayn, K.N.; Denton, N.; Min, J.L.; Zondervan, K.T.; Fleckner, J.; *et al.* Distinct developmental profile of lower-body adipose tissue defines resistance against obesity-associated metabolic complications. *Diabetes* **2014**, *63*, 3785–3797. [CrossRef] [PubMed]

82. Lee, M.S.; Kwun, I.S.; Kim, Y. Eicosapentaenoic acid increases lipolysis through up-regulation of the lipolytic gene expression and down-regulation of the adipogenic gene expression in 3T3-L1 adipocytes. *Genes Nutr.* **2008**, *2*, 327–330. [CrossRef] [PubMed]

83. Todorcevic, M.; Vegusdal, A.; Gjoen, T.; Sundvold, H.; Torstensen, B.E.; Kjaer, M.A.; Ruyter, B. Changes in fatty acids metabolism during differentiation of atlantic salmon preadipocytes; effects of *n*-3 and *n*-9 fatty acids. *Biochim. Biophys. Acta* **2008**, *1781*, 326–335. [CrossRef] [PubMed]

84. Wendel, M.; Heller, A.R. Anticancer actions of ω-3 fatty acids–Current state and future perspectives. *Anticancer Agents Med. Chem.* **2009**, *9*, 457–470. [CrossRef] [PubMed]

85. Prins, J.B.; Walker, N.I.; Winterford, C.M.; Cameron, D.P. Apoptosis of human adipocytes in vitro. *Biochem. Biophys. Res. Commun.* **1994**, *201*, 500–507. [CrossRef] [PubMed]

86. Prins, J.B.; O'Rahilly, S. Regulation of adipose cell number in man. *Clin. Sci.* **1997**, *92*, 3–11. [CrossRef] [PubMed]

87. Nelson-Dooley, C.; Della-Fera, M.A.; Hamrick, M.; Baile, C.A. Novel treatments for obesity and osteoporosis: Targeting apoptotic pathways in adipocytes. *Curr. Med. Chem.* **2005**, *12*, 2215–2225. [CrossRef] [PubMed]

88. Wyllie, A.H. Apoptosis: An overview. *Br. Med. Bull.* **1997**, *53*, 451–465. [CrossRef] [PubMed]

89. Tocher, D.R. Metabolism and functions of lipids and fatty acids in teleost fish. *Rev. Fish. Sci.* **2003**, *11*, 107–184. [CrossRef]

90. Abele, D.; Puntarulo, S. Formation of reactive species and induction of antioxidant defence systems in polar and temperate marine invertebrates and fish. *Comp. Biochem. Physiol. A Mol. Integr. Physiol.* **2004**, *138*, 405–415. [CrossRef] [PubMed]

91. Biondo, P.D.; Brindley, D.N.; Sawyer, M.B.; Field, C.J. The potential for treatment with dietary long-chain polyunsaturated *n*-3 fatty acids during chemotherapy. *J. Nutr. Biochem.* **2008**, *19*, 787–796. [CrossRef] [PubMed]

92. Calviello, G.; Palozza, P.; Maggiano, N.; Piccioni, E.; Franceschelli, P.; Frattucci, A.; Di Nicuolo, F.; Bartoli, G.M. Cell proliferation, differentiation, and apoptosis are modified by *n*-3 polyunsaturated fatty acids in normal colonic mucosa. *Lipids* **1999**, *34*, 599–604. [CrossRef] [PubMed]

93. Todorcevic, M.; Skugor, S.; Ruyter, B. Alterations in oxidative stress status modulate terminal differentiation in atlantic salmon adipocytes cultivated in media rich in *n*-3 fatty acids. *Comp. Biochem. Physiol. B Biochem. Mol. Biol.* **2010**, *156*, 309–318. [CrossRef] [PubMed]

94. Maassen, J.A.; Romijn, J.A.; Heine, R.J. Fatty acid-induced mitochondrial uncoupling in adipocytes as a key protective factor against insulin resistance and β cell dysfunction: Do adipocytes consume sufficient amounts of oxygen to oxidise fatty acids? *Diabetologia* **2008**, *51*, 907–908. [CrossRef] [PubMed]

95. Bouwman, F.G.; Wang, P.; van Baak, M.; Saris, W.H.; Mariman, E.C. Increased β-oxidation with improved glucose uptake capacity in adipose tissue from obese after weight loss and maintenance. *Obesity* **2014**, *22*, 819–827. [CrossRef] [PubMed]

96.   Couet, C.; Delarue, J.; Ritz, P.; Antoine, J.M.; Lamisse, F. Effect of dietary fish oil on body fat mass and basal fat oxidation in healthy adults. *Int. J. Obes. Relat. Metab. Disord.* **1997**, *21*, 637–643. [CrossRef] [PubMed]

97.   Lorente-Cebrian, S.; Bustos, M.; Marti, A.; Martinez, J.A.; Moreno-Aliaga, M.J. Eicosapentaenoic acid stimulates amp-activated protein kinase and increases visfatin secretion in cultured murine adipocytes. *Clin. Sci.* **2009**, *117*, 243–249. [CrossRef] [PubMed]

98.   Flachs, P.; Rossmeisl, M.; Kuda, O.; Kopecky, J. Stimulation of mitochondrial oxidative capacity in white fat independent of UCP1: A key to lean phenotype. *Biochim. Biophys. Acta* **2013**, *1831*, 986–1003. [CrossRef] [PubMed]

99.   Zhao, M.; Chen, X. Eicosapentaenoic acid promotes thermogenic and fatty acid storage capacity in mouse subcutaneous adipocytes. *Biochem. Biophys. Res. Commun.* **2014**, *450*, 1446–1451. [CrossRef] [PubMed]

100. Hosogai, N.; Fukuhara, A.; Oshima, K.; Miyata, Y.; Tanaka, S.; Segawa, K.; Furukawa, S.; Tochino, Y.; Komuro, R.; Matsuda, M.; *et al.* Adipose tissue hypoxia in obesity and its impact on adipocytokine dysregulation. *Diabetes* **2007**, *56*, 901–911. [CrossRef] [PubMed]

101. Trayhurn, P.; Wood, I.S. Adipokines: Inflammation and the pleiotropic role of white adipose tissue. *Br. J. Nutr.* **2004**, *92*, 347–355. [CrossRef] [PubMed]

102. Wood, I.S.; de Heredia, F.P.; Wang, B.; Trayhurn, P. Cellular hypoxia and adipose tissue dysfunction in obesity. *Proc. Nutr. Soc.* **2009**, *68*, 370–377. [CrossRef] [PubMed]

103. Ye, J.; Gao, Z.; Yin, J.; He, Q. Hypoxia is a potential risk factor for chronic inflammation and adiponectin reduction in adipose tissue of *ob/ob* and dietary obese mice. *Am. J. Physiol. Endocrinol. Metab.* **2007**, *293*, E1118–E1128. [CrossRef] [PubMed]

104. Todoric, J.; Loffler, M.; Huber, J.; Bilban, M.; Reimers, M.; Kadl, A.; Zeyda, M.; Waldhausl, W.; Stulnig, T.M. Adipose tissue inflammation induced by high-fat diet in obese diabetic mice is prevented by *n*-3 polyunsaturated fatty acids. *Diabetologia* **2006**, *49*, 2109–2119. [CrossRef] [PubMed]

105. Fantuzzi, G. Adiponectin and inflammation: Consensus and controversy. *J. Allergy Clin. Immunol.* **2008**, *121*, 326–330. [CrossRef] [PubMed]

106. Romacho, T.; Glosse, P.; Richter, I.; Elsen, M.; Schoemaker, M.H.; van Tol, E.A.; Eckel, J. Nutritional ingredients modulate adipokine secretion and inflammation in human primary adipocytes. *Nutrients* **2015**, *7*, 865–886. [CrossRef] [PubMed]

107. Lorente-Cebrian, S.; Perez-Matute, P.; Martinez, J.A.; Marti, A.; Moreno-Aliaga, M.J. Effects of eicosapentaenoic acid (EPA) on adiponectin gene expression and secretion in primary cultured rat adipocytes. *J. Physiol. Biochem.* **2006**, *62*, 61–69. [CrossRef] [PubMed]

108. Murata, M.; Kaji, H.; Takahashi, Y.; Iida, K.; Mizuno, I.; Okimura, Y.; Abe, H.; Chihara, K. Stimulation by eicosapentaenoic acids of leptin mrna expression and its secretion in mouse 3T3-L1 adipocytes *in vitro*. *Biochem. Biophys. Res. Commun.* **2000**, *270*, 343–348. [CrossRef] [PubMed]

109. Perez-Matute, P.; Marti, A.; Martinez, J.A.; Fernandez-Otero, M.P.; Stanhope, K.L.; Havel, P.J.; Moreno-Aliaga, M.J. Eicosapentaenoic fatty acid increases leptin secretion from primary cultured rat adipocytes: Role of glucose metabolism. *Am. J. Physiol. Regul. Integr. Comp. Physiol.* **2005**, *288*, R1682–R1688. [CrossRef] [PubMed]

110. Reseland, J.E.; Haugen, F.; Hollung, K.; Solvoll, K.; Halvorsen, B.; Brude, I.R.; Nenseter, M.S.; Christiansen, E.N.; Drevon, C.A. Reduction of leptin gene expression by dietary polyunsaturated fatty acids. *J. Lipid Res.* **2001**, *42*, 743–750. [PubMed]

111. Aranceta, J.; Perez-Rodrigo, C. Recommended dietary reference intakes, nutritional goals and dietary guidelines for fat and fatty acids: A systematic review. *Br. J. Nutr.* **2012**, *107*, S8–S22. [CrossRef] [PubMed]

14

Omega-3 Fatty Acids in Modern Parenteral Nutrition: A Review of the Current Evidence

Stanislaw Klek

Stanley Dudrick's Memorial Hospital, General Surgery Unit, Skawina 32-050, Poland; klek@poczta.onet.pl

Academic Editors: Lindsay Brown, Bernhard Rauch and Hemant Poudyal

Abstract: Intravenous lipid emulsions are an essential component of parenteral nutrition regimens. Originally employed as an efficient non-glucose energy source to reduce the adverse effects of high glucose intake and provide essential fatty acids, lipid emulsions have assumed a larger therapeutic role due to research demonstrating the effects of omega-3 and omega-6 polyunsaturated fatty acids (PUFA) on key metabolic functions, including inflammatory and immune response, coagulation, and cell signaling. Indeed, emerging evidence suggests that the effects of omega-3 PUFA on inflammation and immune response result in meaningful therapeutic benefits in surgical, cancer, and critically ill patients as well as patients requiring long-term parenteral nutrition. The present review provides an overview of the mechanisms of action through which omega-3 and omega-6 PUFA modulate the immune-inflammatory response and summarizes the current body of evidence regarding the clinical and pharmacoeconomic benefits of intravenous n-3 fatty acid-containing lipid emulsions in patients requiring parenteral nutrition.

Keywords: parenteral nutrition; omega-3 fatty acids; omega-3 PUFA; lipid emulsions

1. Introduction

Intravenous (IV) lipid emulsions (LE) are an integral component of parenteral nutrition (PN) regimens. The earliest LE, subsequently referred to as "first generation" LE, were derived from soybean or cottonseed oil. Soybean oil is rich in omega-6 (n-6) polyunsaturated fatty acids (PUFA) and provides high amounts of linoleic acid (LA) and moderate amounts of α-linolenic acid (ALA), with an n-6/n-3 ratio of approximately 7:1 [1–5]. These early emulsions, which were primarily used as an efficient non-glucose energy source to reduce the adverse effects of high dextrose intake, have two main functions: to provide a source of energy and supply essential fatty acids [6].

While the cottonseed oil-based LE (Lipomul, USA) has been permanently removed from the market [6], the soybean oil-based LE Intralipid® (Fresenius Kabi, Germany) has been used worldwide since its introduction in 1962 and has been proven to be a safe and well tolerated emulsion [3,7–10]. However, a potential disadvantage with existing soybean oil emulsions is their relatively high content of n-6 PUFA (polyunsaturated fatty acids), in particular LA [2,11,12]. The emergence of evidence suggesting that n-6 polyunsaturated fatty acids might be pro-inflammatory and immunosuppressive led to the development of more complex lipid emulsions consisting of a mixture of different oils [13]. As a result, the latest generation of n-3 fatty acid-containing LE provide a more balanced combination of n-6 and n-3 fatty acids, with an n-6/n-3 ratio in the range of 2:1–4:1 [14,15]. For this reason, second and third generation IVLE contain not only soybean oil but alternative lipid sources such as medium-chain triglycerides (MCT), olive oil and/or fish oil/n-3 fatty acids [2,5]. In particular, n-3 fatty acid-containing IVLE have received considerable attention due to their ability to modulate key metabolic functions, including inflammatory response, coagulation, and cell signaling [5].

The present review provides a brief overview of the mechanisms of action and the role of n-6 and n-3 PUFA in modulating the immune-inflammatory response. The subsequent sections summarize the health benefits associated with n-3 long-chain (LC)-PUFA as well as the available evidence regarding the clinical and economic advantages of PN with n-3 fatty acids.

2. Classification and Mechanisms of Action

Fatty acids are classified according to their structure, carbon chain length (short, medium, or long), degree of saturation (number of double bonds), and the location of double bonds (counted from the methyl carbon of the hydrocarbon chain) [2–6]. As a common structural feature of all n-3 PUFAs, the double bond closest to the methyl terminus of the acyl chain of the fatty acid is located on carbon 3 [16]. The parent fatty acid of the n-3 family is ALA. The active ingredients in fish oil are the n-3 LC-PUFAs, eicosapentaenoic acid (EPA, C20:5 n-3) and docosahexaenoic acid (DHA, C22:6 n-3), as well as the n-6 LC-PUFA arachidonic acid (AA, C20:4 n-6). All are involved in the generation of pro- and anti-inflammatory lipid mediators. While AA exerts a pro-inflammatory effect, EPA and DHA have the ability to reduce inflammation through anti-inflammatory and immunomodulatory mechanisms [13,17–19].

The oil obtained from the flesh of oily fish or livers of lean fish is commonly referred to as "fish oil" and it has the distinctive characteristic of being rich in n-3 LC-PUFAs [1]. The effects of emulsions described as "fish oil rich" or "n-3-rich/containing" are attributable to the LC-PUFAs EPA, DHA, and in some cases ALA. Various oily fish contain different amounts of n-3 fatty acids, as do the various fish oils. This also applies to the content of EPA and DHA in enteral and parenteral products; hence, it is important to analyze the ingredients of PN admixtures to ensure they provide the appropriate amount of EPA and DHA.

In Europe there are currently three available IVLE products containing n-3 LC-PUFAs: Omegaven® (Fresenius Kabi, Germany), Lipoplus®/Lipidem® (B. Braun, Germany), and SMOFlipid® (Fresenius Kabi, Germany). Omegaven® is a 10% fish oil emulsion supplement. Lipoplus® contains a mix of 50% MCT, 40% soybean oil, and 10% fish oil, and SMOFlipid® is a 4-oil mixture of 30% soybean oil, 30% MCT, 25% olive oil, and 15% fish oil.

3. Fatty Acids: An Overview of Clinical Impact

Fatty acids represent not only a significant energy source and a human body energy store, but they are also necessary for proper biologic function. Fatty acids are key structural components of cell membranes (phospholipids), assuring membrane integrity and fluidity. They also serve as precursors of bioactive mediators such as eicosanoids (prostaglandins, leukotrienes, and thromboxanes) and steroid hormones (cholesterol) [1]. Finally, lipids regulate the expression of a variety of genes and modulate cell signaling pathways (apoptosis, inflammation, and cell-mediated immune responses). Therefore, lipids can modulate metabolic processes at local, regional, and distant sites [1].

3.1. Fatty Acids and Immune-Inflammatory Response

Inflammation is part of the complex physiological response to harmful stimuli such as pathogens, damaged cells, toxins, and irritants [19]. The primary functions of inflammation are to eliminate the initial cause of injury, launch defense mechanisms, remove necrotic cells and tissues, and initiate tissue repair [1,19]. Properly regulated inflammation represents an efficient physiological mechanism that protects the host from infection and other insults and is thus essential to health. Conversely, excessive pathological inflammation may cause irreparable damage to host tissues and ultimately lead to sepsis—the complex systemic inflammatory host response to an infection [20].

Inflammation can be classified as either acute or chronic according to the duration of the response. It can also be categorized according to the intensity of the process. In 1992, the American College of Chest Physicians and the Society of Critical Care Medicine introduced definitions for systemic inflammatory response syndrome (SIRS), sepsis, severe sepsis, septic shock, and multiple organ dysfunction syndrome [21]. SIRS is nonspecific and can be caused by ischemia, inflammation, trauma, infection, or multiple combined insults. It is defined as two or more of the following: temperature >38 °C (100.4 °F) or <36 °C (96.8 °F), heart rate >90 beats per minute and/or respiratory rate >20 breaths per minute or arterial carbon dioxide tension (PaCO2) <32 mm Hg [21]. It is important to recognize that SIRS is not always related to infection; accordingly, it cannot be treated the same way. Sepsis, by contrast, always stems from infection; indeed, it is defined as the presence of harmful bacteria and bacterial toxins in blood and tissues (sepsis = SIRS + infection). Severe sepsis is a condition in which there is organ dysfunction, hypotension, or hypoperfusion. If it progresses, septic shock may develop, potentially leading to multiple organ dysfunction syndrome (formerly known as multiple organ failure) and death.

During critical illness, increased production of reactive oxygen species and inflammatory mediators occurs along with a reduction in antioxidant activity, which is partly due to preexisting nutritional deficiencies and/or suboptimal provision of clinical nutrition [6]. This state of imbalance can cause tissue damage and may play an important role in the development of sepsis and multiple organ failure [6]. Therefore, the primary goals of treatment in critically ill patients should be to decrease the pro-inflammatory response during the catabolic phase of illness and enhance immune defense mechanisms. PN should always be considered as part of any such intervention if enteral intervention is impossible or insufficient [22]. The n-3 fatty acids EPA and DHA exhibit strong anti-hyperinflammatory and immunomodulatory effects via direct and indirect mechanisms and may thus be of benefit in patients at risk of hyperinflammation and sepsis [2,13,16].

The incorporation of PUFA into the phospholipids of cell membranes ensures the maintenance of membrane fluidity and the adequate function of membrane proteins. Through the formation of membrane rafts, n-3 PUFA are also involved in the inhibition of tumor growth [23,24]. The ratio of n-6/n-3 PUFA released from the hydrolysis of membrane phospholipids influences the synthesis of eicosanoid mediators such as prostaglandins (PGs), thromboxanes (TXs), and leukotrienes (LTs). The n-6 PUFA AA gives rise to 2-series PGs, TXs, 5-hydroxy-eicosatetraenoic acid (HETE), and 4-series LTs, thereby contributing to the inflammatory process and suppressing cell-mediated immunity [25–28]. Conversely, enzymatic conversion of the n-3 fatty acid EPA results in the production of 3-series PGs and TXs and 5-series LTs, all of which are less potent than the AA-derived mediators [16,24,28].

The recent discovery of families of novel pro-resolving lipid mediators such as resolvins, protectins, maresins, and lipoxins has shed new light on the role of n-3 PUFAs in the inflammatory process [29–32]. Pro-resolving lipid mediators derived from EPA are designated resolvins of the E series (RvE), while those derived from DHA are designated resolvins of the D series (RvD) [33]. The latter include the neuroprotectins/protectins (NPD1/PD1) and the maresins (MaR). These mediators have been shown to limit neutrophilic infiltration and enhance macrophage resolution responses, thus playing a role in diseases characterized by excessive uncontrolled inflammation [34–41]. Notably, their generation is linked to the fatty acid composition of cellular membranes and can therefore be effectively increased with n-3 fatty acid supplementation [37].

Exposure of inflammatory cells to n-3 PUFA *in vitro* attenuates chemotaxis of human neutrophils and monocytes and decreases expression of certain adhesion molecules on the surface of monocytes, macrophages, lymphocytes, and endothelial cells [20]. By coupling with surface or intracellular "fatty acid receptors", the LC-PUFA or their oxidized derivatives can regulate gene expression via the activation of transcription factors such as peroxisome proliferator-activated receptor (PPAR)-γ and nuclear factor-kappa B (NF-κB). N-3 LC-PUFA also modulate the inflammatory processes by inhibiting the production of pro-inflammatory cytokines and other pro-inflammatory proteins induced via activation of NF-κB in response to exogenous inflammatory stimuli. It appears that this effect is at least partly mediated by G-protein coupled cell surface receptors [20,24]. Consequently, the use of EPA and DHA leads to a more balanced immune response, which may result in faster resolution of inflammation [4,13,17,18].

4. Physiological Effects and Associated Health Benefits of *n*-3 LC-PUFA

4.1. Cardioprotective, Antihypertensive, and Antithrombotic Effects

In animal models of atherogenesis, *n*-3 fatty acids inhibit the hepatic synthesis of triglycerides [1]. EPA and DHA partly replace AA in membrane phospholipids; therefore, *n*-3 fatty acids may improve membrane structure, ligand/receptor binding, enzyme secretion, antigen presentation, and activation of intracellular signaling pathways [1]. By reducing the availability of AA-derived fatty acids as a substrate for eicosanoid synthesis by cyclooxygenase and lipoxygenase in platelets, monocytes, and macrophages, EPA and DHA delay platelet aggregation and progression of atherogenesis [10].

Consuming *n*-3 PUFA from fish oil is beneficial in the prevention of cardiovascular disease (CVD) and associated complications, as demonstrated by randomized control trials (RCTs) investigating secondary prevention in heart disease patients as well as epidemiological studies in populations that traditionally consume large quantities of sea fish as a part of their daily diet (e.g., Inuit) [42,43]. Potential underlying mechanisms include the inhibition of thrombogenesis and cytokine-dependent inflammation [42]. At total doses >3 g/day, EPA + DHA reduces CVD risk factors by decreasing plasma triglycerides, blood pressure, platelet aggregation, and inflammation and improving vascular reactivity [43].

4.2. Anticancer and Anti-Cachectic Effects and Inhibition of Tumor Growth

N-3 PUFA have been shown to attenuate cell growth and induce apoptosis in a variety of human cancer cell lines such as colonic, pancreatic, prostate, and breast cancer [44]. Through their effects on eicosanoid metabolism, *n*-3 PUFA may also decrease "sprouting angiogenesis", suppress endothelial cell proliferation, decrease tumor micro-vessel density, and even decrease tumor growth [45–49]. Research indicates that *n*-3 fatty acids act synergistically with chemotherapeutic agents and may also be used to enhance tumor radiosensitivity [50–52]. In patients with cancer-related cachexia, the pro-inflammatory state can be modulated by suppressing the inflammatory milieu and the release of pro-inflammatory mediators such as cytokines and prostaglandins by means of fish oil-based preparations, thus allowing nutrition to have an anabolic effect [53]. The underlying mechanisms for these effects include the incorporation of *n*-3 fatty acids into biological membranes as well as the modulation of the expression of proteins involved in the regulation of cell cycle and apoptosis, such as Bcl-2, Bax, and c-Myc [23,45,54]. More studies are needed, however, to fully assess the effects of *n*-3 PUFA in cancer treatment and prevention.

4.3. Visual and Cognitive Development

N-3 PUFA may reduce the risk of neurological disorders by influencing neuronal membranes and the activities of membrane-bound enzymes, receptors, and transporters [55]. Moreover, EPA and DHA can affect neurotransmission, including dopaminergic, noradrenergic, serotoninergic, and GABAergic neurotransmission in specific brain regions [56,57]. DHA, together with AA, is crucial for the development and maintenance of normal structure and function of the central nervous system (CNS). During fetal development DHA is taken up via the placenta and accumulates in the brain where it is required for the proper function of cholinergic neurotransmission [57–60]. Additionally, DHA may protect the brain from free radical and reactive oxygen species by enhancing the activity of cerebral catalase and glutathione peroxidase [61]. DHA may also be important for the efficient regeneration of axons and dendrites following neuronal injury [55].

The putative effects of *n*-3 PUFA on CNS function are mediated not only through an effect on the physicochemical properties of neural membranes but also through activation of transcription factors such as PPAR-γ [62]. AA, EPA, and DHA play a major role in protecting neuronal cells in the brain via inhibition of tumor necrosis factor (TNF)-α synthesis, thereby augmenting acetylcholine and endothelial nitric oxide (NO) formation and enhancing glucose uptake by neuronal cells, resulting in improved memory [53]. Epidemiological data suggest that a low dietary intake of *n*-3 LC-PUFA is a risk factor for Alzheimer disease [63]. Notably, studies have shown that the intake of fish oil lowers the risk of dementia by reducing the synthesis of proinflammatory cytokines and inhibiting the activities of phospholipase A2 and caspase A1 [64,65].

The effects of EPA and ethyl-EPA intake in schizophrenic patients have been investigated in a number of RCTs [63]. Overall, the results suggest a potential benefit; however, due to the limited size and duration of the studies it remains unknown whether the benefit is clinically meaningful. Research also suggests that n-3 LC-PUFA may confer a benefit in certain cases of depression; however, the routine use of n-3 LC-PUFA for the treatment of major depression cannot yet be recommended. Further research is necessary to establish the efficacy, appropriate dosing, and active components (EPA, DHA, or both) of n-3 LC-PUFA in patients with major depression [55].

4.4. Lipid Metabolism and Insulin Sensitivity

Fish oil supplementation has been shown to produce a clinically significant, dose-dependent reduction in fasting blood triglycerides and normalize serum lipid concentrations, including high density lipoproteins (HDL) and low density lipoproteins (LDL), in patients with hyperlipidemia [66]. Fish oil may also be beneficial in individuals with diabetes mellitus. In patients with type 2 diabetes, fish oil lowers triglycerides and raises LDL cholesterol [67]. However, additional studies are needed to gain a more comprehensive understanding of the role of fish oil supplementation in type 2 diabetes.

4.5. Inflammatory Disease

Due to their ability to regulate inflammatory processes and cellular responses, n-3 fatty acids have the potential to affect the development and progression of a multitude of diseases associated with an inflammatory state, including rheumatoid arthritis, Crohn's disease, ulcerative colitis, type-1 diabetes, cystic fibrosis, asthma, allergic disease, chronic obstructive pulmonary disease, psoriasis, and multiple sclerosis (reviewed in [20,68,69]). In a rat model of experimental colitis [70], administration of an n-3 PUFA-enriched parenteral LE decreased colonic concentrations of pro-inflammatory mediators and attenuated the morphological and inflammatory consequences of colitis. Although the current state of knowledge is insufficient to support a clear recommendation for the use of n-3 PUFA in patients with inflammatory bowel disease, emerging evidence suggests a potential benefit. Clinical decisions regarding the use of fish oil in such patients should be informed by due consideration of the available evidence.

4.6. Immune Function

Among other effects, n-3 fatty acids inhibit immune and inflammatory functions by decreasing lymphocyte proliferation, cytokine production, natural killer (NK) cell cytotoxicity, and antibody production [71]. Additionally, n-3 fatty acids suppress neutrophil chemotactic responsiveness to leukotriene B4 [71,72], reduce antigen-presenting capability, and decrease expression of major histocompatibility complex II (MHC II) molecules of mononuclear phagocytes [73]. DHA has been shown to partly restore the oxygen-dependent bactericidal mechanisms of monocytes [74], and neutrophils treated with EPA and DHA showed enhanced antiparasitic activity against Plasmodium falciparum [75].

Reports on the effects of different n-3 fatty acids on cytokine secretion and immune cell activity are somewhat inconsistent. In mice fed a diet rich in EPA, plasma concentrations of TNF-α were increased [76], whereas others have demonstrated decreased TNF-α secretion by neutrophils in DHA-fed human volunteers [77]. Purasiri et al. [78] observed decreased production of interleukin-1 (IL)-1, IL-2, TNF-α, and interferon-γ by human neutrophils treated with n-3 fatty acids, while Chavali et al. [76] reported decreased expression of IL-6 and IL-10 by endothelial cells and monocytes in mice fed an EPA-enriched diet [76]. Diets rich in n-3 fatty acids have been shown to inhibit lymphocyte activation and modulate antibody production by B-lymphocytes [71]. Conversely, the proliferative response to T-cell mitogens was increased by n-3 fatty acids in an animal model of autoimmune disease [79]. In a rat model of antibody-mediated autoimmune disease, diets low in fat, deficient in essential fatty acids, or rich in fish omega-3 fatty acids were associated with a better prognosis and higher survival [80]. In general, *n*-3 PUFA inhibit NK cell and lymphokine-activated killer cell activities. DHA feeding inhibited NK cell activity in healthy men [77]; however, a diet rich in *n*-3 fatty acids augmented NK cell cytotoxicity in healthy rats [81].

N-3 and *n*-6 PUFA differentially influence the plasma free fatty acid profile, with consequent effects on neutrophil functions [82]. In an open-label randomized study of septic patients with markedly reduced neutrophil function, patients receiving *n*-6 lipid infusions experienced persistent or worsening abnormalities in plasma free fatty acids and impaired neutrophil function, while patients receiving *n*-3 lipid infusions showed a rapid switch in the plasma free fatty acid fraction to a predominance of EPA and DHA over AA, with rapid incorporation of *n*-3 fatty acids into mononuclear leukocyte membranes and subsequent suppression of pro-inflammatory cytokine generation. Additionally, neutrophil function was significantly improved following administration of *n*-3 LE [82].

Collectively, these findings suggest that *n*-3 PUFA have a favorable effect on immunocompetence and inflammation and may therefore reduce the risk of clinical sequelae in critically ill septic patients.

5. N-3 Fatty Acids in Parenteral Nutrition—Clinical Benefits

5.1. Preservation of Hepatocellular Integrity During Long-Term PN in Adults and Children

Patients with critical illness, compromised gastrointestinal tract, sepsis, or recurrent infection who require prolonged PN therapy are at high risk of developing hepatic complications [83–85]. The long-term use of IVLE, especially at doses exceeding 1g/kg of body weight per day, is thought to play a role in the etiology of intestinal failure-associated liver disease (IFALD) [7,86]. Emerging evidence suggests that reducing the amount of *n*-6 fatty acids from soybean oil by partial replacement with *n*-3 PUFA from fish oil may improve parameters of liver function in parenterally fed adult and pediatric patients [87–93]. Thus, replacing a pure soybean oil emulsion by an LE containing soybean oil, MCT, olive oil, and fish oil (resulting in a lower *n*-6/*n*-3 fatty acid ratio of ~2.5:1) appears to be a promising approach [7]. Indeed, the available evidence supports the use of *n*-3 PUFA in PN, infused either as a part of the basic LE or added separately (as a fish oil emulsion supplement). Studies evaluating both short- and long-term use of *n*-3 PUFA-containing LE have demonstrated preserved hepatic integrity and improvements in parameters of liver function in adult and pediatric patients [7,89,90,94]. Klek *et al.* investigated the safety and tolerability of a soybean/MCT/olive oil/fish oil emulsion in patients with intestinal failure receiving long-term PN. After four weeks of treatment, measures of liver function (alanine transaminase [ALT], aspartate transaminase [AST], and total bilirubin) were significantly improved in patients who received the soybean/MCT/olive oil/fish oil emulsion compared with controls who received a conventional soybean oil emulsion [7]. Parenteral infusion of *n*-3 PUFA from fish oil has also been repeatedly shown to be effective in reversing PN-associated cholestasis in children when administered alone or in combination with a soybean oil-based lipid emulsion [95–99].

5.2. Critical Illness

According to the European Society for Clinical Nutrition and Metabolism (ESPEN) definition, a critically ill patient is a patient developing an intensive inflammatory response with failure of at least one organ (Sequential Organ Failure Assessment (SOFA) score >4) necessitating support of organ function during an ICU episode expected to be longer than three days [100]. Patients admitted to the intensive care unit (ICU) only for monitoring (typical ICU stay <3 days) are therefore not representative ICU patients. The aforementioned acute inflammatory conditions, SIRS, sepsis, and septic shock represent the range of abnormalities during critical illness.

Numerous studies in ICU patients confirm the clinical value of *n*-3 PUFA in critically ill patients. In a multicenter study in 661 critically ill patients with a Simplified Acute Physiology II Score

(SAPS II) >32, Heller *et al.* demonstrated that IV fish oil improved survival compared with that predicted by the SAPS II score and reduced infection rates, antibiotic requirements, and length of stay in a dose-dependent manner [101]. Consistent with these findings, Mayer *et al.* concluded, based on a review of the available evidence, that inclusion of *n*-3 fatty acids in PN improves immunologic parameters and length of stay in surgical patients [102]. Finally, in a recent comprehensive meta-analysis of studies evaluating the use of *n*-3 PUFA in ICU patients, Manzanares *et al.* analyzed data from 10 RCTs involving 733 patients and showed that the use of fish oil-containing LE was associated with significantly fewer infectious complications (RR 0.64; 95% CI, 0.44–0.92; $p = 0.02$) [103]. Trends toward a reduction in the number of days on mechanical ventilation (weighted mean difference [WMD] -1.14; 95% CI, -2.67 to 0.38; $p = 0.14$; heterogeneity I2 = 0%) and the length of hospital stay (WMD -3.71; 95% CI, -9.31 to 1.88; $p = 0.19$) were also reported. However, there was no significant effect on ICU length of stay (WMD -1.42; 95% CI, -4.53 to 1.69; $p = 0.37$) or mortality (RR 0.90; 95% CI, 0.67–1.20; $p = 0.46$; heterogeneity I2 = 0%). In a subgroup analysis of trials including patients who received IV *n*-3 PUFA in combination with enteral nutrition (EN) [104–107], a trend toward a reduction in mortality was observed (RR 0.69; 95% CI, 0.40–1.18; $p = 0.18$; heterogeneity I2 = 35%) [103].

According to the ESPEN Guidelines on Parenteral Nutrition in Intensive Care, the addition of EPA and DHA to lipid emulsions has demonstrable effects on cell membranes and inflammatory processes, and fish oil-enriched LEs likely decrease the length of hospital stay in critically ill patients (grade B) [100]. Canadian recommendations endorse the use of second generation LE when PN is indicated [108].

5.3. Oncology

Preclinical studies have demonstrated that *n*-3 PUFA can be effective in preventing the initiation and progression of cancer cells [45]. In the clinical setting, it was recently shown that fish oil-supplemented PN may help to reduce inflammation and stabilize energy expenditure in patients with pancreatic cancer [49]. In the same study, fish oil also improved patients' quality of life (QOL) by reducing cachexia, increasing appetite, and increasing performance status. In a separate study, fish oil-containing LE combined with gemcitabine improved the effectiveness of anti-cancer therapy in patients with advanced pancreatic cancer by decreasing gemcitabine resistance and improving QOL [49]. However, referring to a systematic review of the published studies evaluating EPA in cancer patients by Dewey *et al.* [109], ESPEN concluded that there was no benefit associated with the oral administration of EPA in patients with consolidated cachexia [110].

In recent years several well-designed clinical studies assessing the effect of nutritional intervention with EPA/fish oil in conjunction with antineoplastic therapy have been published. Positive results have be shown with regard to increased energy/protein intake and gain/maintenance of body weight/lean body mass (LBM) [111–113], with evidence to suggest a potential effect on several domains of health-related quality of life (HRQOL) [113]. Ma *et al.* recently published a systematic review examining the effects of *n*-3 fatty acids in patients with unresectable pancreatic cancer and reported a significant increase in body weight and LBM as well as a significant decrease in resting energy expenditure and improved overall survival (130–259 days *vs.* 63–130 days) in patients who consumed an oral nutrition supplement enriched with *n*-3 fatty acids compared to those who consumed conventional nutrition [114]. The review concluded that *n*-3 fatty acids are safe and appear to exert a positive effect on clinical outcomes and survival in pancreatic cancer patients.

5.4. Surgery

Recent studies have shown that the use of LE containing an increased dosage of *n*-3 PUFA may improve outcomes in surgical patients [115–120]. Among the clinical benefits observed in these studies were improvements in liver function tests [115,116], improvements in measures of immunologic function and inflammatory response [117,118], decreased length of hospitalization [116,119,120], and a reduced risk of clinical complications [116]. Moreover, the benefits of *n*-3 PUFA were observed when administered preoperatively (three days) [118], postoperatively (seven days) [116,117,119], or during the entire perioperative period [121]. Based on these findings, n-3 PUFA-enriched LE administered as a part of PN appear to confer benefits to selected groups of surgical patients, including those with major trauma or undergoing extended digestive tract resections or liver transplantation [122]. A summary of recent studies evaluating various IVLE formulations in surgical patients is presented in Table 1.

Table 1. Latest studies/meta-analyses evaluating the benefits of n-3 PUFA (polyunsaturated fatty acids) in parenteral nutrition in surgical populations *.

Author	Year	Population	Intervention	Duration	Result
Jiang [117]	2010	Colectomy and rectotomy ($n = 206$)	LCT vs LCT+fish oil	7 days post-surgery	Significant reduction in LOS and SIRS
Wang [115]	2012	Gastrointestinal surgery ($n = 64$)	MCT/LCT vs. LCT+fish oil	5 days post-surgery	Amelioration of liver function and immune status
Han [116]	2012	Major surgery ($n = 38$)	MCT/LCT vs. LCT+fish oil	7 days post-surgery	Reduced postoperative liver dysfunction and infection rate
Zhu [119]	2012	Colectomy and rectotomy ($n = 57$)	LCT vs. fish oil	7 days post-surgery	Reduced LOS
Zhu [120]	2012	Liver transplantation ($n = 98$)	Oral diet vs. standard PN vs fish oil PN	7 days post-surgery	Reduced incidence of liver injury, decreased LOS and infectious complications
Berger [121]	2013	Cardiopulmonary bypass surgery ($n = 28$)	Fish oils vs saline	12 and 2 h before surgery and after surgery	Decreased biological and clinical signs of inflammation
De Miranda Torrinhas [118]	2013	Surgery for gastrointestinal cancer ($n = 63$)	MCT/LCT vs. fish oil	3 days post-surgery	Significant increase in IL-10 levels (day 3), decrease in IL-6 and IL-10 levels (day 6), less decline in leukocyte oxidative burst
Chen [123]	2010	Major abdominal surgery, meta-analysis ($n = 892$)	Fish oil vs. various control emulsions	Various	Decreased LOS in the hospital and ICU, reduced postoperative infection rate, improved liver function
Li [124]	2013	Major surgery, meta-analysis ($n = 1487$)	Fish oil	Various	Decreased infection rate, LOS, and liver dysfunction; no effect on mortality
Pradelli [125]	2012	Subgroup analysis in patients undergoing major abdominal surgery and not admitted to ICU ($n = 740$)	n-3 PUFA-enriched vs. standard lipid emulsions	Various	Significant reduction in the infection rate and LOS
Tian [126]	2013	Surgical patients, meta-analysis ($n = 306$)	Fish oil/LCT/ MCT vs. LCT/olive oil	Various	No significant difference, fish oil less toxic to liver when compared to LCT or olive oil

* Adapted from Klek *et al.* 2015 [122]. Abbreviations: ICU = intensive care unit; LCT = long-chain triglycerides; LOS = length of stay; MCT = medium-chain triglycerides; PN = parenteral nutrition; RCT = randomized clinical trial; SIRS = systemic inflammatory response syndrome.

Several recent meta-analyses evaluating the clinical benefit of n-3 PUFA-enriched PN in surgical patients showed significant reductions in infectious complications [123–127], with three of these meta-analyses reporting a significant reduction in the length of hospital stay in surgical patients who received *n*-3 fatty acid-containing LE compared with controls [125–127].

5.5. Safety and Tolerability during Long-Term Use

Data from available studies confirm the safety and tolerability of *n*-3 PUFA-containing LE during long-term use, regardless of indication [7,91]. In adult patients with stable intestinal failure requiring long-term PN, beneficial effects were observed on parameters of liver function and Vitamin E profile following the administration of a mixed-type LE containing 15% fish oil for four weeks [7]. Safety and tolerability were also demonstrated in 28 children (age, five months to 11 years) with short bowel syndrome, chronic intestinal pseudo-obstruction, or congenital disease of the intestinal mucosa who required home PN for at least four weeks [91]. Finally, a meta-analysis of 23 trials involving 1503 patients found no evidence of deleterious effects or symptoms of intolerance during long-term use of fish oil-containing LE during ICU stay or surgical hospitalization [126].

5.6. Recommended Dosage and Duration of Intervention

According to ESPEN Guidelines on Parenteral Nutrition in Intensive Care, lipids should be an integral part of the regimen to provide energy and essential fatty acids in all patients requiring PN [100]. IVLE (LCT, MCT, or mixed emulsions) can be administered safely at a rate of 0.7–1.5 g/kg over 12 to 24 h [100]. In the previously mentioned multicenter trial by Heller *et al.*, IV fish oil was safe and conferred significant clinical benefits when administered to critically ill adults in doses between 0.1 and 0.2 g/kg/day [101]. Therefore, it seems reasonable to recommend the administration of fish oil in doses higher than 0.1 g/kg/day. Studies in surgical patients showed that while short-term (<5 days) administration of *n*-3 PUFA influences immune parameters and liver function, postoperative administration also reduces complication rates and length of stay [118,119]. While it takes several days for *n*-3 PUFA to be incorporated in host tissues and influence the generation of inflammatory mediators, impairment of host defense mechanisms occurs immediately after surgery. Braga *et al.* [128] thus concluded based on a literature review that *n*-3 PUFA should be given prior to surgery to achieve an optimum effect. In premature infants, a mixed LE with 15% fish oil administered for seven to 14 days showed a potential beneficial effect on cholestasis, *n*-3 fatty acids, and Vitamin E status [90,92,129].

5.7. Cost-Effectiveness

The cost-effectiveness of omega-3 PUFA-enriched LE is an important consideration, as acquisition costs for fish oil-containing LE are comparatively higher than those for pure soybean or MCT/LCT-based emulsions [130]. Nonetheless, pharmacoeconomic analyses support the supplementation of LE with *n*-3 PUFA. Wu *et al.* demonstrated that fish oil-based LE improves clinical outcomes and decreases the overall costs of ICU stay compared with standard LE in Chinese ICU patients (mean savings, ¥10,000) [131]. Additionally, in the most comprehensive analysis of the cost-effectiveness of LE published to date, Pradelli *et al.* analyzed patient outcomes and hospital economic data from Italian, French, German, and UK hospitals using a discrete event simulation scheme and demonstrated that treatment costs were entirely offset by reductions in antibiotic use and the length of hospital stay [132]. Cost savings ranged from €3972 to €4897 per ICU patient and from €561 to €1762 per non-ICU patient [126].

6. Conclusions

Lipids are not only an important energy source, but they also modulate metabolic processes at local, regional, and distant sites. IVLE are undoubtedly an indispensable element of PN regimens. Indeed, there is a strong scientific rationale for *n*-3 PUFA in PN; they improve clinical outcomes in pediatric, surgical, cancer, and critically ill patients as well as patients requiring long-term PN. Finally, LE-containing fish oils have a proven safety and tolerability profile and represent a cost-effective component of PN regimens.

Author Contributions: Stanislaw Klek was responsible for critical data analysis, evaluation of the outcomes, and writing of the manuscript.

References

1. Sobotka, L. *Basics in Clinical Nutrition*, 4th ed.; Galen: Prague, Czech Republic, 2011.
2. Waitzberg, D.L.; Torrinhas, R.S.; Jacintho, T.M. New parenteral lipid emulsions for clinical use. *JPEN J. Parenter. Enteral Nutr.* **2006**, *30*, 351–367. [CrossRef] [PubMed]
3. Wanten, G.J.; Calder, P.C. Immune modulation by parenteral lipid emulsions. *Am. J. Clin. Nutr.* **2007**, *85*, 1171–1184. [PubMed]
4. Calder, P.C. Long-chain *n*-3 fatty acids and inflammation: Potential Application in Surgical and Trauma Patients. *Braz. J. Med. Biol. Res.* **2003**, *36*, 433–446. [CrossRef] [PubMed]
5. Carpentier, Y.A.; Dupont, I.E. Advances in intravenous lipid emulsions. *World J. Surg.* **2000**, *24*, 1493–1497. [CrossRef] [PubMed]
6. Calder, P.C.; Jensen, G.L.; Koletzko, B.V.; Singer, P.; Wanten, G.J. Lipid emulsions in parenteral nutrition of intensive care patients: Current Thinking and Future Directions. *Intensive Care Med.* **2010**, *36*, 735–749. [CrossRef] [PubMed]
7. Klek, S.; Chambrier, C.; Singer, P.; Rubin, M.; Bowling, T.; Staun, M.; Joly, F.; Rasmussen, H.; Strauss, B.J.; Wanten, G.; *et al.* Four-week parenteral nutrition using a third generation lipid emulsion (smoflipid)—A double-blind, randomised, multicentre study in adults. *Clin. Nutr.* **2013**, *32*, 224–231. [CrossRef] [PubMed]
8. Carpentier, Y.A. Intravascular metabolism of fat emulsions: The Arvid Wretlind Lecture, Espen 1988. *Clin. Nutr.* **1989**, *8*, 115–125. [CrossRef]
9. Carneheim, C.; Larsson-Backström, C.; Ekman, L. New fatty acids in the emulsions of the nineties. possibilities and implications. In *Essential Fatty Acids and Total Parenteral Nutrition*; Ghisolfi, J., Ed.; John Libbey Eurotext: Paris, France, 1990; pp. 171–180.
10. Calder, P.C. Hot topics in parenteral nutrition. Rationale for using new lipid emulsions in parenteral nutrition and a review of the trials performed in adults. *Proc. Nutr. Soc.* **2009**, *68*, 252–260. [CrossRef] [PubMed]
11. Krohn, K.; Koletzko, B. Parenteral lipid emulsions in paediatrics. *Curr. Opin. Clin. Nutr. Metab. Care* **2006**, *9*, 319–323. [CrossRef] [PubMed]
12. Hamilton, C.; Austin, T.; Seidner, D.L. Essential fatty acid deficiency in human adults during parenteral nutrition. *Nutr. Clin. Pract.* **2006**, *21*, 387–394. [CrossRef] [PubMed]
13. Calder, P.C. Use of fish oil in parenteral nutrition: Rationale and reality. *Proc. Nutr. Soc.* **2006**, *65*, 264–277. [CrossRef] [PubMed]
14. Mayer, K.; Schaefer, M.B.; Seeger, W. Fish oil in the critically ill: From experimental to clinical data. *Curr. Opin. Clin. Nutr. Metab. Care* **2006**, *9*, 140–148. [CrossRef] [PubMed]
15. Fürst, P.; Kuhn, K.S. Fish oil emulsions: What benefits can they bring? *Clin. Nutr.* **2000**, *19*, 7–14. [CrossRef] [PubMed]
16. Calder, P.C. Omega-3 polyunsaturated fatty acids and inflammatory processes: Nutrition or pharmacology? *Br. J. Clin. Pharmacol.* **2013**, *75*, 645–662. [CrossRef] [PubMed]
17. Mayer, K.; Gokorsch, S.; Fegbeutel, C.; Hattar, K.; Rosseau, S.; Walmrath, D.; Seeger, W.; Grimminger, F. Parenteral nutrition with fish oil modulates cytokine response in patients with sepsis. *Am. J. Respir. Crit Care Med.* **2003**, *167*, 1321–1328. [CrossRef] [PubMed]
18. Calder, P.C. Rationale and use of *n*-3 fatty acids in artificial nutrition. *Proc. Nutr. Soc.* **2010**, *69*, 565–573. [CrossRef] [PubMed]
19. Ferrero-Miliani, L.; Nielsen, O.H.; Andersen, P.S.; Girardin, S.E. Chronic inflammation: Importance of Nod2 and Nalp3 in interleukin-1beta generation. *Clin. Exp. Immunol.* **2007**, *147*, 227–235. [CrossRef] [PubMed]
20. Calder, P.C. Omega-3 fatty acids and inflammatory processes. *Nutrients* **2010**, *2*, 355–374. [CrossRef] [PubMed]
21. Bone, R.C.; Balk, R.A.; Cerra, F.B.; Dellinger, R.P.; Fein, A.M.; Knaus, W.A.; Schein, R.M.; Sibbald, W.J. Definitions for sepsis and organ failure and guidelines for the use of innovative therapies in sepsis. The ACCP/SCCM consensus conference committee. American college of chest physicians/society of critical care medicine. *Chest* **1992**, *101*, 1644–1655. [CrossRef] [PubMed]
22. Singer, P.; Doig, G.; Pichard, C. The truth about nutrition in the icu. *Intensive Care Med.* **2014**, *40*, 252–255. [CrossRef] [PubMed]

23. Calviello, G.; Serini, S.; Piccioni, E. N-3 polyunsaturated fatty acids and the prevention of colorectal cancer: Molecular mechanisms involved. *Curr. Med. Chem.* **2007**, *14*, 3059–3069. [CrossRef] [PubMed]

24. Calder, P.C. Mechanisms of action of (*n*-3) fatty acids. *J. Nutr.* **2012**, *142*, 592S–599S. [CrossRef] [PubMed]

25. Grbic, J.T.; Mannick, J.A.; Gough, D.B.; Rodrick, M.L. The role of prostaglandin E2 in immune suppression following injury. *Ann. Surg.* **1991**, *214*, 253–262. [CrossRef] [PubMed]

26. Ertel, W.; Morrison, M.H.; Meldrum, D.R.; Ayala, A.; Chaudry, I.H. Ibuprofen restores cellular immunity and decreases susceptibility to sepsis following hemorrhage. *J. Surg Res.* **1992**, *53*, 55–61. [CrossRef]

27. Kollef, M.H.; Schuster, D.P. The acute respiratory distress syndrome. *N. Engl. J. Med.* **1995**, *332*, 27–37. [CrossRef] [PubMed]

28. Calder, P.C. The 2008 espen sir david cuthbertson lecture: Fatty acids and inflammation—From the membrane to the nucleus and from the laboratory bench to the clinic. *Clin. Nutr.* **2010**, *29*, 5–12. [CrossRef] [PubMed]

29. Bannenberg, G.L.; Chiang, N.; Ariel, A.; Arita, M.; Tjonahen, E.; Gotlinger, K.H.; Hong, S.; Serhan, C.N. Molecular circuits of resolution: Formation and actions of resolvins and protectins. *J. Immunol.* **2005**, *174*, 4345–4355. [CrossRef] [PubMed]

30. Bannenberg, G.; Arita, M.; Serhan, C.N. Endogenous receptor agonists: Resolving inflammation. *Sci. World J.* **2007**, *7*, 1440–1462. [CrossRef] [PubMed]

31. Bannenberg, G.; Serhan, C.N. Specialized pro-resolving lipid mediators in the inflammatory response: An update. *Biochim. Biophys. Acta* **2010**, *1801*, 1260–1273. [CrossRef] [PubMed]

32. Serhan, C.N. Pro-resolving lipid mediators are leads for resolution physiology. *Nature* **2014**, *510*, 92–101. [CrossRef] [PubMed]

33. Hong, S.; Lu, Y. Omega-3 fatty acid-derived resolvins and protectins in inflammation resolution and leukocyte functions: Targeting novel lipid mediator pathways in mitigation of acute kidney injury. *Front. Immunol.* **2013**, *4*, 13. [CrossRef] [PubMed]

34. Hong, S.; Gronert, K.; Devchand, P.R.; Moussignac, R.L.; Serhan, C.N. Novel docosatrienes and 17s-resolvins generated from docosahexaenoic acid in murine brain, human blood, and glial cells autacoids in anti-inflammation. *J. Biol. Chem.* **2003**, *278*, 14677–14687. [CrossRef] [PubMed]

35. Serhan, C.N.; Hong, S.; Gronert, K.; Colgan, S.P.; Devchand, P.R.; Mirick, G.; Moussignac, R.L. Resolvins: A Family of Bioactive Products of Omega-3 Fatty Acid Transformation Circuits Initiated by Aspirin Treatment that Counter Proinflammation Signals. *J. Exp. Med.* **2002**, *196*, 1025–1037. [CrossRef] [PubMed]

36. Marcheselli, V.L.; Hong, S.; Lukiw, W.J.; Tian, X.H.; Gronert, K.; Musto, A.; Hardy, M.; Gimenez, J.M.; Chiang, N.; Serhan, C.N.; *et al.* Novel docosanoids inhibit brain ischemia-reperfusion-mediated leukocyte infiltration and pro-inflammatory gene expression. *J. Biol. Chem.* **2003**, *278*, 43807–43817. [CrossRef] [PubMed]

37. Serhan, C.N.; Petasis, N.A. Resolvins and protectins in inflammation resolution. *Chem. Rev.* **2011**, *111*, 5922–5943. [CrossRef] [PubMed]

38. Tian, H.; Lu, Y.; Shah, S.P.; Hong, S. Autacoid 14S, 21R-dihydroxy-docosahexaenoic acid counteracts diabetic impairment of macrophage prohealing functions. *Am. J. Pathol.* **2011**, *179*, 1780–1791. [CrossRef] [PubMed]

39. Hisada, T.; Ishizuka, T.; Aoki, H.; Mori, M. Resolvin E1 as a novel agent for the treatment of asthma. *Expert Opin. Ther. Targets* **2009**, *13*, 513–522. [CrossRef]

40. Morita, M.; Kuba, K.; Ichikawa, A.; Nakayama, M.; Katahira, J.; Iwamoto, R.; Watanebe, T.; Sakabe, S.; Daidoji, T.; Nakamura, S.; *et al.* The lipid mediator protectin D1 inhibits influenza virus replication and improves severe influenza. *Cell* **2013**, *153*, 112–125. [CrossRef] [PubMed]

41. Ortigoza, M.B.; Dibben, O.; Maamary, J.; Martinez-Gil, L.; Leyva-Grado, V.H.; Abreu, P., Jr.; Ayllon, J.; Palese, P.; Shaw, M.L. A novel small molecule inhibitor of influenza a viruses that targets polymerase function and indirectly induces interferon. *PLoS Pathog.* **2012**, *8*, e1002668. [CrossRef] [PubMed]

42. Von Schacky, C. Cardiovascular disease prevention and treatment. *Prostaglandins Leukot. Essent. Fatty Acids* **2009**, *81*, 193–198. [CrossRef] [PubMed]

43. Breslow, J.L. N-3 fatty acids and cardiovascular disease. *Am. J. Clin. Nutr.* **2006**, *83*, 1477S–1482S. [PubMed]

44. Wendel, M.; Heller, A.R. Anticancer actions of omega-3 fatty acids—Current state and future perspectives. *Anticancer Agents Med. Chem.* **2009**, *9*, 457–470. [CrossRef] [PubMed]

45. Yang, P.; Jiang, Y.; Fischer, S.M. Prostaglandin E3 metabolism and cancer. *Cancer Lett.* **2014**, *348*, 1–11. [CrossRef] [PubMed]

46. Jing, K.; Wu, T.; Lim, K. Omega-3 polyunsaturated fatty acids and cancer. *Anticancer Agents Med. Chem.* **2013**, *13*, 1162–1177. [CrossRef] [PubMed]

47. Tsuji, M.; Murota, S.I.; Morita, I. Docosapentaenoic acid (22:5, *n*-3) suppressed tube-forming activity in endothelial cells induced by vascular endothelial growth factor. *Prostaglandins Leukot. Essent. Fatty Acids* **2003**, *68*, 337–342. [CrossRef]

48. Calviello, G.; di Nicuolo, F.; Gragnoli, S.; Piccioni, E.; Serini, S.; Maggiano, N.; Tringali, G.; Navarra, P.; Ranelletti, F.O.; Palozza, P. *N*-3 pufas reduce vegf expression in human colon cancer cells modulating the COX-2/PGE2 induced ERK-1 and -2 and HIF-1alpha induction pathway. *Carcinogenesis* **2004**, *25*, 2303–2310. [CrossRef] [PubMed]

49. Arshad, A.; Isherwood, J.; Mann, C.; Cooke, J.; Pollard, C.; Runau, F.; Morgan, B.; Steward, W.; Metcalfe, M.; Dennison, A. Intravenous omega-3 fatty acids plus gemcitabine: Potential to improve response and quality of life in advanced pancreatic cancer. *J. Parenter Enteral Nutr.* **2015**. [CrossRef]

50. Baracos, V.E.; Mazurak, V.C.; Ma, D.W. *N*-3 polyunsaturated fatty acids throughout the cancer trajectory: Influence on disease incidence, progression, response to therapy and cancer-associated cachexia. *Nutr. Res. Rev.* **2004**, *17*, 177–192. [CrossRef] [PubMed]

51. Xue, H.; Sawyer, M.B.; Field, C.J.; Dieleman, L.A.; Baracos, V.E. Nutritional modulation of antitumor efficacy and diarrhea toxicity related to irinotecan chemotherapy in rats bearing the ward colon tumor. *Clin. Cancer Res.* **2007**, *13*, 7146–7154. [CrossRef] [PubMed]

52. Xue, H.; Ren, W.; Denkinger, M.; Schlotzer, E.; Wischmeyer, P.E. Nutrition modulation of cardiotoxicity and anticancer efficacy related to doxorubicin chemotherapy by glutamine and omega-3 polyunsaturated fatty acids. *J. Parenter. Enteral Nutr.* **2015**. [CrossRef]

53. Barber, M.D. The pathophysiology and treatment of cancer cachexia. *Nutr. Clin. Pract.* **2002**, *17*, 203–209. [CrossRef] [PubMed]

54. Chang, W.L.; Chapkin, R.S.; Lupton, J.R. Fish oil blocks azoxymethane-induced rat colon tumorigenesis by increasing cell differentiation and apoptosis rather than decreasing cell proliferation. *J. Nutr.* **1998**, *128*, 491–497. [PubMed]

55. Assisi, A.; Banzi, R.; Buonocore, C.; Capasso, F.; Di Muzio, V.; Michelacci, F.; Renzo, D.; Tafuri, G.; Trotta, F.; Vitocolonna, M.; *et al.* Fish oil and mental health: The role of *n*-3 long-chain polyunsaturated fatty acids in cognitive development and neurological disorders. *Int. Clin. Psychopharmacol.* **2006**, *21*, 319–336. [CrossRef] [PubMed]

56. Chalon, S.; Delion-Vancassel, S.; Belzung, C.; Guilloteau, D.; Leguisquet, A.M.; Besnard, J.C.; Durand, G. Dietary fish oil affects monoaminergic neurotransmission and behavior in rats. *J. Nutr.* **1998**, *128*, 2512–2519. [PubMed]

57. Chalon, S.; Vancassel, S.; Zimmer, L.; Guilloteau, D.; Durand, G. Polyunsaturated fatty acids and cerebral function: Focus on monoaminergic neurotransmission. *Lipids* **2001**, *36*, 937–944. [CrossRef] [PubMed]

58. Hogyes, E.; Nyakas, C.; Kiliaan, A.; Farkas, T.; Penke, B.; Luiten, P.G. Neuroprotective effect of developmental docosahexaenoic acid supplement against excitotoxic brain damage in infant rats. *Neuroscience* **2003**, *119*, 999–1012. [CrossRef]

59. Minami, M.; Kimura, S.; Endo, T.; Hamaue, N.; Hirafuji, M.; Togashi, H.; Matsumoto, M.; Yoshioka, M.; Saito, H.; Watanabe, S.; *et al.* Dietary docosahexaenoic acid increases cerebral acetylcholine levels and improves passive avoidance performance in stroke-prone spontaneously hypertensive rats. *Pharmacol. Biochem. Behav.* **1997**, *58*, 1123–1129. [CrossRef]

60. Xiao, Y.; Li, X. Polyunsaturated fatty acids modify mouse hippocampal neuronal excitability during excitotoxic or convulsant stimulation. *Brain Res.* **1999**, *846*, 112–121. [CrossRef]

61. Hossain, M.S.; Hashimoto, M.; Gamoh, S.; Masumura, S. Antioxidative effects of docosahexaenoic acid in the cerebrum *versus* cerebellum and brainstem of aged hypercholesterolemic rats. *J. Neurochem.* **1999**, *72*, 1133–1138. [CrossRef] [PubMed]

62. Issemann, I.; Prince, R.A.; Tugwood, J.D.; Green, S. The peroxisome proliferator-activated receptor:Retinoid x receptor heterodimer is activated by fatty acids and fibrate hypolipidaemic drugs. *J. Mol. Endocrinol.* **1993**, *11*, 37–47. [CrossRef] [PubMed]

63. Kyle, D.J.; Schaefer, E.; Patton, G.; Beiser, A. Low serum docosahexaenoic acid is a significant risk factor for alzheimer's dementia. *Lipids* **1999**, *34*, S245. [CrossRef] [PubMed]

64. Akiyama, H.; Barger, S.; Barnum, S.; Bradt, B.; Bauer, J.; Cole, G.M.; Cooper, N.R.; Eikelenboom, P.; Emmerling, M.; Fiebich, B.L.; *et al.* Inflammation and Alzheimer's disease. *Neurobiol. Aging* **2000**, *21*, 383–421. [CrossRef]

65. Boston, P.F.; Bennett, A.; Horrobin, D.F.; Bennett, C.N. Ethyl-EPA in alzheimer's disease—A pilot study. *Prostaglandins Leukot. Essent. Fatty Acids* **2004**, *71*, 341–346. [CrossRef] [PubMed]

66. Eslick, G.D.; Howe, P.R.; Smith, C.; Priest, R.; Bensoussan, A. Benefits of fish oil supplementation in hyperlipidemia: A systematic review and meta-analysis. *Int. J. Cardiol.* **2009**, *136*, 4–16. [CrossRef] [PubMed]

67. Montori, V.M.; Farmer, A.; Wollan, P.C.; Dinneen, S.F. Fish oil supplementation in type 2 diabetes: A quantitative systematic review. *Diabetes Care* **2000**, *23*, 1407–1415. [CrossRef] [PubMed]

68. Spite, M. Deciphering the role of *n*-3 polyunsaturated fatty acid-derived lipid mediators in health and disease. *Proc. Nutr. Soc.* **2013**, *72*, 441–450. [CrossRef] [PubMed]

69. Miles, E.A.; Calder, P.C. Influence of marine *n*-3 polyunsaturated fatty acids on immune function and a systematic review of their effects on clinical outcomes in rheumatoid arthritis. *Br. J. Nutr.* **2012**, *107*, S171–S184. [CrossRef] [PubMed]

70. Campos, F.G.; Waitzberg, D.L.; Logulo, A.F.; Torrinhas, R.S.; Teixeira, W.G.; Habr-Gama, A. Immunonutrition in experimental colitis: Beneficial effects of omega-3 fatty acids. *Arq. Gastroenterol.* **2002**, *39*, 48–54. [CrossRef] [PubMed]

71. Pompeia, C.; Lopes, L.R.; Miyasaka, C.K.; Procopio, J.; Sannomiya, P.; Curi, R. Effect of fatty acids on leukocyte function. *Braz.J. Med. Biol. Res.* **2000**, *33*, 1255–1268. [CrossRef] [PubMed]

72. Calder, P.C. Immunoregulatory and anti-inflammatory effects of *n*-3 polyunsaturated fatty acids. *Braz. J. Med. Biol. Res.* **1998**, *31*, 467–490. [CrossRef] [PubMed]

73. Hughes, D.A.; Pinder, A.C. *N*-3 polyunsaturated fatty acids modulate the expression of functionally associated molecules on human monocytes and inhibit antigen-presentation *in vitro*. *Clin. Exp. Immunol.* **1997**, *110*, 516–523. [CrossRef] [PubMed]

74. Zheng, L.; Zomerdijk, T.P.; van den Barselaar, M.T.; Geertsma, M.F.; Van Furth, R.; Nibbering, P.H. Arachidonic acid, but not its metabolites, is essential for fcgammar-stimulated intracellular killing of staphylococcus aureus by human monocytes. *Immunology* **1999**, *96*, 90–97. [CrossRef] [PubMed]

75. Kumaratilake, L.M.; Ferrante, A.; Robinson, B.S.; Jaeger, T.; Poulos, A. Enhancement of neutrophil-mediated killing of plasmodium falciparum asexual blood forms by fatty acids: Importance of fatty acid structure. *Infect. Immun.* **1997**, *65*, 4152–4157. [PubMed]

76. Chavali, S.R.; Weeks, C.E.; Zhong, W.W.; Forse, R.A. Increased production of tnf-alpha and decreased levels of dienoic eicosanoids, IL-6 and IL-10 in mice fed menhaden oil and juniper oil diets in response to an intraperitoneal lethal dose of lps. *Prostaglandins Leukot. Essent. Fatty Acids* **1998**, *59*, 89–93. [CrossRef]

77. Kelley, D.S.; Taylor, P.C.; Nelson, G.J.; Schmidt, P.C.; Ferretti, A.; Erickson, K.L.; Yu, R.; Chandra, R.K.; Mackey, B.E. Docosahexaenoic acid ingestion inhibits natural killer cell activity and production of inflammatory mediators in young healthy men. *Lipids* **1999**, *34*, 317–324. [CrossRef] [PubMed]

78. Purasiri, P.; McKechnie, A.; Heys, S.D.; Eremin, O. Modulation *in vitro* of human natural cytotoxicity, lymphocyte proliferative response to mitogens and cytokine production by essential fatty acids. *Immunology* **1997**, *92*, 166–172. [CrossRef] [PubMed]

79. Fernandes, G.; Bysani, C.; Venkatraman, J.T.; Tomar, V.; Zhao, W. Increased tgf-beta and decreased oncogene expression by omega-3 fatty acids in the spleen delays onset of autoimmune disease in b/w mice. *J. Immunol.* **1994**, *152*, 5979–5987. [PubMed]

80. Miyasaka, C.K.; Mendonca, J.R.; Silva, Z.L.; de Sousa, J.A.; Tavares de Lima, W.; Curi, R. Modulation of hypersensitivity reaction by lipids given orally. *Gen. Pharmacol.* **1999**, *32*, 597–602. [CrossRef]

81. Robinson, L.E.; Field, C.J. Dietary long-chain (*n*-3) fatty acids facilitate immune cell activation in sedentary, but not exercise-trained rats. *J. Nutr.* **1998**, *128*, 498–504. [PubMed]

82. Mayer, K.; Fegbeutel, C.; Hattar, K.; Sibelius, U.; Kramer, H.J.; Heuer, K.U.; Temmesfeld-Wollbruck, B.; Gokorsch, S.; Grimminger, F.; Seeger, W. Omega-3 *vs.* Omega-6 lipid emulsions exert differential influence on neutrophils in septic shock patients: Impact on plasma fatty acids and lipid mediator generation. *Intensive Care Med.* **2003**, *29*, 1472–1481. [CrossRef] [PubMed]

83. Gabe, S.; Culkin, A. Abnormal liver function tests in the parenteral nutrition fed patient. *Frontline Gastroenterol.* **2010**, *1*, 98–104. [CrossRef]

84. Lindor, K.D.; Fleming, C.R.; Abrams, A.; Hirschkorn, M.A. Liver function values in adults receiving total parenteral nutrition. *JAMA* **1979**, *241*, 2398–2400. [CrossRef] [PubMed]

85. Staun, M.; Pironi, L.; Bozzetti, F.; Baxter, J.; Forbes, A.; Joly, F.; Jeppesen, P.; Moreno, J.; Hebuterne, X.; Pertkiewicz, M.; *et al.* Espen guidelines on parenteral nutrition: Home parenteral nutrition (HPN) in adult patients. *Clin. Nutr.* **2009**, *28*, 467–479. [CrossRef] [PubMed]

86. Goulet, O.; Joly, F.; Corriol, O.; Colomb-Jung, V. Some new insights in intestinal failure-associated liver disease. *Curr. Opin. Organ. Transplant.* **2009**, *14*, 256–261. [CrossRef] [PubMed]

87. Antebi, H.; Mansoor, O.; Ferrier, C.; Tetegan, M.; Morvan, C.; Rangaraj, J.; Alcindor, L.G. Liver function and plasma antioxidant status in intensive care unit patients requiring total parenteral nutrition: Comparison of 2 fat emulsions. *J. Parenter. Enteral Nutr.* **2004**, *28*, 142–148. [CrossRef]

88. Heller, A.R.; Rossel, T.; Gottschlich, B.; Tiebel, O.; Menschikowski, M.; Litz, R.J.; Zimmermann, T.; Koch, T. Omega-3 fatty acids improve liver and pancreas function in postoperative cancer patients. *Int. J. Cancer* **2004**, *111*, 611–616. [CrossRef] [PubMed]

89. Piper, S.N.; Schade, I.; Beschmann, R.B.; Maleck, W.H.; Boldt, J.; Rohm, K.D. Hepatocellular integrity after parenteral nutrition: Comparison of a fish-oil-containing lipid emulsion with an olive-soybean oil-based lipid emulsion. *Eur. J. Anaesthesiol.* **2009**, *26*, 1076–1082. [CrossRef] [PubMed]

90. Tomsits, E.; Pataki, M.; Tolgyesi, A.; Fekete, G.; Rischak, K.; Szollar, L. Safety and efficacy of a lipid emulsion containing a mixture of soybean oil, medium-chain triglycerides, olive oil, and fish oil: A randomised, double-blind clinical trial in premature infants requiring parenteral nutrition. *J. Pediatr. Gastroenterol. Nutr.* **2010**, *51*, 514–521. [CrossRef] [PubMed]

91. Goulet, O.; Antebi, H.; Wolf, C.; Talbotec, C.; Alcindor, L.G.; Corriol, O.; Lamor, M.; Colomb-Jung, V. A new intravenous fat emulsion containing soybean oil, medium-chain triglycerides, olive oil, and fish oil: A single-center, double-blind randomized study on efficacy and safety in pediatric patients receiving home parenteral nutrition. *J. Parenter. Enteral Nutr.* **2010**, *34*, 485–495. [CrossRef] [PubMed]

92. Rayyan, M.; Devlieger, H.; Jochum, F.; Allegaert, K. Short-term use of parenteral nutrition with a lipid emulsion containing a mixture of soybean oil, olive oil, medium-chain triglycerides, and fish oil: A randomized, double-blind study in preterm infants. *JPEN* **2012**, *36*, 81S–94S. [CrossRef] [PubMed]

93. D'Ascenzo, R.; Savini, S.; Biagetti, C.; Bellagamba, M.P.; Marchionni, P.; Pompilio, A.; Cogo, P.E.; Carnielli, V.P. Higher docosahexaenoic acid, lower arachidonic acid and reduced lipid tolerance with high doses of a lipid emulsion containing 15% fish oil: A randomized clinical trial. *Clin. Nutr.* **2014**, *33*, 1002–1009. [CrossRef] [PubMed]

94. De Meijer, V.E.; Gura, K.M.; Meisel, J.A.; Le, H.D.; Puder, M. Parenteral fish oil monotherapy in the management of patients with parenteral nutrition-associated liver disease. *Arch. Surg.* **2010**, *145*, 547–551. [CrossRef] [PubMed]

95. Diamond, I.R.; Sterescu, A.; Pencharz, P.B.; Kim, J.H.; Wales, P.W. Changing the paradigm: Omegaven for the treatment of liver failure in pediatric short bowel syndrome. *J. Pediatr. Gastroenterol. Nutr.* **2009**, *48*, 209–215. [CrossRef] [PubMed]

96. Gura, K.M.; Duggan, C.P.; Collier, S.B.; Jennings, R.W.; Folkman, J.; Bistrian, B.R.; Puder, M. Reversal of parenteral nutrition-associated liver disease in two infants with short bowel syndrome using parenteral fish oil: Implications for future management. *Pediatrics* **2006**, *118*, e197–e201. [CrossRef] [PubMed]

97. Gura, K.M.; Lee, S.; Valim, C.; Zhou, J.; Kim, S.; Modi, B.P.; Arsenault, D.A.; Strijbosch, R.A.; Lopes, S.; Duggan, C.; *et al.* Safety and efficacy of a fish-oil-based fat emulsion in the treatment of parenteral nutrition-associated liver disease. *Pediatrics* **2008**, *121*, e678–e686. [CrossRef] [PubMed]

98. Ekema, G.; Falchetti, D.; Boroni, G.; Tanca, A.R.; Altana, C.; Righetti, L.; Ridella, M.; Gambarotti, M.; Berchich, L. Reversal of severe parenteral nutrition-associated liver disease in an infant with short bowel syndrome using parenteral fish oil (omega-3 fatty acids). *J. Pediatr. Surg.* **2008**, *43*, 1191–1195. [CrossRef] [PubMed]

99. Beken, S.; Dilli, D.; Fettah, N.D.; Kabatas, E.U.; Zenciroglu, A.; Okumus, N. The influence of fish-oil lipid emulsions on retinopathy of prematurity in very low birth weight infants: A randomized controlled trial. *Early Hum. Dev.* **2014**, *90*, 27–31. [CrossRef] [PubMed]

100. Singer, P.; Berger, M.M.; Van den, B.G.; Biolo, G.; Calder, P.; Forbes, A.; Griffiths, R.; Kreyman, G.; Leverve, X.; Pichard, C.; *et al.* Espen guidelines on parenteral nutrition: Intensive care. *Clin. Nutr.* **2009**, *28*, 387–400. [CrossRef] [PubMed]

101. Heller, A.R.; Rossler, S.; Litz, R.J.; Stehr, S.N.; Heller, S.C.; Koch, R.; Koch, T. Omega-3 fatty acids improve the diagnosis-related clinical outcome. *Crit. Care Med.* **2006**, *34*, 972–979. [CrossRef] [PubMed]

102. Mayer, K.; Seeger, W. Fish oil in critical illness. *Curr. Opin. Clin. Nutr. Metab. Care* **2008**, *11*, 121–127. [CrossRef] [PubMed]

103. Manzanares, W.; Langlois, P.L.; Dhaliwal, R.; Lemieux, M.; Heyland, D.K. Intravenous fish oil lipid emulsions in critically ill patients: An updated systematic review and meta-analysis. *Crit. Care* **2015**, *19*, 167. [CrossRef] [PubMed]

104. Gupta, A.; Govil, D.; Bhatnagar, S.; Gupta, S.; Goyal, J.; Patel, S.; Baweja, H. Efficacy and safety of parenteral omega 3 fatty acids in ventilated patients with acute lung injury. *Indian J. Crit. Care Med.* **2011**, *15*, 108. [CrossRef] [PubMed]

105. Khor, B.S.; Liaw, S.J.; Shih, H.C.; Wang, L.S. Randomized, double blind, placebo-controlled trial of fish-oil-based lipid emulsion infusion for treatment of critically ill patients with severe sepsis. *Asian J. Surg.* **2011**, *34*, 1–10. [CrossRef]

106. Hall, T.C.; Bilku, D.K.; Al-Leswas, D.; Neal, C.P.; Horst, C.; Cooke, J.; Metcalfe, M.S.; Dennison, A.R. A randomized controlled trial investigating the effects of parenteral fish oil on survival outcomes in critically ill patients with sepsis: A pilot study. *J. Parenter. Enteral Nutr.* **2015**, *39*, 301–312. [CrossRef] [PubMed]

107. Burkhart, C.S.; Dell-Kuster, S.; Siegemund, M.; Pargger, H.; Marsch, S.; Strebel, S.P.; Steiner, L.A. Effect of *n*-3 fatty acids on markers of brain injury and incidence of sepsis-associated delirium in septic patients. *Acta Anaesthesiol. Scand.* **2014**, *58*, 689–700. [CrossRef] [PubMed]

108. Dhaliwal, R.; Cahill, N.; Lemieux, M.; Heyland, D.K. The canadian critical care nutrition guidelines in 2013: An update on current recommendations and implementation strategies. *Nutr. Clin. Pract.* **2014**, *29*, 29–43. [CrossRef] [PubMed]

109. Dewey, A.; Baughan, C.; Dean, T.; Higgins, B.; Johnson, I. Eicospentaenoic acid (EPA, an omega-3 fatty acid from fish oils) for the treatment of cancer cachexia (review). *Cochrane Database Syst. Rev.* **2010**. [CrossRef]

110. Bozzetti, F.; Arends, J.; Lundholm, K.; Micklewright, A.; Zurcher, G.; Muscaritoli, M. Espen guidelines on parenteral nutrition: Non-surgical oncology. *Clin. Nutr.* **2009**, *28*, 445–454. [CrossRef] [PubMed]

111. Sanchez-Lara, K.; Turcott, J.G.; Juarez-Hernandez, E.; Nunez-Valencia, C.; Villanueva, G.; Guevara, P.; de la Torre-Vallejo, M.; Mohar, A.; Arrieta, O. Effects of an oral nutritional supplement containing eicosapentaenoic acid on nutritional and clinical outcomes in patients with advanced non-small cell lung cancer: Randomised trial. *Clin. Nutr.* **2014**, *33*, 1017–1023. [CrossRef] [PubMed]

112. van der Meij, B.S.; Langius, J.A.; Spreeuwenberg, M.D.; Slootmaker, S.M.; Paul, M.A.; Smit, E.F.; van Leeuwen, P.A. Oral nutritional supplements containing *n*-3 polyunsaturated fatty acids affect quality of life and functional status in lung cancer patients during multimodality treatment: An RCT. *Eur. J. Clin. Nutr.* **2012**, *66*, 399–404. [CrossRef] [PubMed]

113. Trabal, J.; Leyes, P.; Forga, M.; Maurel, J. Potential usefulness of an EPA-enriched nutritional supplement on chemotherapy tolerability in cancer patients without overt malnutrition. *Nutr. Hosp.* **2010**, *25*, 736–740. [PubMed]

114. Ma, Y.J.; Yu, J.; Xiao, J.; Cao, B.W. The consumption of omega-3 polyunsaturated fatty acids improves clinical outcomes and prognosis in pancreatic cancer patients: A systematic evaluation. *Nutr. Cancer* **2015**, *67*, 112–118. [CrossRef] [PubMed]

115. Wang, J.; Yu, J.C.; Kang, W.M.; Ma, Z.Q. Superiority of a fish oil-enriched emulsion to medium-chain triacylglycerols/long-chain triacylglycerols in gastrointestinal surgery patients: A randomized clinical trial. *Nutrition* **2012**, *28*, 623–629. [CrossRef] [PubMed]

116. Han, Y.Y.; Lai, S.L.; Ko, W.J.; Chou, C.H.; Lai, H.S. Effects of fish oil on inflammatory modulation in surgical intensive care unit patients. *Nutr. Clin. Pract.* **2012**, *27*, 91–98. [CrossRef] [PubMed]

117. Jiang, Z.M.; Wilmore, D.W.; Wang, X.R.; Wei, J.M.; Zhang, Z.T.; Gu, Z.Y.; Wang, S.; Han, S.M.; Jiang, H.; Yu, K. Randomized clinical trial of intravenous soybean oil alone *versus* soybean oil plus fish oil emulsion after gastrointestinal cancer surgery. *Br. J. Surg.* **2010**, *97*, 804–809. [CrossRef] [PubMed]

118. de Miranda Torrinhas, R.S.; Santana, R.; Garcia, T.; Cury-Boaventura, M.F.; Sales, M.M.; Curi, R.; Waitzberg, D.L. Parenteral fish oil as a pharmacological agent to modulate post-operative immune response: A randomized, double-blind, and controlled clinical trial in patients with gastrointestinal cancer. *Clin. Nutr.* **2013**, *32*, 503–510. [CrossRef] [PubMed]

119. Zhu, M.W.; Tang, D.N.; Hou, J.; Wei, J.M.; Hua, B.; Sun, J.H.; Cui, H.Y. Impact of fish oil enriched total parenteral nutrition on elderly patients after colorectal cancer surgery. *Chin. Med. J. (Engl.)* **2012**, *125*, 178–181.

120. Zhu, X.; Wu, Y.; Qiu, Y.; Jiang, C.; Ding, Y. Effects of omega-3 fish oil lipid emulsion combined with parenteral nutrition on patients undergoing liver transplantation. *J. Parenter. Enteral Nutr.* **2013**, *37*, 68–74. [CrossRef] [PubMed]

121. Berger, M.M.; Delodder, F.; Liaudet, L.; Tozzi, P.; Schlaepfer, J.; Chiolero, R.L.; Tappy, L. Three short perioperative infusions of *n*-3 pufas reduce systemic inflammation induced by cardiopulmonary bypass surgery: A Randomized Controlled Trial. *Am. J. Clin. Nutr.* **2013**, *97*, 246–254. [CrossRef] [PubMed]

122. Klek, S.; Waitzberg, D.L. Intravenous lipids in adult surgical patients. In *Intravenous Lipid Emulsions*; Calder, P.C., Waitzberg, D.L., Koletzko, B., Eds.; Karger: Basel, Switzerland, 2015; Volume 112, pp. 115–119.

123. Chen, B.; Zhou, Y.; Yang, P.; Wan, H.W.; Wu, X.T. Safety and efficacy of fish oil-enriched parenteral nutrition regimen on postoperative patients undergoing major abdominal surgery: A Meta-Analysis of Randomized Controlled Trials. *J. Parenter. Enteral Nutr.* **2010**, *34*, 387–394. [CrossRef] [PubMed]

124. Li, N.N.; Zhou, Y.; Qin, X.P.; Chen, Y.; He, D.; Feng, J.Y.; Wu, X.T. Does intravenous fish oil benefit patients post-surgery? A meta-analysis of randomised controlled trials. *Clin. Nutr.* **2014**, *33*, 226–239. [CrossRef] [PubMed]

125. Pradelli, L.; Mayer, K.; Muscaritoli, M.; Heller, A.R. *N*-3 fatty acid-enriched parenteral nutrition regimens in elective surgical and icu patients: A Meta-Analysis. *Crit. Care* **2012**, *16*, R184. [CrossRef] [PubMed]

126. Tian, H.; Yao, X.; Zeng, R.; Sun, R.; Tian, H.; Shi, C.; Li, L.; Tian, J.; Yang, K. Safety and efficacy of a new parenteral lipid emulsion (SMOF) for surgical patients: A systematic review and meta-analysis of randomized controlled trials. *Nutr. Rev.* **2013**, *71*, 815–821. [CrossRef] [PubMed]

127. Wei, C.; Hua, J.; Bin, C.; Klassen, K. Impact of lipid emulsion containing fish oil on outcomes of surgical patients: Systematic Review of Randomized Controlled Trials from Europe and Asia. *Nutrition* **2010**, *26*, 474–481. [CrossRef] [PubMed]

128. Braga, M.; Wischmeyer, P.E.; Drover, J.; Heyland, D.K. Clinical evidence for pharmaconutrition in major elective surgery. *J. Parenter. Enteral Nutr.* **2013**, *37*, 66S–72S. [CrossRef] [PubMed]

129. Skouroliakou, M.; Konstantinou, D.; Agakidis, C.; Delikou, N.; Koutri, K.; Antoniadi, M.; Karagiozoglou-Lampoudi, T. Cholestasis, bronchopulmonary dysplasia, and lipid profile in preterm infants receiving MCT/omega-3-PUFA-containing or soybean-based lipid emulsions. *Nutr. Clin. Pract.* **2012**, *27*, 817–824. [CrossRef] [PubMed]

130. Klek, S.; Kulig, J.; Szczepanik, A.M.; Jedrys, J.; Kolodziejczyk, P. The clinical value of parenteral immunonutrition in surgical patients. *Acta Chir. Belg.* **2005**, *105*, 175–179. [PubMed]

131. Wu, G.H.; Gao, J.; Ji, C.Y.; Pradelli, L.; Xi, Q.L.; Zhuang, Q.L. Cost and effectiveness of omega-3 fatty acid supplementation in chinese iCU patients receiving parenteral nutrition. *Clinicoecon. Outcomes Res.* **2015**, *7*, 369–375. [PubMed]

132. Pradelli, L.; Eandi, M.; Povero, M.; Mayer, K.; Muscaritoli, M.; Heller, A.R.; Fries-Schaffner, E. Cost-effectiveness of omega-3 fatty acid supplements in parenteral nutrition therapy in hospitals: A Discrete Event Simulation Model. *Clin. Nutr.* **2014**, *33*, 785–792. [CrossRef] [PubMed]

15

Mechanisms Involved in the Improvement of Lipotoxicity and Impaired Lipid Metabolism by Dietary α-Linolenic Acid Rich *Salvia hispanica* L (Salba) Seed in the Heart of Dyslipemic Insulin-Resistant Rats

Agustina Creus, María R. Ferreira, María E. Oliva and Yolanda B. Lombardo *

Department of Biochemistry, School of Biochemistry, University of Litoral, Ciudad Universitaria, Paraje El Pozo, CC 242, (3000) Santa Fe, Argentina; agustinacreus@gmail.com (A.C.); mrferreira@fbcb.unl.edu.ar (M.R.F.); meoliva@fbcb.unl.edu.ar (M.E.O.)
* Correspondence: ylombard@fbcb.unl.edu.ar

Academic Editors: Lindsay Brown, Bernhard Rauch and Hemant Poudyal

Abstract: This study explores the mechanisms underlying the altered lipid metabolism in the heart of dyslipemic insulin-resistant (IR) rats fed a sucrose-rich diet (SRD) and investigates if chia seeds (rich in α-linolenic acid 18:3, *n*-3 ALA) improve/reverse cardiac lipotoxicity. Wistar rats received an SRD-diet for three months. Half of the animals continued with the SRD up to month 6. The other half was fed an SRD in which the fat source, corn oil (CO), was replaced by chia seeds from month 3 to 6 (SRD+chia). A reference group consumed a control diet (CD) all the time. Triglyceride, long-chain acyl CoA (LC ACoA) and diacylglycerol (DAG) contents, pyruvate dehydrogenase complex (PDHc) and muscle-type carnitine palmitoyltransferase 1 (M-CPT1) activities and protein mass levels of M-CPT1, membrane fatty acid transporter (FAT/CD36), peroxisome proliferator activated receptor α (PPARα) and uncoupling protein 2 (UCP2) were analyzed. Results show that: (a) the hearts of SRD-fed rats display lipotoxicity suggesting impaired myocardial lipid utilization; (b) Compared with the SRD group, dietary chia normalizes blood pressure; reverses/improves heart lipotoxicity, glucose oxidation, the increased protein mass level of FAT/CD36, and the impaired insulin stimulated FAT/CD36 translocation to the plasma membrane. The enhanced M-CPT1 activity is markedly reduced without similar changes in protein mass. PPARα slightly decreases, while the UCP2 protein level remains unchanged in all groups. Normalization of dyslipidemia and IR by chia reduces plasma fatty acids (FAs) availability, suggesting that a different milieu prevents the robust translocation of FAT/CD36. This could reduce the influx of FAs, decreasing the elevated M-CPT1 activity and lipid storage and improving glucose oxidation in cardiac muscles of SRD-fed rats.

Keywords: α-linolenic acid (ALA); cardiac muscle; lipotoxicity; dyslipidemia; insulin resistance; high-sucrose diet

1. Introduction

Metabolic syndrome (MS) is a complex metabolic disorder influenced by genetic and environmental factors [1]. In Western societies, the high increase of MS, including cardiovascular disease (CVD), seems to be due to changes in lifestyle (e.g., increased consumption of food high in refined sugar and decreased physical activities). CVD represents a major cause of premature death in Western countries [2]. Therefore, there is growing interest in identifying novel therapeutic approaches including a particular focus on nutrition and dietary interventions.

Cardiac energy metabolic shifts occur as a normal response to diverse physiological and dietary conditions and as a component of the pathophysiological processes that accompany heart disease. It is well established that insulin and fatty acids (FAs) are important modulators of cardiac substrate utilization [3]. In the heart, there is a fine-tuning of high rates of myocellular FAs uptake and of mitochondrial fatty acid oxidation. When the rate of FA delivery to the heart increases (e.g., diabetes, high fat feeding) it may cause a mismatch between FA uptake and oxidation leading to excessive intracellular storage of the bio-active lipid intermediates within the cardiomyocytes that could subsequently lead to cardiac dysfunction [4,5]. Accordingly, several studies have shown that lipids accumulate in the heart of diabetic animals [6,7]. Myocardial FA uptake is largely regulated by the membrane fatty acid transporter (FAT/CD36) [8]. Chiu et al. [9] showed that a myocardial lipid accretion due to an increase of fat uptake leads to myocyte apoptosis and cardiomyopathy. An enhanced long-chain acyl CoA (LC ACoA) uptake and channeling into triglycerides was observed in the heart of obese Zucker rats [10]. The accumulation of triglyceride is likely toxic to the myocardium and has been linked with insulin resistance (IR) and cardiac dysfunction [6,11]. Besides, it is generally acknowledged that dietary factors, among them FAs, up-regulated the transcription of genes encoding for proteins involved in cardiac FA transport and metabolism, most likely through the activation of peroxisome proliferator activated receptor α (PPARα) (e.g., expression of muscle-type carnitine palmitoyltransferase 1 (M-CPT1) [12,13].

On the other hand, high sucrose, high fructose and/or high fat diets have been used to induce metabolic and physiological alterations in rodents, mimicking several aspects of the MS in humans such as dyslipidemia, IR and adiposity [14]. Furthermore, we have previously demonstrated that the cardiac muscle of rats chronically fed a sucrose-rich diet (SRD) showed a significant increase of lipid storage accompanied by a significant reduction of basal and insulin stimulated glucose uptake and metabolism (isolated perfusion according to Langendorff's recirculating mode), as well as in the activities of key enzymes involved in glucose metabolism [15,16].

Epidemiological data show that a high intake of n-3 polyunsaturated fatty acids (n-3 PUFAs) from fish is associated with a lower incidence of heart failure and cardio protective function [17]. Moreover, different epidemiological and clinical studies have suggested that a high concentration of dietary α-linolenic acid 18:3 n-3, (ALA) is associated with a decreased risk of CVD [18,19]. Recent studies carried out in rats by Folino et al. [20] showed that ALA protects against cardiac injury and remodeling induced by beta-adrenergic over stimulation, and that a protective role is played by β_2 adrenergic receptors which mediate the activation of the Src kinase-phosphatidylinositol-3-kinase protective pathway. The seeds of Salvia hispanica L, commonly known as chia seeds, contain the richest botanical oil source of ALA and high amounts of fiber and minerals. Poudyal et al. [21,22] have recently shown that the administration of chia oil improved heart left ventricular dimensions, contractility, volume and stiffness as well as hypertension, glucose tolerance and insulin sensitivity in rats fed a high fat-high fructose diet. In this line, recent studies of our group have demonstrated that the administration of chia seeds as a dietary source of fat in rats fed an SRD reversed dyslipidemia and IR, improved adipose tissue dysfunction and glucose and lipid metabolism in the skeletal muscle [23–25]. However, the effect of chia seeds on myocardial substrate utilization has been only partially investigated in this experimental model [21,22].

Thus, the aims of the present study were the following: (i) to further explore the mechanisms underlying the impaired lipid metabolism in the heart muscle of dyslipidemic insulin-resistant rats fed an SRD; (ii) to investigate if chia seeds as a dietary intervention could improve or even revert cardiac lipotoxicity. To achieve these goals: (a) we analyzed the protein mass levels of FAT/CD36 both at basal conditions and under insulin stimulation and the mitochondrial oxidation of LC ACoA by the activity and protein mass levels of the enzyme M-CPT1; (b) since the effect of FAs or FA derivatives in cardiac myocytes are considered to be PPARα mediated, we measured the protein mass level of this receptor; (c) we evaluated the protein mass levels of uncoupling protein 2 (UCP2), which plays a major role in the mitochondrial FAs flux. Additionally, the activities of the pyruvate dehydrogenase complex

(PDHc) and lipid storage were assessed. The study was conducted in rats fed an SRD during 6 months, during which permanent dyslipidemia, IR, abnormal glucose homeostasis and visceral adiposity were present before the source of dietary fat, corn oil (CO), was replaced by an isocaloric amount of chia seeds for the last three months of the experimental period in half of the animals.

2. Materials and Methods

2.1. Animals

Male Wistar rats initially weighing 180–190 g purchased from the National Institute of Pharmacology (Buenos Aires, Argentina) were housed in an animal room under controlled temperature (22 ± 1 °C), humidity and airflow, with a fixed (12 h) light–dark cycle (lights on from 07:00 to 19:00 h) and with free access to water and food. Adequate measures were taken to minimize the pain or discomfort of the rats and we used the smallest number of animals as possible. The animal protocols were evaluated and approved by the Human and Animal Research Investigation Committee of the School of Biochemistry, University of Litoral, Argentina (FONCyT-PICT #945/2012).

2.2. Experimental Design

The rats ($n = 60$) were initially fed with a standard non-purified diet (Ralston Purina, St Louis, MO, USA). After one week of acclimation, the rats were randomly divided into two separate groups and were fed a semi-synthetic diet. The control group ($n = 20$) received a control diet (CD) containing corn starch (60% energy), protein (17% energy) and CO as sources of fat (23% energy) throughout the experimental period (6 months). The other group ($n = 40$) received the same semi-synthetic diet with the sucrose as the carbohydrate source (SRD). After 3 months, the animals in the SRD group were randomly divided into two subgroups. The rats in the first subgroup continued with the SRD diet for up to 6 months of feeding. The second subgroup received the Salba seed (chia) as the source of dietary fat (SRD + chia) for the next 3 months. The carbohydrates, proteins, fibers, vitamins and mineral contents in the chia seed of SRD + chia group were balanced with the CD and SRD groups, according to the amount of these nutrients present in the chia seeds. A detailed composition of each diet is described in Table 1. The fatty acid composition of each experimental diet is shown in Table 2. The preparation and handling of diets have been reported elsewhere [23,24]. All diets provided approximately 17 kJ/g of food.

Table 1. Composition of experimental diets [1].

Diet Ingredients	Control Diet (CD)		Sucrose-Rich Diet (SRD)		SRD+chia Seed (SRD+chia)	
	% w/w	% Energy	% w/w	% Energy	% w/w	% Energy
Carbohydrates						
Corn starch	58.0	60.0	2.5	2.6	–	–
Sucrose	–	–	55.5	57.4	55.5	57.4
Chia seed [2]	–	–	–	–	2.5	2.6
Fat						
Corn oil	10.5	23.0	10.5	23.0	0.1	0.2
Chia seed	–	–	–	–	10.4	22.8
Protein						
Casein (vitamin free)	16.3	17.0	16.3	17.0	8.6	9.0
Chia seed	–	–	–	–	7.7	8.0

[1] The compositions of experimental diets are based on the AIN-93M diet. All diets contain by weight: salt mix 3.5% (AIN-93Mx); vitamin mix 1% (AIN-93Vx); choline chloride 0.2%; methionine 0.3%; fiber 10%–11%; [2] Chia seed (variety Salba; Salvia *hispánica* L.): 362 g/Kg diet. Chia composition (g/100 g chia seed): carbohydrate 37.45; insoluble fiber 81% of total of carbohydrates; fat 30.23; protein 21.19. Mineral composition (mg/100 g chia seed): Na 103.15; K 826.15; Ca 589.60; Fe 11.90; Mg 77.0; P 604.0; Zn 5.32; Cu 1.66; Mn 1.36.

Table 2. Total fatty acid composition of experimental diets (g/kg diet).

Fatty Acids [1]	CD and SRD	SRD+chia Seed
16:0	10.92	6.96
18:0	2.73	2.42
18:1 n-9	33.71	7.39
18:2 n-6	54.10	19.85
18:3 n-3	0.80	67.26
20:1 n-9	0.47	0.36
Total saturated	13.65	9.38
Monounsaturated	34.18	7.75
Polyunsaturated		
n-6	54.10	19.85
n-3	0.80	67.26
n-6/n-3	67.62	0.295

[1] Other minor fatty acids have been excluded.

The body weight and energy intake of each animal were recorded twice per week throughout the experimental period in all groups and subgroups of rats. In a separate experiment, the individual caloric intake and weight gain of eight animals in each group and subgroup were assessed twice a week. At the end of the experimental period, food was removed at 07:00 h (end of the dark period) and unless otherwise indicated, experiments were performed under feed conditions.

2.3. Analytical Methods

Rats from the three dietary groups were anaesthetized with intraperitoneal sodium pentobarbital (60 mg/kg body weight). Blood samples were obtained from the jugular vein, collected in tubes containing sodium EDTA as anticoagulant and rapidly centrifuged. Plasma was either immediately assayed or stored at −20 °C. Plasma triglycerides, cholesterol, glucose and free fatty acids and immunoreactive insulin were determined as previously described [25]. Epididymal, retroperitoneal and omental adipose tissues were removed and weighed. The visceral adiposity index (%) was calculated as shown elsewhere [25]. The heart muscle was totally removed; then, it was weighed and the left ventricle was separated. The heart tissue was immediately frozen and stored at temperature of liquid N_2. Heart weight was normalized relative to the tibia length at the time of removal. The homogenate of frozen muscle powder was used to determine triglyceride [26], LC ACoA [27] and diacylglycerol (DAG) content [28].

2.4. Determination of Blood Pressure

Blood pressure was measured in the three dietary groups in conscious animals maintained at 28 °C in a restraining tube, at the beginning, at 3 months and at the end of the experimental period using a CODA™ Monitor of tail-cuff non-invasive blood pressure system (Kent Scientific Corporation, Torrington, CT, USA). The values are reported as the average of 8 individual measurements.

2.5. Enzymatic Activity Assays of CPT and PDHc

Heart M-CPT1 enzyme activities were measured as reported by Ling *et al.* [29] with some modifications. Frozen tissue was homogenized in buffer (20 mM HEPES pH 7.4, 140 mM KCl, 10 mM EDTA and 5 mM $MgCl_2$) and after centrifugation; the mitochondrial pellet was resuspended in a homogenization buffer. Protein concentration was measured by the Bradford assay (Bio-Rad reagent). To determine the total CPT activity, 100 μg of protein were added in a reaction buffer (20 mM HEPES pH 7.4, 220 mM sucrose, 40 mM KCl, 1 mM EGTA, 0.1 mM 5,5′-dithio-bis(2-nitrobenzoic acid) (DTNB) and 40 μM palmitoyl CoA). In addition, 1 mM of L-carnitine was added to start the reaction. The rate of appearance of CoASH-DTNB was monitored at 412 nm at 37 °C. CPT2 activity was measured under the same conditions in the presence of 10 μM of malonyl CoA (M-CPT1 inhibitor). The M-CPT1 activity was calculated as the difference between total CPT and CPT2 activities. The M-CPT1 activity was expressed as the amount of CoASH released per min per mg of protein. The extract and assay of the PDHc activity from the heart muscle were measured as previously described [15].

2.6. Determination of FAT/CD36 Protein Mass Level (Euglycemic-Hyperinsulinemic Clamp Studies)

The heart muscles of six rats from the CD, SRD and SRD+chia groups were rapidly removed (time 0 of clamp study) and stored at −80 °C for the determination of the FAT/CD36 protein levels. Immediately, in the other six rats from each dietary group, an infusion of highly purified porcine neutral insulin (Actrapid, Novo Nordisk,) was administered at 0.8 units/(kg × h) for 120 min. Glycemia was maintained at a euglycemic level by infusing glucose at a variable rate. The glucose infusion rate (GIR) during the second hour of the clamp study was taken as the net steady state of the whole body glucose. At the end of the clamp period, the heart muscle of each dietary group was rapidly removed for determination of the FAT/CD36 protein mass levels (for details see ref. [30]). Plasma membrane fractions from heart muscle were prepared according to the method of Rodnick et al. [31]. Briefly, the muscle was homogenized in ice-cold buffer (20 mM HEPES pH 7.4, 1 mM EDTA, 250 mM sucrose and 5 μL/mL protease inhibitor cocktail (Sigma, St. Louis, MO, USA)) and the homogenate was centrifuged at 3000× g at 4 °C. The supernatant was centrifuged at 184,000× g at 4 °C. The resulting pellet (membrane fraction) was resuspended in buffer and stored at −80 °C until the assay. Protein concentrations were quantified by the Bradford assay (Bio-Rad reagent). Proteins were separated by SDS-PAGE and transferred to PVDF membranes. The membranes were probed with a specific antibody (rabbit polyclonal anti-CD36 from Santa Cruz Biotechnology, Inc., Santa Cruz, CA, USA). The blot was incubated with horseradish peroxidase-linked secondary antibody (Santa Cruz Biotechnology) followed by chemiluminescence detection according to the manufacturer's instruction (Pierce Biotechnology, Rockford, IL, USA). The protein levels were normalized to actin. The intensity of the bands was quantified by National Institutes of Health (NIH) imaging software (Bethesda, MD, USA). The relationship between the amount of the sample subjected to immunoblotting and the signal intensity observed was linear under the conditions described above.

2.7. Determination of M-CPT1 and PPARα Protein Mass Levels

Frozen heart powder was homogenized in a lysis buffer (10 mM Tris-HCl pH 7.4, 150 mM NaCl, 1 mM EGTA, 1 mM EDTA, 1% Triton X-100 and 5 μL/mL protease inhibitor cocktail (Sigma)) as described by Bogazzi et al. [32]. After 30 min incubation on ice, the lysates were centrifuged at 4 °C and supernatants were stored at −80 °C. The protein content was quantified by the Bradford assay. Total protein samples (100 μg/lane) were resolved on SDS-PAGE, transferred to PVDF membranes and probed with specific antibodies (rabbit polyclonal anti M-CPT1 or rabbit polyclonal anti-PPARα from Santa Cruz Biotechnology, Inc.). The blots were incubated with horseradish peroxidase-linked secondary antibody (Santa Cruz Biotechnology) followed by chemiluminescence detection as described above. The protein levels were normalized to actin.

2.8. Determination of UCP2 Protein Mass Level

The mitochondrial fraction from the heart muscle was carried out according to the method described by Pecqueur et al. [33]. Briefly, the tissue was homogenized at 4 °C in a TES buffer (10 mM Tris pH 7.5, 1 mM EDTA, 250 mM sucrose and 5 μL/mL protease inhibitor cocktail (Sigma)). After centrifugation, the mitochondrial pellet was resuspended in TES buffer and stored at −80 °C. The protein content was quantified by the Bradford assay. Protein samples (50 μg protein/lane) were resolved by SDS-PAGE and transferred to PVDF membranes. The membranes were probed with a specific antibody (goat polyclonal anti-UCP2 from Santa Cruz Biotechnology, Inc.). The blot was incubated with horseradish peroxidase-linked secondary antibody (Santa Cruz Biotechnology) followed by chemiluminescence detection as described above. The protein levels were normalized to actin.

2.9. Statistical Analysis

Sample sizes were calculated on the basis of measurements previously made with rats fed either a CD or SRD [16,25,30] considering an 80% power as described by Glantz [34]. Results were expressed as mean with their standard errors. The homogeneity of variances were tested using Barlett's test. The statistical significance between groups was determined by one way analysis of variance (ANOVA) with one factor (diet) followed by the Newman Keul's multiple comparison *post hoc* test [35]. Differences having *p* values lower than 0.05 were considered to be statistically significant. Statistical analyses were performed using GraphPad Prism version 5.00 for Windows (San Diego, CA, USA). All reported *p* values are 2-sided.

3. Results

3.1. Body Weight, Energy Intake and Visceral Adiposity Index

Body weight and energy intake were carefully monitored in all groups of rats through the experimental period. As previously shown [25], a significant increase in body weight and energy intake occurred in rats fed an SRD from month 3 to 6 compared to those fed a CD (Table 3). A similar energy intake was recorded in both SRD and SRD+chia groups during the last three months of the experimental period while body weight at month 6 was slightly lower without statistical differences in the latter group. As in our previous report [24], SRD-fed rats showed a significant increase of the visceral adiposity index compared to the CD group. The chia seed enriched diet significantly reduced the aforementioned index, which reached values similar to those of the CD group.

Table 3. Body weight, energy intake and adiposity index of rats fed a control diet (CD), sucrose-rich diet (SRD) or SRD + chia seed (SRD + chia) [1].

Diet	Body Weight (g)		Energy Intake (kJ/Day)	Diet	Body Weight (g)	Energy Intake (kJ/Day)	Visceral Adiposity Index (%)
	Initial	3 Months	Initial to 3 Months		6 Months	3 to 6 Months	6 Months
CD (8)	184.3 ± 2.6	414.5 ± 5.5	294.5 ± 12.5	CD (8)	476.3 ± 7.6 [b]	292.0 ± 7.2 [b]	4.1 ± 0.3 [b]
SRD (16)	186.0 ± 1.6	428.0 ± 6.0	292.0 ± 7.2	SRD (8)	545.0 ± 10.0 [a]	374.0 ± 9.5 [a]	6.2 ± 0.4 [a]
				SRD+chia (8)	524.0 ± 7.3 [a]	356.5 ± 13.0 [a]	4.5 ± 0.2 [b]

[1] Values are expressed as mean ± SEM, () number of rats. Values in a column that do not share the same superscript letter (a, b) are significantly different *p* < 0.05 when one variable at a time was compared by the Newman Keul's test.

3.2. Total and Relative Heart Weight and Systolic Blood Pressure

Total heart weights recorded at the end of experimental period in each dietary group showed a significant increase in SRD-fed rats compared with the CD-fed rats. SRD + chia did not modify heart weight. Conversely, relative heart weights as g/100 g body weight or by the length of the tibia (mg/mm) were similar in all dietary groups (Table 4). SRD feeding increased systolic blood pressure throughout the six-month feeding protocol with values at three and six months significantly higher compared to those observed in the CD-fed group. Chia seeds in the SRD group normalized systolic blood pressure after three months of treatment reaching values similar to those of the CD group (Table 4).

Table 4. Total and relative heart weight at the end of the experimental period and systolic blood pressure of rats fed a control diet (CD), sucrose-rich diet (SRD) or SRD + chia seed (SRD + chia) [1].

	CD	SRD	SRD+chia
Heart tissue			
Total wet weight, g	1.24 ± 0.01 [b] (8)	1.31 ± 0.03 [a] (8)	1.28 ± 0.02 [a] (8)
g wet weight/100 g body weight	0.260 ± 0.003 (8)	0.250 ± 0.004 (8)	0.250 ± 0.005 (8)
mg wet weight/mm tibia length	27.2 ± 1.0 (8)	30.1 ± 1.3 (8)	28.3 ± 1.0 (8)
Systolic blood pressure, mmHg			
Initial	115.0 ± 4.6 (8)	116.0 ± 2.4 (16)	
3 months	123.3 ± 1.0 [b] (8)	130.9 ± 1.2 [a] (16)	
6 months	120.2 ± 4.8 [b] (8)	138.4 ± 1.6 [a] (8)	118.8 ± 1.6 [b] (8)

[1] Values are expressed as mean ± SEM, () number of rats. Values in a line that do not share the same superscript letter (a, b) are significantly different $p < 0.05$ when one variable at a time was compared by the Newman Keul's test.

3.3. Plasma Metabolites, Insulin Levels and GIR

Confirming previous studies [25], the changes observed after three or six months of SRD on plasma triglyceride, free fatty acids and glucose concentration were similar and both significantly different from those of the CD groups to which the data from SRD + chia were similar (Table 5). No statistical differences in plasma insulin levels were observed at the end of the experimental period between the three dietary groups. Furthermore, the significant decrease of the GIR recorded in the SRD-fed group returned to values similar to those obtained in the CD-fed rats in the SRD + chia group (Figure 1).

Table 5. Plasma metabolites of rats fed a control diet (CD), sucrose-rich diet (SRD) or SRD + chia seed (SRD+chia) [1].

Diet	Time on Diet (Months)	Triglyceride (mM)	Free Fatty Acids (μM)	Cholesterol (mM)	Glucose (mM)	Insulin (μU/mL)
CD	3	0.69 ± 0.04 [b]	300.1 ± 16.0 [b]	1.85 ± 0.10 [b]	6.5 ± 0.2 [b]	64.1 ± 3.2
SRD	3	1.98 ± 0.08 [a]	716.0 ± 8.1 [a]	3.21 ± 0.14 [a]	7.9 ± 0.1 [a]	60.1 ± 4.2
CD	6	0.72 ± 0.03 [b]	335.0 ± 13.0 [b]	1.92 ± 0.11 [b]	6.6 ± 0.1 [b]	62.0 ± 2.9
SRD	6	2.06 ± 0.17 [a]	760.4 ± 16.3 [a]	3.60 ± 0.04 [a]	8.3 ± 0.1 [a]	65.0 ± 3.2
SRD+chia	3 to 6	0.72 ± 0.05 [b]	363.0 ± 35.4 [b]	1.75 ± 0.21 [b]	6.9 ± 0.1 [b]	67.4 ± 6.5

[1] Values are expressed as mean ± SEM, $n = 6$. Values in a column that do not share the same superscript letter (a, b) are significantly different $p < 0.05$ when one variable at a time was compared by the Newman Keul's test.

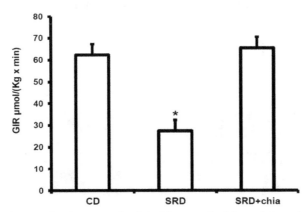

Values are mean, with their standard errors depicted by vertical bars (six animals per group).* $p < 0.05$ SRD *vs.* CD and SRD + chia.

Figure 1. GIR during euglycemic-hyperinsulinemic clamp in rats fed a control diet (CD), sucrose-rich diet (SRD) or SRD + chia seed (SRD + chia).

3.4. Heart Muscle Metabolites Concentrations and PDHc Activity

Table 6 depicts significant increases of lipid storage (triglycerides, LC ACoA and DAG) levels within the cardiac muscle of SRD-fed rats. The present data show that in the SRD + chia seed group, neither parameter differed from those of the CD group at the end of the experimental period. Moreover, the administration of chia seed (SRD+chia) was able to revert the reduced active form of PDHc (PDHa) observed in the SRD-fed group reaching values similar to those of the control group (CD). The total PDHc activity expressed per gram of wet tissue did not differ between the groups (data not shown).

Table 6. Intramyocardial lipid accumulation and PDHc activity of rats fed a control diet (CD), sucrose-rich diet (SRD) or SRD + chia seed (SRD + chia) at the end of the experimental period [1].

	CD	SRD	SRD+chia
Triglyceride (µmol/g wet tissue)	3.60 ± 0.22 [b]	6.03 ± 0.34 [a]	4.44 ± 0.60 [b]
LC ACoA (nmol/g wet tissue)	31.4 ± 5.5 [b]	68.0 ± 4.0 [a]	45.8 ± 5.5 [b]
DAG (nmol/g wet tissue)	250.8 ± 19.5 [b]	355.3 ± 15.4 [a]	276.6 ± 24.0 [b]
PDHa (% of total PDHc)	59.7 ± 5.8 [a]	26.6 ± 4.6 [b]	45.1 ± 4.9 [a]

[1] Values are expressed as mean $\pm$ SEM, $n = 6$. Values in a line that do not share the same superscript letter (a, b) are significantly different $p < 0.05$ when one variable at a time was compared by the Newman Keul's test.

3.5. FAT/CD36 Protein Mass Level in Heart Muscle at the Beginning and at the End of the Euglycemic-Hyperinsulinemic Clamp Studies

Figure 2 shows the protein mass level of FAT/CD36 at the beginning (0 min) and at the end of the clamp. The immunoblottting of the heart muscle revealed a single 90 KDa band consistent with FAT/CD36. Each gel contained an equal number of samples from rats fed a CD, SRD and SRD + chia at 0 min and 120 min of euglycemic hyperinsulinemic clamp (Figure 2, top panel). After the densitometry of immunoblots, FAT/CD36 at the beginning of the clamp was normalized to 100%, and both the SRD and SRD + chia groups at the beginning as well as the three dietary groups at the end of the study were expressed relative to this. At the beginning of the clamp, the qualitative and quantitative analysis of the Western blot showed a significant increase ($p < 0.05$) in the relative abundance of FAT/CD36 in the SRD-fed rats compared to the CD and SRD+chia groups. The latter reached values similar to those of the CD group. At the end of the clamp study, insulin stimulated the translocation of FAT/CD36 to the sarcolemma in the CD-fed rats that showed a significant ($p < 0.05$) increase of their protein mass level, while in the heart of SRD-fed rats, insulin did not further recruit FAT/CD36 to the sarcolemma under the same experimental conditions. Moreover, changes induced by the SRD were reverted by the chia seed enriched diet (Figure 2 bottom panel).

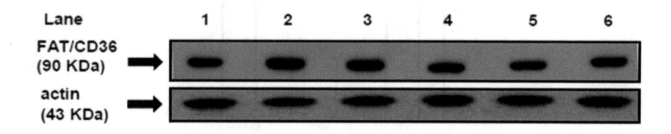

Figure 2. *Cont.*

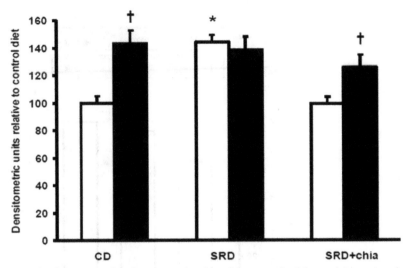

Values are mean, with their standard errors depicted by vertical bars (six animals per group) and expressed as percentage relative to the control diet at 0 min of the clamp. * $p < 0.05$ SRD at 0 min *vs.* CD and SRD+chia at 0 min of the clamp. † $p < 0.05$ CD and SRD+chia at 120 min *vs.* CD and SRD+chia at 0 min of the clamp.

Figure 2. Heart protein mass levels of FAT/CD36 at the beginning (0 min) and under the insulin stimulation at the end (120 min) of the clamp studies in rats fed a control diet (CD), a sucrose-rich diet (SRD) or SRD + chia seed (SRD + chia). Top panel: a representative immunoblot of heart FAT/CD36 of rats fed CD, SRD and SRD + chia. Molecular marker is shown on the right. Lane 1, CD 0 min; lane 2, CD 120 min; lane 3, SRD 0 min; lane 4, SRD 120 min; lane 5, SRD + chia 0 min; lane 6, SRD + chia 120 min. Bottom panel: densitometric immunoblot analysis of heart FAT/CD36 protein mass level of rats fed CD, SRD or SRD + chia at the beginning (0 min □) and at the end (120 min ■) of clamp studies.

3.6. M-CPT1 Activity and Protein Mass Level

Figure 3a shows the cardiac muscle activity of the M-CPT1 in the three dietary groups. Compared with the CD-fed group, a three-fold increase of the mitochondrial M-CPT1 activity was observed in the heart of rats fed an SRD. The M-CPT1 activity was significantly reduced under the administration of chia seed. However, values were still higher than those recorded in the CD-fed rats. The CPT2 activity remained similar in the three dietary groups. Immunoblotting of cardiac muscle M-CPT1 revealed a single 75 KDa band consistent with M-CPT1. Each gel contained an equal number of samples from rats fed a CD, SRD and SRD+chia (Figure 3b top panel). After densitometry of immunoblots the M-CPT1 of the CD group was normalized to 100%, and both the SRD and SRD+chia groups were expressed relative to this. The qualitative and quantitative abundance of the Western blot showed that M-CPT1 protein mass level significantly increased ($p < 0.05$) in the heart muscle of the SRD group when compared with rats fed a CD (Figure 3b bottom panel). Interestingly, although the enzymatic activity of M-CPT1 decreased when chia seed replaced CO as a source of fat in the SRD, the relative abundance of M-CPT1 was still significantly higher.

a

Oxidative enzyme activity [nmol/(mg protein x min)]	CD	SRD	SRD+chia
M-CPT1	8.80 ± 0.74^c	22.10 ± 1.93^a	14.80 ± 2.10^b
CPT2	11.3 ± 1.0	12.8 ± 1.0	11.0 ± 1.0

Figure 3. *Cont.*

b

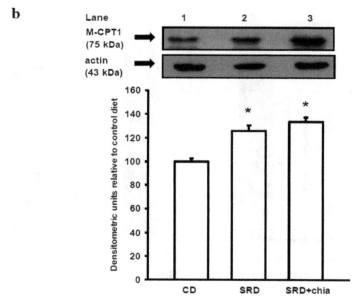

Values are mean, with their standard errors depicted by vertical bars (six animals per group) and expressed as percentage relative to the control diet. * $p < 0.05$ SRD and SRD + chia *vs.* CD.

Figure 3. (**a**) Heart enzyme activities of M-CPT1 and CPT2 in rats fed a control diet (CD), sucrose-rich diet (SRD) or SRD+chia seed (SRD+chia). Values are expressed as mean ± SEM (six animals per group). Values in a line that do not share the same superscript letter (**a**, **b**, **c**) are significantly different ($p < 0.05$) when one variable at time was compared by the Newman Keul's test; (**b**) Top panel: a representative immunoblot of heart M-CPT1 protein mass level of rats fed CD, SRD and SRD + chia. Molecular marker is shown on the right. Lane 1, CD; lane 2, SRD; lane 3, SRD + chia. Bottom panel: densitometric immunoblot analysis of heart M-CPT1 protein mass level of rats fed CD, SRD or SRD + chia.

3.7. PPARα Protein Mass Level

We examined the protein mass level of PPARα, since this receptor is considered a master regulator of FAs metabolism in several organs including the heart. The immunoblotting of the cardiac muscle revealed a single 55KDa band consistent with PPARα. Each gel contained an equal number of samples from the CD, SRD and SRD + chia groups (Figure 4 top panel). After the densitometry of immunoblots, the PPARα of the CD group was normalized to 100%, and both the SRD and SRD + chia groups were expressed relative to this. The qualitative and quantitative abundance of the Western blot showed that the relative abundance of the PPARα protein mass level significantly increased ($p < 0.05$) in the hearts of both the SRD and SRD + chia groups, although the protein mass level was slightly lower without statistical differences in the latter group (Figure 4 bottom panel). On the other hand, we measured the protein mass levels of UCP2 since this uncoupling protein could be regulated by increased FA concentration through PPARα activation. The qualitative and quantitative analysis of the Western blots showed that the relative abundance of mitochondrial UCP2 protein mass level was similar in the hearts of the three dietary groups. Values were as follows: (mean ± SEM, $n = 6$); CD 100 ± 3.2; SRD 103.8 ± 2.5 and SRD + chia 95.7 ± 5.3, p NS.

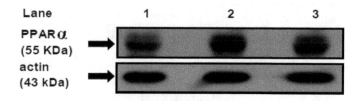

Figure 4. *Cont.*

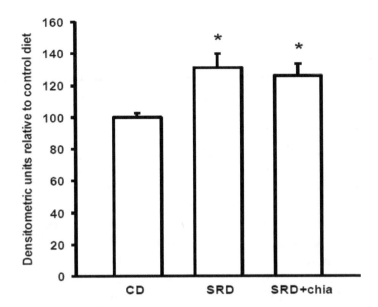

Figure 4. Heart protein mass level of PPARα in rats fed a control diet (CD), sucrose-rich diet (SRD) or SRD + chia seed (SRD + chia). Top panel: a representative immunoblot of heart PPARα of rats fed a CD, SRD and SRD + chia. Molecular marker is shown on the right. Lane 1 CD; lane 2 SRD; lane 3 SRD + chia. Bottom panel: densitometric immunoblot analysis of heart PPARα protein mass level of rats fed CD, SRD or SRD + chia.. Values are mean, with their standard errors depicted by vertical bars (6 animals per group) and expressed as percentage relative to the control diet. * $p < 0.05$ SRD and SRD + chia *vs.* CD.

4. Discussion

The present study provides new information on the mechanisms involved in heart muscle lipotoxicity in dyslipemic insulin resistant rats fed an SRD and explores the possible beneficial effects of dietary chia supplementation on reversed or improved pre-exiting impaired cardiac lipid metabolism. Disruption of the sensitive balance between FAs and glucose in the heart and increased intramyocellular fat contents and fatty acid metabolites are likely to play a pivotal role in the development of insulin resistance, cardiac lipotoxicity and heart dysfunction [36]. FAT/CD36 plays a pivotal role in governing myocardial FAs uptake [8]. In the present work, the increased intracellular LC ACoA in the heart of SRD-fed rats is accompanied by a significant increase of protein mass level of FAT/CD36 in the plasma membrane, suggesting that the enhanced amount of FAT/CD36 on sarcolemma elicits an increased rate of FAs uptake. In this regard, an increased availability of plasma free fatty acids and triglyceride levels is recorded in the SRD-fed group. Moreover, despite a significant increase of both the M-CPT1 activity and its protein mass level, triglyceride accumulates in the heart of this dietary group. It is possible that the increased flux of FAs to the heart exceeds the mitochondrial oxidative capacity leading to an increase of FAs storage into the triglyceride pool. The dynamic equilibrium between triglyceride stores and their metabolites cause accumulation of DAG and ceramide during prolonged long-chain fatty acid (LCFA) influx. Although in the present study we did not measure the level of ceramide, our previous results [16] and the present data show an increase of DAG concentration in the heart of rats fed an SRD. Both metabolites are implicated in counteracting insulin signaling, reducing insulin responsiveness and altering its ability to regulate substrate handling [4]. In this regard, the present data show that insulin stimulated the cell surface recruitment of FAT/CD36 in the heart of CD-fed rats. However, insulin was unable to further recruit FAT/CD36 to the sarcolemma in the heart of SRD-fed rats that was completely insensitive to the stimulus of the hormone. Similarly, in cardiac myocytes from obese Zucker rats, Coort *et al.* [10] reported that insulin failed to alter the sub cellular localization of FAT/CD36 and the rate of LCFA uptake and triglyceride esterification. Besides, in cardiamyocytes of Wistar rats in which a high-fat diet induced cardiac contractile dysfunction,

Ouwens *et al.* [5] demonstrated that a permanent presence of FAT/CD36 in the sarcolemma membrane resulted in the enhancement of LCFA uptake and myocardial triglyceride accumulation.

PPARα and its co-activator PPARγ co-activator 1 alpha (PGC-1α) play an important role in the transcriptional regulation of cardiac energy metabolism, and the effect of FAs in cardiac myocytes is considered to be PPARα mediated [37]. Several lines of evidence suggested that LCFAs that induce the gene expression of M-CPT1 and other enzymes in the cellular fatty acid utilization pathway are namely mediated by PPARα transcriptional control [13]. LCFAs: linoleic acid 18:2 *n*-6, ALA and docosahexaenoic acid 22:6, *n*-3 (DHA) among them, and a variety of related compounds serve as PPARα ligands [38]. In this context, the present study shows a significant increase of the relative abundance of the protein mass level of PPARα and the mitochondrial M-CPT1 activity in the heart of SRD-fed rats. These results suggest that a chronic high exposure to Fas, which enhances their uptake, induces the activation of PPARα protein expression that, in turn, encodes the proteins responsible for FAs oxidation, M-CPT1 among others. Since an increase of intramyocardial lipids is observed in the SRD heart, it is possible that a disruption of the balance between lipid oxidation-storage occurs in the heart muscle of this dyslipemic insulin-resistant model. In this vein, Buchanam *et al.* [39] have documented an increased PPARα and PGC-1α expression in murine insulin-resistant hearts. A high fat diet also activates PPARα in the heart and stimulates expression of key proteins involved in fatty acid oxidation [40].

It is well known that dietary *n*-3 PUFAs, mainly eicosapentaenoic acid 20:5, *n*-3 (EPA) and DHA, improve cardiac function [17]. ALA could be a valuable source of *n*-3 long-chain FAs via elongase/desaturase activities. Dietary ALA exerts a protective effect on the CVD [18]. In this regard, and confirming previous results, the present work demonstrates a reversion of dyslipidemia, abnormal glucose homeostasis and whole body peripheral insulin insensitivity when dietary chia seed replaced CO in the SRD-fed rats. The reverse of dyslipidemia by chia seed led to a significant reduction of lipid storage in the heart of SRD-fed rats, reaching values similar to those observed in the heart of CD-fed rats. Moreover, at basal conditions (beginning of the clamp study) a decrease of FAT/CD36 protein mass level suggests that a different milieu (decreased plasma lipids levels) prevented the robust relocations of fatty acid translocase to the sarcolemma, which was otherwise seen in the cardiac muscle of SRD-fed rats and, therefore, reduced the influx of FAs. Furthermore, the heart of dietary chia-fed rats was sensitive to the stimulus of insulin. As in the CD-fed group, the hormone significantly induced the translocation of FAT/CD36 to the plasma membrane. Recently, in isolated rat cardiomyocytes incubated under insulin resistance evoking conditions, Franekova *et al.* [41] demonstrated that the inclusion of EPA and DHA to the medium prevented the persistent translocation of CD36 to the sarcolemma and protected the metabolic and functional properties of the cardiomyocytes. In this regard, we previously demonstrated that the administration of dietary fish oil to SRD-fed rats was able to reverse heart muscle lipotoxicity and benefit key enzyme activities involved in the glucose metabolism [16]. At present, we are unaware of other studies concerning the effect of the long-term consumption of dietary chia and/or ALA on lipid metabolism in the cardiac muscle of SRD-fed rats. However, the reversion of the impaired glucose oxidation, as well as the accretion of triglyceride and fatty acid derivatives, the normalization of the enhanced sarcolemmal FAT/CD36 and the significantly reduced mitochondrial oxidative flux suggests that dietary chia seeds could improve the altered balance of heart fuel utilization. Interestingly, compared with CD-fed rats the protein mass level of the nuclear receptor PPARα and the activity of its target enzyme M-CPT1 were still higher in the heart of the SRD + chia group. Our results do not provide data on the mechanisms underlying the effect of chia seed on this nuclear receptor but it was shown that ALA and DHA, among others, are natural occurring ligands of PPARα in the heart [38]. In this regard, it has been demonstrated by our group [23] and others [21,42] that chia seeds change the plasma fatty acid profile increasing ALA, EPA, docosapentaenoic acid 22:5, *n*-3 (DPA) and DHA levels as well as the *n*-3/*n*-6 FAs ratio in rats fed an SRD, a control diet, or a high fat, high fructose diet. Thus, we do not discard the possibility that the different plasma FA profiles to which the heart was exposed could contribute to this finding.

On the other hand, an increase of FAs could induce UCP2 expression through PPARα activation in adult rat cardiomyocytes [43]. Besides, an increase of UCP2 and PPARα was recorded in the heart of ob/ob mice [39]. However, under the present experimental protocol, our results showed that the mitochondrial protein mass levels of UCP2 were similar in the three experimental groups. Besides, we are unaware of any other studies that evaluated the potential role of UCP2 in altering myocardial substrate in the heart muscle of SRD rats, and the effect of either chia seeds or oil upon UCP2. Further studies will be needed to evaluate this matter.

Chia seeds were able to decrease the systolic blood pressure that developed in the SRD-fed rats. In this regard, Poudyal et al. [21], in rats fed a high fructose-high fat diet, recorded that chia seed normalized systolic blood pressure increasing DPA and DHA contents in FAs of the heart, and Rousseau et al. [44] showed a decrease in blood pressure and increased DHA and EPA in cardiac phospholipids in rats fed a high fructose diet supplemented with either DHA or EPA. Interestingly, we observed an increase of DHA and ALA in the FA phospholipids of cardiac membrane in the SRD + chia group (data not shown). Moreover, Vuksan et al. [45] showed that a long-term supplementation with Salba (S. hispanica L) attenuates systolic blood pressure and emerging cardiovascular risk factors, safely beyond conventional therapy, while maintaining good glycemic and lipid control in well-controlled type-2 diabetic patients.

5. Conclusions

In brief, this study demonstrated that the lipotoxicity present in the heart of SRD-fed rats, an experimental model of dyslipidemia and insulin resistance, is accompanied by changes involving lipid metabolism suggesting an impaired myocardial lipid utilization. In this scenario, and for the first time, this work also provides new information concerning the possible mechanisms underlying the beneficial effects of dietary chia seeds on lipid cardiac metabolism and glucose oxidation. Although caution is warranted before extrapolating results from rodents to humans, chia seeds may serve as an alternative dietary strategy in the management of these metabolic alterations susceptible to dietary manipulation.

Acknowledgments: The authors wish to thank Silvia Rodriguez and Walter Daru for their skillful technical assistance and Adriana Chicco for her valuable suggestions throughout the development of this study. The present study was carried out with the financial support of Agencia Nacional de Promoción Científica y Tecnológica (ANPCyT) (grants PICT 945 BID OC/AR 2011) and University of Litoral (CAI+D 50120110100058 LI-2012).The authors thank Agrisalba S. A. Buenos Aires, Argentina for providing the chia seeds Salba.

Author Contributions: Agustina Creus was involved in the design of the experimental protocol and performed the experiments. María R. Ferreira was involved in the analysis of protein mass levels and contributes of the analysis of the results. María E. Oliva was involved on the determination of plasma and tissues metabolites. Yolanda B. Lombardo designs the experimental protocol, wrote the manuscripts and discussed it with the whole group of authors.

References

1. Pollex, R.L.; Hegele, R.A. Genetic determinants of the metabolic syndrome. *Nat. Clin. Pract. Cardiovasc. Med.* **2006**, *3*, 482–489. [CrossRef] [PubMed]
2. Gaziano, T.A.; Bitton, A.; Anand, S.; Abrahams-Gessel, S.; Murphy, A. Growing epidemic of coronary heart disease in low- and middle- income countries. *Curr. Probl. Cardiol.* **2010**, *35*, 72–115. [CrossRef] [PubMed]
3. Mazumder, P.K.; O'Neill, B.T.; Roberts, M.W.; Buchanan, J.; Yun, U.J.; Cooksey, R.C.; Boudina, S.; Abel, E.D. Impaired cardiac efficiency and increased fatty acid oxidation in insulin-resistant Ob/Ob mouse hearts. *Diabetes* **2004**, *53*, 2366–2374. [CrossRef] [PubMed]
4. Glatz, J.F.; Angin, Y.; Steinbusch, L.K.; Schwenk, R.W.; Luiken, J.J. CD36 as a target to prevent cardiac lipotoxicity and insulin resistance. *Prostaglandins Leukot. Essent. Fatty Acids* **2013**, *88*, 71–77. [CrossRef] [PubMed]
5. Ouwens, D.M.; Diamant, M.; Fodor, M.; Habets, D.D.; Pelsers, M.M.; El, H.M.; Dang, Z.C.; van den Brom, C.E.; Vlasblom, R.; Rietdijk, A.; et al. Cardiac contractile dysfunction in insulin-resistant rats fed a high-fat diet is associated with elevated CD36-mediated fatty acid uptake and esterification. *Diabetologia* **2007**, *50*, 1938–1948. [CrossRef] [PubMed]

6.   Zhou, Y.T.; Grayburn, P.; Karim, A.; Shimabukuro, M.; Higa, M.; Baetens, D.; Orci, L.; Unger, R.H. Lipotoxic heart disease in obese rats: Implications for human obesity. *Proc. Natl. Acad. Sci. USA* **2000**, *97*, 1784–1789. [CrossRef] [PubMed]

7.   Paulson, D.J.; Crass, M.F., III. Endogenous triacylglycerol metabolism in diabetic heart. *Am. J. Physiol.* **1982**, *242*, H1084–H1094. [PubMed]

8.   Van Oort, M.M.; van Doorn, J.M.; Bonen, A.; Glatz, J.F.; van der Horst, D.J.; Rodenburg, K.W.; Luiken, J.J. Insulin-induced translocation of CD36 to the plasma membrane is reversible and shows similarity to that of GLUT4. *Biochim. Biophys. Acta* **2008**, *1781*, 61–71. [CrossRef] [PubMed]

9.   Chiu, H.C.; Kovacs, A.; Ford, D.A.; Hsu, F.F.; Garcia, R.; Herrero, P.; Saffitz, J.E.; Schaffer, J.E. A novel mouse model of lipotoxic cardiomyopathy. *J. Clin. Investig.* **2001**, *107*, 813–822. [CrossRef] [PubMed]

10.   Coort, S.L.; Hasselbaink, D.M.; Koonen, D.P.; Willems, J.; Coumans, W.A.; Chabowski, A.; van der Vusse, G.J.; Bonen, A.; Glatz, J.F.; Luiken, J.J. Enhanced sarcolemmal FAT/CD36 content and triacylglycerol storage in cardiac myocytes from obese Zucker rats. *Diabetes* **2004**, *53*, 1655–1663. [CrossRef] [PubMed]

11.   Finck, B.N.; Han, X.; Courtois, M.; Aimond, F.; Nerbonne, J.M.; Kovacs, A.; Gross, R.W.; Kelly, D.P. A critical role for PPARalpha-mediated lipotoxicity in the pathogenesis of diabetic cardiomyopathy: Modulation by dietary fat content. *Proc. Natl. Acad. Sci. USA* **2003**, *100*, 1226–1231. [CrossRef] [PubMed]

12.   Barger, P.M.; Kelly, D.P. PPAR signaling in the control of cardiac energy metabolism. *Trends Cardiovasc. Med.* **2000**, *10*, 238–245. [CrossRef]

13.   Brandt, J.M.; Djouadi, F.; Kelly, D.P. Fatty acids activate transcription of the muscle carnitine palmitoyltransferase I gene in cardiac myocytes via the peroxisome proliferator-activated receptor alpha. *J. Biol. Chem.* **1998**, *273*, 23786–23792. [CrossRef] [PubMed]

14.   Lombardo, Y.B.; Chicco, A.G. Effects of dietary polyunsaturated *n*-3 fatty acids on dyslipidemia and insulin resistance in rodents and humans. A review. *J. Nutr. Biochem.* **2006**, *17*, 1–13. [CrossRef] [PubMed]

15.   Montes, M.; Chicco, A.; Lombardo, Y.B. The effect of insulin on the uptake and metabolic fate of glucose in isolated perfused hearts of dyslipemic rats. *J. Nutr. Biochem.* **2000**, *11*, 30–37. [CrossRef]

16.   D'Alessandro, M.E.; Chicco, A.; Lombardo, Y.B. Dietary fish oil reverses lipotoxicity, altered glucose metabolism, and nPKCepsilon translocation in the heart of dyslipemic insulin-resistant rats. *Metabolism* **2008**, *57*, 911–919. [CrossRef] [PubMed]

17.   Jump, D.B.; Depner, C.M.; Tripathy, S. Omega-3 fatty acid supplementation and cardiovascular disease. *J. Lipid Res.* **2012**, *53*, 2525–2545. [CrossRef] [PubMed]

18.   Djousse, L.; Arnett, D.K.; Carr, J.J.; Eckfeldt, J.H.; Hopkins, P.N.; Province, M.A.; Ellison, R.C. Dietary linolenic acid is inversely associated with calcified atherosclerotic plaque in the coronary arteries: The National Heart, Lung, and Blood Institute Family Heart Study. *Circulation* **2005**, *111*, 2921–2926. [CrossRef] [PubMed]

19.   Mozaffarian, D.; Ascherio, A.; Hu, F.B.; Stampfer, M.J.; Willett, W.C.; Siscovick, D.S.; Rimm, E.B. Interplay between different polyunsaturated fatty acids and risk of coronary heart disease in men. *Circulation* **2005**, *111*, 157–164. [CrossRef] [PubMed]

20.   Folino, A.; Sprio, A.E.; di Scipio, F.; Berta, G.N.; Rastaldo, R. Alpha-linolenic acid protects against cardiac injury and remodeling induced by beta-adrenergic overstimulation. *Food Funct.* **2015**, *6*, 2231–2239. [CrossRef] [PubMed]

21.   Poudyal, H.; Panchal, S.K.; Ward, L.C.; Waanders, J.; Brown, L. Chronic high-carbohydrate, high-fat feeding in rats induces reversible metabolic, cardiovascular, and liver changes. *Am. J. Physiol. Endocrinol. Metab.* **2012**, *302*, E1472–E1482. [CrossRef] [PubMed]

22.   Poudyal, H.; Panchal, S.K.; Ward, L.C.; Brown, L. Effects of ALA, EPA and DHA in high-carbohydrate, high-fat diet-induced metabolic syndrome in rats. *J. Nutr. Biochem.* **2013**, *24*, 1041–1052. [CrossRef] [PubMed]

23.   Chicco, A.G.; D'Alessandro, M.E.; Hein, G.J.; Oliva, M.E.; Lombardo, Y.B. Dietary chia seed (Salvia *hispanica* L.) rich in alpha-linolenic acid improves adiposity and normalises hypertriacylglycerolaemia and insulin resistance in dyslipaemic rats. *Br. J. Nutr.* **2009**, *101*, 41–50. [CrossRef] [PubMed]

24.   Rossi, A.S.; Oliva, M.E.; Ferreira, M.R.; Chicco, A.; Lombardo, Y.B. Dietary chia seed induced changes in hepatic transcription factors and their target lipogenic and oxidative enzyme activities in dyslipidaemic insulin-resistant rats. *Br. J. Nutr.* **2013**, *109*, 1617–1627. [CrossRef] [PubMed]

25. Oliva, M.E.; Ferreira, M.R.; Chicco, A.; Lombardo, Y.B. Dietary salba (Salvia *hispanica* L) seed rich in alpha-linolenic acid improves adipose tissue dysfunction and the altered skeletal muscle glucose and lipid metabolism in dyslipidemic insulin-resistant rats. *Prostaglandins Leukot. Essent. Fatty Acids* **2013**, *89*, 279–289. [CrossRef] [PubMed]

26. Laurell, S. A method for routine determination of plasma triglycerides. *Scan. J. Clin. Lab. Investig.* **1966**, *18*, 668–672. [CrossRef]

27. Lowenstein, J.M. Citric Acid cycle. In *Methods in Enzymology*; Academic Press: New York, NY, USA, 1969; pp. 450–468.

28. Schmitz-Peiffer, C.; Browne, C.L.; Oakes, N.D.; Watkinson, A.; Chisholm, D.J.; Kraegen, E.W.; Biden, T.J. Alterations in the expression and cellular localization of protein kinase C isozymes ε and θ are associated with insulin resistance in skeletal muscle of the high-fat-fed rat. *Diabetes* **1997**, *46*, 169–178. [CrossRef] [PubMed]

29. Ling, B.; Aziz, C.; Alcorn, J. Systematic evaluation of key L-carnitine homeostasis mechanisms during postnatal development in rat. *Nutr. Metab (Lond.)* **2012**, *9*, 66. [CrossRef] [PubMed]

30. Chicco, A.; D'Alessandro, M.E.; Karabatas, L.; Pastorale, C.; Basabe, J.C.; Lombardo, Y.B. Muscle lipid metabolism and insulin secretion are altered in insulin-resistant rats fed a high sucrose diet. *J. Nutr.* **2003**, *133*, 127–133. [PubMed]

31. Rodnick, K.J.; Slot, J.W.; Studelska, D.R.; Hanpeter, D.E.; Robinson, L.J.; Geuze, H.J.; James, D.E. Immunocytochemical and biochemical studies of GLUT4 in rat skeletal muscle. *J. Biol. Chem.* **1992**, *267*, 6278–6285. [PubMed]

32. Bogazzi, F.; Raggi, F.; Ultimieri, F.; Russo, D.; D'Alessio, A.; Manariti, A.; Brogioni, S.; Manetti, L.; Martino, E. Regulation of cardiac fatty acids metabolism in transgenic mice overexpressing bovine GH. *J. Endocrinol.* **2009**, *201*, 419–427. [CrossRef] [PubMed]

33. Pecqueur, C.; Alves-Guerra, M.C.; Gelly, C.; Levi-Meyrueis, C.; Couplan, E.; Collins, S.; Ricquier, D.; Bouillaud, F.; Miroux, B. Uncoupling protein 2, *in vivo* distribution, induction upon oxidative stress, and evidence for translational regulation. *J. Biol. Chem.* **2001**, *276*, 8705–8712. [CrossRef] [PubMed]

34. Glantz, S.A. *Primer of Biostatistics*; McGraw Hill: New York, NY, USA, 2005.

35. Snedecor, G.W.; Cochran, W.G. *Factorial Experiments, in Statistical Methods Applied to Experimental in Agriculture and Biology*; Iowa State University Press: Ames, IA, USA, 1967; pp. 339–350.

36. Chess, D.J.; Stanley, W.C. Role of diet and fuel overabundance in the development and progression of heart failure. *Cardiovasc. Res.* **2008**, *79*, 269–278. [CrossRef] [PubMed]

37. Duncan, J.G. Peroxisome proliferator activated receptor-alpha (PPARalpha) and PPAR gamma coactivator-1alpha (PGC-1alpha) regulation of cardiac metabolism in diabetes. *Pediatr. Cardiol.* **2011**, *32*, 323–328. [CrossRef] [PubMed]

38. Georgiadi, A.; Boekschoten, M.V.; Muller, M.; Kersten, S. Detailed transcriptomics analysis of the effect of dietary fatty acids on gene expression in the heart. *Physiol. Genom.* **2012**, *44*, 352–361. [CrossRef] [PubMed]

39. Buchanan, J.; Mazumder, P.K.; Hu, P.; Chakrabarti, G.; Roberts, M.W.; Yun, U.J.; Cooksey, R.C.; Litwin, S.E.; Abel, E.D. Reduced cardiac efficiency and altered substrate metabolism precedes the onset of hyperglycemia and contractile dysfunction in two mouse models of insulin resistance and obesity. *Endocrinology* **2005**, *146*, 5341–5349. [CrossRef] [PubMed]

40. Stanley, W.C.; Dabkowski, E.R.; Ribeiro, R.F., Jr.; O'Connell, K.A. Dietary fat and heart failure: Moving from lipotoxicity to lipoprotection. *Circ. Res.* **2012**, *110*, 764–776. [CrossRef] [PubMed]

41. Franekova, V.; Angin, Y.; Hoebers, N.T.; Coumans, W.A.; Simons, P.J.; Glatz, J.F.; Luiken, J.J.; Larsen, T.S. Marine omega-3 fatty acids prevent myocardial insulin resistance and metabolic remodeling as induced experimentally by high insulin exposure. *Am. J. Physiol. Cell Physiol.* **2015**, *308*, C297–C307. [CrossRef] [PubMed]

42. Ayerza, R.; Coates, W. Ground chia seed and chia oil effects on plasma lipids and fatty acids in the rat. *J. Endocrinol.* **2005**, *25*, 995–1003. [CrossRef]

43. Li, N.; Wang, J.; Gao, F.; Tian, Y.; Song, R.; Zhu, S.J. The role of uncoupling protein 2 in the apoptosis induced by free fatty acid in rat cardiomyocytes. *J. Cardiovasc. Pharmacol.* **2010**, *55*, 161–167. [CrossRef] [PubMed]

44. Rousseau, D.; Helies-Toussaint, C.; Moreau, D.; Raederstorff, D.; Grynberg, A. Dietary *n*-3 PUFAs affect the blood pressure rise and cardiac impairments in a hyperinsulinemia rat model *in vivo*. *Am. J. Physiol. Heart Circ. Physiol.* **2003**, *285*, H1294–H1302. [CrossRef] [PubMed]

45. Vuksan, V.; Whitham, D.; Sievenpiper, J.L.; Jenkins, A.L.; Rogovik, A.L.; Bazinet, R.P.; Vidgen, E.; Hanna, A. Supplementation of conventional therapy with the novel grain Salba (Salvia *hispanica* L.) improves major and emerging cardiovascular risk factors in Type 2 diabetes: Results of a randomized controlled trial. *Diabetes Care* **2007**, *30*, 2804–2810. [CrossRef] [PubMed]

Permissions

All chapters in this book were first published by MDPI; hereby published with permission under the Creative Commons Attribution License or equivalent. Every chapter published in this book has been scrutinized by our experts. Their significance has been extensively debated. The topics covered herein carry significant findings which will fuel the growth of the discipline. They may even be implemented as practical applications or may be referred to as a beginning point for another development.

The contributors of this book come from diverse backgrounds, making this book a truly international effort. This book will bring forth new frontiers with its revolutionizing research information and detailed analysis of the nascent developments around the world.

We would like to thank all the contributing authors for lending their expertise to make the book truly unique. They have played a crucial role in the development of this book. Without their invaluable contributions this book wouldn't have been possible. They have made vital efforts to compile up to date information on the varied aspects of this subject to make this book a valuable addition to the collection of many professionals and students.

This book was conceptualized with the vision of imparting up-to-date information and advanced data in this field. To ensure the same, a matchless editorial board was set up. Every individual on the board went through rigorous rounds of assessment to prove their worth. After which they invested a large part of their time researching and compiling the most relevant data for our readers.

The editorial board has been involved in producing this book since its inception. They have spent rigorous hours researching and exploring the diverse topics which have resulted in the successful publishing of this book. They have passed on their knowledge of decades through this book. To expedite this challenging task, the publisher supported the team at every step. A small team of assistant editors was also appointed to further simplify the editing procedure and attain best results for the readers.

Apart from the editorial board, the designing team has also invested a significant amount of their time in understanding the subject and creating the most relevant covers. They scrutinized every image to scout for the most suitable representation of the subject and create an appropriate cover for the book.

The publishing team has been an ardent support to the editorial, designing and production team. Their endless efforts to recruit the best for this project, has resulted in the accomplishment of this book. They are a veteran in the field of academics and their pool of knowledge is as vast as their experience in printing. Their expertise and guidance has proved useful at every step. Their uncompromising quality standards have made this book an exceptional effort. Their encouragement from time to time has been an inspiration for everyone.

The publisher and the editorial board hope that this book will prove to be a valuable piece of knowledge for researchers, students, practitioners and scholars across the globe.

List of Contributors

Ya-Hui Huang
Graduate Institute of Clinical Medicine, College of Medicine, Taipei Medical University, Taipei 11031, Taiwan
Department of Dietetics and Nutrition, Heping Fuyou Branch, Taipei City Hospital, Taipei 10065, Taiwan

Wan-Chun Chiu
School of Nutrition and Health Sciences, College of Nutrition, Taipei Medical University, Taipei 11031, Taiwan
Research Center of Geriatric Nutrition, College of Nutrition, Taipei Medical University, Taipei 11031, Taiwan

Yuan-Pin Hsu
Graduate Institute of Clinical Medicine, College of Medicine, Taipei Medical University, Taipei 11031, Taiwan
Emergency Department, Wan Fang Hospital, Taipei Medical University, Taipei 11696, Taiwan

Yen-Li Lo
Department of Biomedical Engineering, National Yang-Ming University, Taipei 11221, Taiwan

Yuan-Hung Wang
Graduate Institute of Clinical Medicine, College of Medicine, Taipei Medical University, Taipei 11031, Taiwan
Department of Medical Research, Shuang Ho Hospital, Taipei Medical University, New Taipei City 23561, Taiwan

Barbara Troesch and Ines Warnke
Nutrition Science and Advocacy, DSM Nutritional Products, 4303 Kaiseraugst, Switzerland

Manfred Eggersdorfer
Department of Internal Medicine, University Medical Center Groningen, 9713 GZ Groningen, The Netherlands

Alessandro Laviano
Department of Translational and Precision Medicine, Sapienza University, 00185 Rome, Italy

Yves Rolland
Gérontopôle de Toulouse, Institut du Vieillissement, INSERM 1027, Centre Hospitalo-Universitaire de Toulouse, 31300 Toulouse, France

A. David Smith
Department of Pharmacology, University of Oxford, Oxford OX1 2JD, UK

Arved Weimann
Clinic for General, Visceral and Oncological Surgery, St. Georg gGmbH Clinic, 04129 Leipzig, Germany

Philip C. Calder
Faculty of Medicine, University of Southampton and NIHR Southampton Biomedical Research Centre, University Hospital Southampton NHS Foundation Trust and University of Southampton, Southampton SO16 6YD, UK

Woojung Yang, Jae-woo Lee and Yonghwan Kim
Department of Family Medicine, Chungbuk National University Hospital, Cheongju 28644, Korea

Jong Hun Lee
Department of Food Science and Biotechnology, Gachon University, Seongnam 13120, Korea

Hee-Taik Kang
Department of Family Medicine, Chungbuk National University Hospital, Cheongju 28644, Korea
Department of Family Medicine, Chungbuk National University College of Medicine, Cheongju 28644, Korea

Homer S. Black
Department of Dermatology, Baylor College of Medicine, Houston, TX 77030, USA

Lesley E. Rhodes
Photobiology Unit, Dermatology Centre, University of Manchester, Salford Royal Hospital, Manchester M6 8HD, UK

Georgia Lenihan-Geels
Wageningen University and Research Centre, 6708 PB Wageningen, the Netherlands

Karen S. Bishop and Lynnette R. Ferguson
Auckland Cancer Society Research Centre, University of Auckland, Auckland 1142, New Zealand

Grace G. Abdukeyum
Division of Medical and Exercise Science, School of Medicine, Faculty of Science Medicine and Health, University of Wollongong, Wollongong NSW 2522, Australia

Alice J. Owen
Centre of Cardiovascular Research & Education in Therapeutics, School of Public Health & Preventive Medicine, Monash University, Melbourne VIC 3004, Australia

Theresa A. Larkin and Peter L. McLennan
Centre for Human and Applied Physiology, Graduate School of Medicine, School of Medicine, Faculty of Science Medicine and Health, University of Wollongong, Wollongong NSW 2522, Australia

Donatella D'Eliseo
Department of Molecular Medicine, Istituto Pasteur-Fondazione Cenci Bolognetti, Sapienza University of Rome, 00161 Rome, Italy
Department of Ecological and Biological Sciences (DEB), La Tuscia University, Largo dell'Università, 01100 Viterbo, Italy

Francesca Velotti
Department of Ecological and Biological Sciences (DEB), La Tuscia University, Largo dell'Università, 01100 Viterbo, Italy

Michael E.R. Dugan, Payam Vahmani, Manuel Juárez, Nuria Prieto and Jennifer L. Aalhus
Agriculture and Agri-Food Canada, Lacombe Research Centre, Lacombe T4L 1W1, AB, Canada

Tyler D. Turner
Josera GmbH & Co. KG, Kleinheubach 63924, Germany

Cletos Mapiye
Department of Animal Sciences, Stellenbosch University, Stellenbosch 7602, South Africa

Angela D. Beaulieu
Prairie Swine Centre, Inc., Saskatoon S7H 3J8, SK, Canada

Ruurd T. Zijlstra
Department of Agricultural, Food and Nutritional Sciences, University of Alberta, Edmonton T6G 2R3, AB, Canada

John F. Patience
Department of Animal Science, Iowa State University, Ames, IA 50011-3150, USA

Alicia I. Leikin-Frenkel
The Sackler Faculty of Medicine, Tel Aviv University, Tel Aviv 69978, Israel
Bert Strassburger Lipid Center, Sheba, Tel Hashomer, Ramat Gan 52621, Israel

Jennifer L. Watts
School of Molecular Biosciences and Center for Reproductive Biology, College of Veterinary Medicine, Washington State University, Pullman, WA 99164, USA

Paola Bozzatello, Elena Brignolo, Elisa De Grandi and Silvio Bellino
Centre for Personality Disorders, Department of Neuroscience, University of Turin, 10126 Turin, Italy

Mandi M. Hopkins, Zhihong Zhang, Ze Liu and Kathryn E. Meier
Department of Pharmaceutical Sciences, College of Pharmacy, Washington State University, Spokane, WA 99163, USA

Marijana Todorčević and Leanne Hodson
Oxford Centre for Diabetes, Endocrinology and Metabolism, University of Oxford, Churchill Hospital, OX3 7LE Oxford, UK

Stanislaw Klek
Stanley Dudrick's Memorial Hospital, General Surgery Unit, Skawina 32-050, Poland

Agustina Creus, María R. Ferreira, María E. Oliva and Yolanda B. Lombardo
Department of Biochemistry, School of Biochemistry, University of Litoral, Ciudad Universitaria, Paraje El Pozo, CC 242, (3000) Santa Fe, Argentina

Index

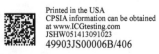

9 781646 465873